Volume 2
The Mouth and Perioral Tissues

Clinical Dentistry
in health and disease

Volume 1: The Dental Patient   Professor Crispian Scully

Volume 2: The Mouth and Perioral Tissues   Professor Crispian Scully

Volume 3: The Dentition and Dental Care   Professor Richard J. Elderton

Volume 4: Orthodontics and Occlusal Management   Professor William C. Shaw

CLINICAL DENTISTRY
in health and disease

Co-ordinating Editor: Professor David K. Mason
Dean, Glasgow Dental
Hospital and School

Volume 2
The Mouth and Perioral Tissues

Edited by

Crispian Scully,
BSc, BDS, PhD, FDSRCPS, MRCPath, MD

Professor, Head of Clinical Dental School and Head of Department,
University Department of Oral Medicine, Surgery and Pathology,
Bristol Dental School and Hospital

Heinemann Medical Books

Heinemann Medical Books
An imprint of Heinemann Professional Publishing Ltd
Halley Court, Jordan Hill, Oxford OX2 8EJ

OXFORD   LONDON   SINGAPORE   NAIROBI
IBADAN   KINGSTON

First published 1989

British Library Cataloguing in Publication Data
The Mouth and perioral tissues.
  1. Dentistry. Periodontics—For dental
  hygiene
  I. Scully, C. (Crispian)
  III. Series
  617.6′32
ISBN 0 433 00055 4

Filmset by Eta Services (Typesetters) Ltd, Beccles, Suffolk
and printed by Butler & Tanner Ltd, Frome

Contents

Contributors

BRIAN AVERY BDS MBBS FDS FRCS
Consultant, Department of Oral and Maxillofacial
Surgery, Middlesborough General Hospital, Ayresome
Green Lane, Middlesborough

JOHN W. EVESON BDS FDS PhD MRCPath
Consultant and Senior Lecturer, University Department
of Oral Medicine, Surgery and Pathology, Bristol Dental
School and Hospital, Lower Maudlin Street, Bristol

PHILIP J. LAMEY BSc BDS MBChB DDS FDS
Consultant and Senior Lecturer, University Department
of Oral Medicine and Pathology, Glasgow Dental
Hospital and School, Glasgow

JOHN D. LANGDON MBBS BDS FDS FRCS
Consultant and Senior Lecturer, Department of Oral and
Maxillofacial Surgery, King's College Hospital, Denmark
Hill, London

ROBERT ORD FDS FRCS
Consultant, Department of Oral and Maxillofacial
Surgery, Sunderland District General Hospital,
Sunderland

STEPHEN R. PORTER BSc BDS PhD FDSRCS
Lecturer, University Department of Oral Medicine,
Surgery and Pathology, Bristol Dental School and
Hospital, Lower Maudlin Street, Bristol

STEPHEN S. PRIME BDS FDS PhD
Consultant and Senior Lecturer, University Department
of Oral Medicine, Surgery and Pathology, Bristol Dental
School and Hospital, Lower Maudlin Street, Bristol

JOHN RAYNE FDS DPhil DOrth
Consultant, Department of Oral Surgery, John Radcliffe
Hospital, Headington, Oxford

CRISPIAN SCULLY BSc BDS MBBS PhD FDS
MRCPath MD
Professor, Consultant and Head of Department,
University Department of Oral Medicine, Surgery and
Pathology, Bristol Dental School and Hospital, Lower
Maudlin Street, Bristol

ROGER G. SMITH BDS MDS FDS
Consultant and Senior Lecturer, University Department
of Oral Medicine, Surgery and Pathology, Bristol Dental
School and Hospital, Lower Maudlin Street, Bristol

BERNARD SPECULAND BDS MDS FDS FFD
FRACDS DOS
Consultant, Department of Oral and Maxillofacial
Surgery, Dudley Road Hospital, Birmingham

PETER WARD-BOOTH BDS MBBS FDS FRCS
Consultant, Department of Oral and Maxillofacial
Surgery, Sunderland District General Hospital,
Sunderland

D. WIESENFELD MDSc FDS FRACDS (OMS)
Consultant, Lewis House, 766 Elizabeth Street,
Melbourne, Australia

Preface

The diagnosis and treatment of patients with diseases of the mouth and associated structures have advanced remarkably since dentistry became recognized as a specialty in its own right. Today's dental surgeon is seeing a progressive change in the philosophy of dental care, with increasing emphasis on prevention of oral disease along with a deeper involvement in integrating the management of the patient as a total being. Interlinked with these changes in attitude are changes in the pattern of oral disease and systemic problems related to dental care.

We have seen on the one hand a slowly declining incidence of dental caries while on the other the appearance of new diseases such as AIDS.

This book is the product mainly of a number of younger workers in the field with most of whom the Editor has personally worked. They have a progressive approach to the teaching of dentistry and attempt to give a contemporary and practical view, unrestricted by the somewhat artificial boundaries of the various disciplines within. Where possible a symptomatic and clinical approach has been used since patients present in that way.

The book is designed to help mainly undergraduate students of dentistry but should also be useful to those in medicine and to postgraduates.

The curriculum is now so full that one sympathizes with the vast amount of knowledge that undergraduates must assimilate. However, study and qualification at a postgraduate level are now accepted as essential for those who wish to work in one of the dental specialties and the realist accepts that vocational training is desirable even for those who wish to be 'generalists'.

The text is aimed mainly at those who have completed training in the basic sciences and human diseases, as well as pharmacology, and a degree of knowledge and understanding is assumed.

The text does not attempt to give details of the finer points of histochemistry, immunology, microbiology, medicine, surgery or pathology, other than those that are required for a basic understanding of disease. Furthermore, this text is not a comprehensive coverage of oral surgery, oral medicine and oral pathology, since some aspects, such as disorders of the teeth and periodontium, and facial deformities are covered in other volumes in this series.

One of the main difficulties facing dental undergraduates is the acquisition of knowledge and understanding in such a way as to achieve a realistic approach to patient care: many uncommon conditions need to be understood and yet most of dental practice deals with the common and perhaps less exotic disorders. Only clinical experience will reinforce the fact of life that 'swallows are more common than eagles', and this cannot be acquired (nor clinical examinations passed!) by sitting in the library. The clinic is where the action is.

Furthermore, it is impossible without a photographic memory to retain all the facts, and often the best way to learn is from basic principles, using a skeleton of facts on which to build the whole.

This is a synopsis of the subject that should give a foundation for further study. There is inevitably a degree of overlap between chapters and a minor degree of repetition where important points are being made. The final section is designed to help revision. We hope there are no serious omissions; most apparent deficiencies are covered by sections in the other volumes.

C. Scully, 1989

Acknowledgements

The encouragement of Professor David K. Mason has, as always, been most welcome. Dr Richard Barling has been an enthusiastic supporter and adviser whose pleasant and courteous approach has encouraged us to keep to schedule.

Some of the illustrations appear in colour in *Colour Atlas of Stomatology* (C. Scully and S. Flint), and we are grateful to Martin Dunitz for permission to use them here.

I am as always grateful to Professor R. A. Cawson for his frequent and stimulating discussions and his forebearance when I sometimes adopt or adapt his original ideas, and to my various publishers, especially Wrights and *British Dental Journal*, for permission to adapt material. I am grateful to Hugh Levers for assistance in proof-reading.

Section I
Diseases in Bones and Joints

Chapter

1
Congenital disorders

STRUCTURE OF BONE

All bones consist of an external cortical and internal cancellous type. The basic structure both of cortical and cancellous bone comprises blood vessels (Haversian canals) surrounded by successive layers (lamellae) of bone tissue. Between the lamellae lie the osteocytes. In cortical bone this lamellated structure is extremely dense, forming a thick outer protective surface, while in cancellous bone thin plates of bone tissue (trabeculae) form a series of spaces to contain the bone marrow.

Bone tissue is composed of an organic element, principally collagen, and mineral–hydroxyapatite. During bone formation organic tissue is laid down first; and this **osteoid** then mineralizes and hardens due to deposition of hydroxyapatite crystals (cf. tooth formation).

Collagen serves a mechanical supportive role in bone and many other tissues (Chapter 11). Ten main collagen types have been described (types I–X). The most common and widespread are known as **interstitial** collagens (types I, II, III) and are found in bone, cartilage, tendon and skin. Type IV collagen forms the main collagenous component of the lamina densa of **basement membranes**. The other collagen types appear at present to be of lesser clinical importance.

Some congenital disorders of bones and joints are caused by collagen defects. For example, defects of type I collagen underly osteogenesis imperfecta (p. 7), Marfan's syndrome (p. 11) and a subtype of Ehlers–Danlos syndrome (type VII) (p. 11). Other subtypes of Ehlers–Danlos syndrome are caused by defects of type III collagen, and it is possible that a type II collagen defect underlies achondroplasia (p. 4).

CONGENITAL DISORDERS OF BONE AND JOINTS

There are many rare congenital disorders but only the more common and relevant are dealt with here.

Torus palatinus

This is a common benign exostosis seen in the centre of the vault of the palate (Fig. 1.1). It is of variable size and may have a smooth or nodular surface. The torus is

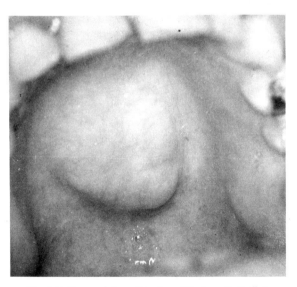

Fig. 1.1 *Torus palatinus. (Courtesy of Professor C. Scully.)*

more common in mongoloid races and may become more apparent with increasing age. Tori rarely cause any problem but occasionally interfere with denture construction.

Torus mandibularis

Although there is no association with torus palatinus, the torus mandibularis is also seen most commonly in mongoloids and is more obvious with increasing age. The tori are usually located bilaterally, lingual to the mandibular premolars (Fig. 1.2).

Achondroplasia (chondrodystrophia fetalis)

Achondroplasia is the most common form of short-limbed dwarfism. It is a genetic disorder, transmitted in an autosomal dominant manner. Endochondral ossification is reduced. However, up to 80% of achondroplasts have normal parents and are thought to be the consequence of a recent genetic mutation. Until recently it was assumed that achondroplasia frequently led to death *in utero* but this is no longer thought to be true. Indeed most achondroplasts have a normal lifespan.

Affected patients are dwarfs having disproportionately short limbs, bowed legs, lordosis (excessive curvature

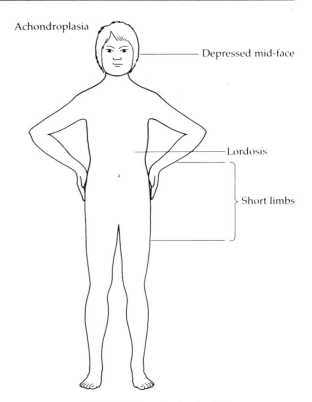

Fig. 1.3 Features of achondroplasia.

of the spine) prominent buttocks and abdomen, and trident hands with relatively short fingers. The skull is relatively large, having prominent frontal, occipital and parietal bones. The middle third of the face is hypoplastic and the nasal bridge depressed (Fig. 1.3). The foramen magnum is often narrow and spinal cord compression can occur at this and lower levels. Joints can be of limited mobility and the pelvic inlet narrow. Thus pregnant achondroplastic females may require a caesarian section for childbirth.

Dental aspects

Aside from the earlier mentioned facial features, achondroplasts may have a class III type malocclusion due to mid-face hypoplasia. Congenital absence of teeth has been observed in some affected patients. There may be an increased susceptibility to recurrent upper respiratory tract infections and, as a consequence of deficient growth of the maxilla, nasal intubation for general anaesthesia may be difficult. Thus antibiotic cover may be required before oral surgery is undertaken.

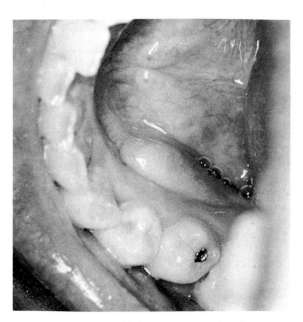

Fig. 1.2 Torus mandibularis. (Courtesy of Professor C. Scully.)

Cleidocranial dysplasia (Marie–Sainton syndrome)

Cleidocranial dysplasia is an inherited bone disorder transmitted primarily in an autosomal dominant manner although occasionally it can arise spontaneously. It is characterized by defective development and ossification mainly of the skull, clavicles and pelvis (Table 1.1). The clinical consequences of cleidocranial dysplasia are minimal: patients are of a mildly reduced stature, can

Cleidocranial dysplasia

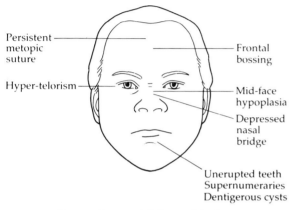

Persistent metopic suture

Hyper-telorism

Frontal bossing

Mid-face hypoplasia

Depressed nasal bridge

Unerupted teeth
Supernumeraries
Dentigerous cysts

Fig. 1.4 *Features of cleidocranial dysplasia.*

approximate the shoulders (Fig. 1.4) and may suffer recurrent dislocation of the shoulder, elbow and hip joints (Fig. 1.5). Because of a narrow pelvic inlet (Fig. 1.6), caesarian section may be required for childbirth.

Table 1.1
Principal clinical features of cleidocranial dysplasia

Skull	Persistent, enlarged fontanelles
	Widened sutures
	Multiple wormian bones
	Parietal, temporal and frontal bone enlargement (bossing)
	Reduced or absent paranasal sinuses
	Class III skeletal appearance
	Enlarged foramen magnum
	Hypertelorism
	Depressed nasal bridge
Shoulders*	Partial or total aplasia of one or both clavicles
	Small, deformed scapulae
Pelvis	Hypoplastic pelvis
Other	Shortening of distal phalanges
	Scoliosis

* The shoulder joint is hypermobile and clavicles defective, thus patients can bring their shoulders forward almost to touch in midline.

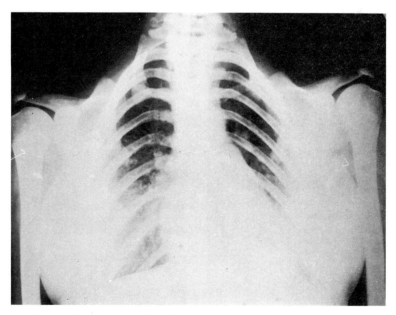

Fig. 1.5 *Cleidocranial dysplasia showing the typical feature of aplasia of the clavicles. (Courtesy of Professor C. Scully.)*

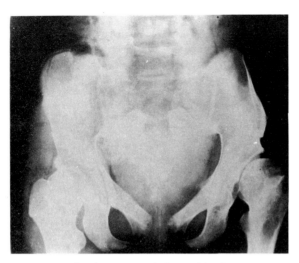

Fig. 1.6 *Pelvic deformities in cleidocranial dysplasia. (Courtesy of Professor C. Scully.)*

Dental aspects

As a consequence of enlargement of the frontal, parietal and temporal bones, affected patients have enlarged heads, sutures close late and there are multiple wormian bones (Fig. 1.7 and 1.8). Depression of the nasal bridge, hypertelorism (wide spacing of the eyes) and a tendency towards a class III skeletal appearance are other facial features of cleidocranial dysplasia (Fig. 1.8). The palate may be high, arched and narrow.

Eruption of permanent teeth is retarded and dentigerous cysts are frequently found. Supernumerary teeth are common in cleidocranial dysplasia, especially in the anterior mandible. The crowns of the teeth are normal, but the roots can be short, thin and lack acellular cement (Fig. 1.9).

Patients with cleidocranial dysplasia do not have major medical problems that complicate routine dental treatment.

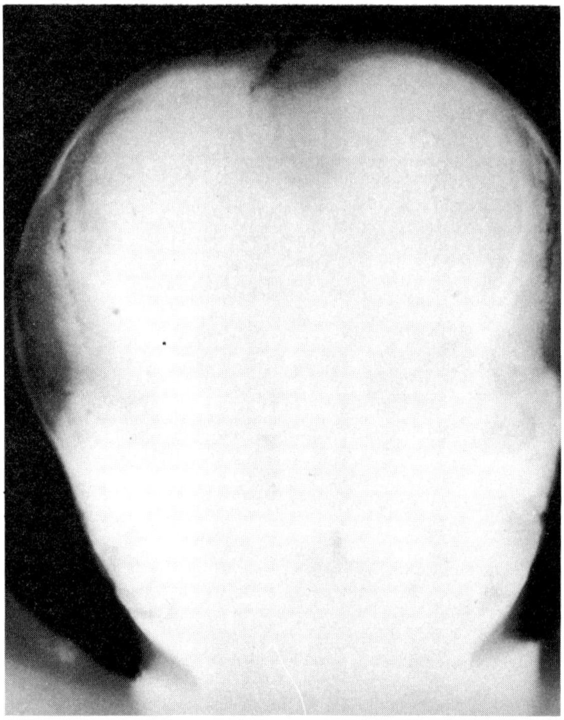

Fig. 1.7 *Delayed closure of sutures, and multiple wormian bones in cleidocranial dysplasia. (Courtesy of Professor C. Scully.)*

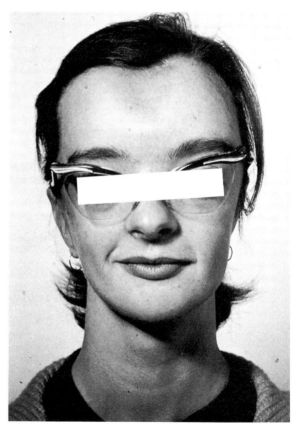

Fig. 1.8 *Facial features of cleidocranial dysplasia. (Courtesy of B. Beeching.)*

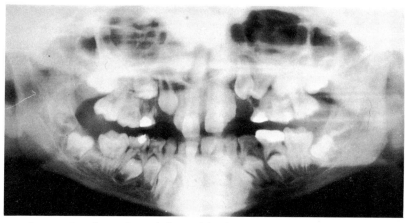

Fig. 1.9 *Dental anomalies in cleidocranial dysplasia. (Courtesy of Professor C. Scully.)*

Osteogenesis imperfecta (fragilitas ossium: brittle bone syndrome)

Osteogenesis imperfecta is the term given to a group of inherited bone disorders characterized by excessive bone fragility and a number of extraskeletal connective tissue disorders. Based upon genetic and clinical features, there are at least four types of osteogenesis imperfecta (Table 1.2).

Bone defects

The severity of bone fragility is highly variable. In type II osteogenesis imperfecta the fragility can be so extreme as to cause death *in utero* or shortly after birth. Affected children may have multiple rib fractures (giving a 'beaded' radiographic appearance) and shortened concertina-like long bones. The skulls of such children are soft and have multiple wormian bones. Patients with severe skeletal involvement who do survive into childhood and early adulthood are usually of short stature, have grossly deformed limbs and often cannot walk. These children also have enlarged heads and deformities of the spine and trunk.

Patients with mild osteogenesis imperfecta have few skeletal anomalies and are of normal stature. Fracture of limb bones following mild injury is the most common skeletal problem of such patients.

Table 1.2
Clinical subtypes of osteogenesis imperfecta

Type	Inheritance*	Main clinical features
I	AD	Blue sclera Presenile deafness Variable bone fragility
II	AR	Multiple fractures causing death *in utero* or shortly after birth
III	AD	Variable bone fragility Affected patients usually have white sclera
IV	AD or X-linked	Variable bone fragility Affected patients usually have white sclera

* AD = autosomal dominant, AR = autosomal recessive.

Ocular problems

Blue sclera are seen in up to 90% of all osteogenesis imperfecta patients. Their clinical significance is unpredictable. The intensity of colour is not proportional to the degree of skeletal deformity and may disappear in early childhood.

The exact cause of the blue colour is unknown, but scleral thinness causing increased visibility of the pigmented choroid and/or increased deposition of mucopolysaccharide ground substance within the sclera are possible causes. (Blue sclera can also be seen in healthy infants and in patients with Ehlers–Danlos syndrome (p. 11) or Marfan's syndrome (p. 11).)

Deafness

Deafness is a common problem of *mild* osteogenesis imperfecta and is due to defective conduction of sound through the external and middle ear as a direct consequence of deformity of the associated bones.

Skin

The skin of osteogenesis imperfecta patients can be smooth, soft and fragile; it scars following trauma and often gives rise to keloids (hypertrophic scars).

Lax ligaments

Weakness and laxity of ligaments can cause hypermobility and recurrent dislocation of joints.

Other aspects

Cardiovascular problems such as floppy valves (predisposing to infective endocarditis) and an increased bleeding tendency are rare clinical aspects of osteogenesis imperfecta.

The current treatment of osteogenesis imperfecta is unsatisfactory. Hormones (calcitonin), vitamins (e.g. vitamin C or D), fluoride and flavonoids have, to date, been of little value and in most instances surgical interventions to treat fractures and correct skeletal deformities are the only effective treatment measures. Correction of extraskeletal problems, physiotherapy and splinting of limbs are also important in the management of osteogenesis imperfecta.

Dental aspects

Dentinogenesis imperfecta is the main oral manifestation. The deciduous dentition is more severely affected than the permanent. The teeth are translucent and brown or purplish in colour (Figs. 1.10 and 32.6). Enamel is rapidly lost from affected teeth as a result of either a defective dentino-enamel junction or dentine. The teeth become discoloured, and attrition rapidly causes loss of clinical crowns though the pulp is usually obliterated by secondary dentine (Figs. 1.11 and 1.12). Restorative procedures in dentinogenesis imperfecta are complicated by softness of the dentine.

Facial fractures are uncommon in osteogenesis imper-

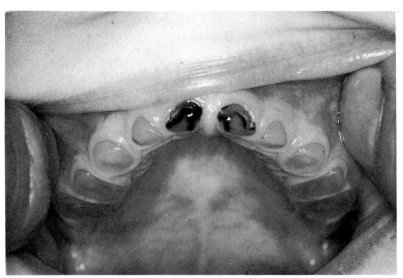

Fig. 1.10 *Dentinogenesis imperfecta showing gross attrition. (Courtesy of Professor C. Scully.)*

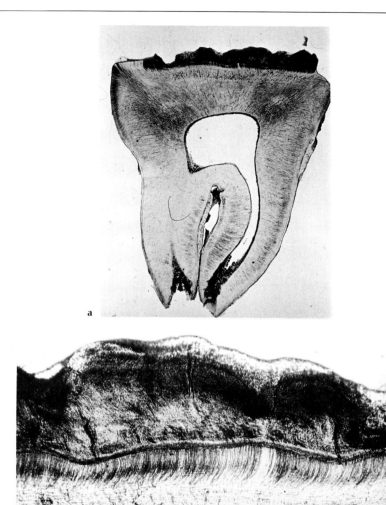

Fig. 1.11 *Dentinogenesis imperfecta: (a) ground section showing loss of dentine; (b) higher power photomicrograph. (Courtesy of Professor C. Scully.)*

fecta but when extracting teeth extra care must be taken to avoid fracture of the maxilla or mandible. General anaesthesia may be complicated by chest deformities (especially common in severe osteogenesis imperfecta) and cardiac valvular deformities. The latter will necessitate antibiotic cover to prevent infective endocarditis (Volume 1).

Osteopetrosis (marble bone disease; Albers–Schönberg disease)

Osteopetrosis is a rare disorder characterized by increased bone density with replacement of normal medullary bone by irregular avascular bone. Haemopoietic marrow is replaced by bone, and thus extramedullary

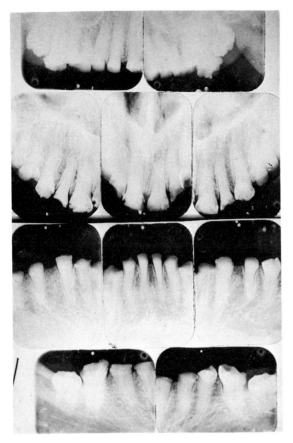

Fig. 1.12 *Dentinogenesis imperfecta: attrition, and oblitera-tion of pulp with secondary dentine. (Courtesy of Professor C. Scully.)*

Table 1.3
Clinical features of osteopetrosis

Autosomal dominant	Autosomal recessive
Rarely fatal	Usually fatal
Recurrent bone fractures	Recurrent bone fractures
Mild anaemia	Anaemia, thrombocytopenia
Hepatosplenomegaly	Hepatosplenomegaly
Cranial nerve palsies	Cranial nerve palsies
	Hydrocephalus
	Recurrent respiratory and intestinal infections

sites such as the liver, spleen and lymph nodes develop haemopoietic function.

Osteopetrosis is inherited in an autosomal dominant or recessive manner. The clinical features of each variant are summarized in Table 1.3. Patients with the autosomal dominant form have good general health and a normal lifespan.

There is no effective treatment for the recessive form of osteopetrosis. Regular blood transfusions, steroids and splenectomy may correct the anaemia; cranial nerve decompression may be necessary and, if hydrocephalus develops, ventricular shunts may be required. However, most affected children die in the first decade of life, usually as a consequence of overwhelming infection or haemorrhage.

Dental aspects

The jaws, particularly the maxilla, are thickened and sclerotic (Fig. 1.13) and the paranasal sinuses are often reduced in size. If the child is hydrocephalic, there may be evidence of macrocephaly. Recurrent sinusitis and cranial nerve palsies (especially II, III, V, VII and VIII) are other orofacial problems of osteopetrosis. Children with the recessive form may have teeth with hypoplastic enamel, shortened roots and an increased susceptibility to caries. Eruption of teeth can be delayed or absent.

As a consequence of the sclerotic bone, dental extrac-tions can be difficult and the mandible also liable to fracture. The reduced vascularity of bone predisposes to postextraction osteomyelitis and thus all dental surgical procedures should be as atraumatic as possible and carried out under antibiotic cover. If the patient is regularly

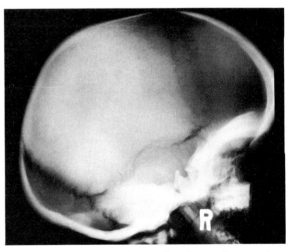

Fig. 1.13 *Osteopetrosis showing dense bones. (Courtesy of Professor C. Scully.)*

receiving corticosteroid therapy for anaemia, steroid cover may be required before complex dental procedures are undertaken (Volume 1).

Marfan's syndrome (arachnodactyly)

Marfan's syndrome is an autosomal dominant disorder characterized by disproportionately long extremities (arachnodactyly), dislocation of the lens of the eye, thoracic defects, articular defects and cardiovascular problems such as aortic aneurysms and mitral valve regurgitation (predisposing to infective endocarditis). Affected patients may be taller than the average for their age or family and, as a result of excessive rib growth, can have an anteriorly (pigeon-breast) or posteriorly (pectus excavatum) displaced sternum. Other skeletal anomalies of Marfan's syndrome include flat feet and kyphoscoliosis (forward and lateral curvature of the spine) (Fig. 1.14).

Dental aspects

A high-arched palate and bifid uvula are the most consistent oral manifestations of Marfan's syndrome; recurrent dislocation of the temporomandibular joint and multiple dental cysts being less common. Dental treatment may require antibiotic cover and alteration of anticoagulant therapy (if the patient has a prosthetic heart valve and is anticoagulated).

Ehlers–Danlos syndrome

Ehlers–Danlos syndrome is a clinically heterogeneous disorder in which the major clinical features are skin hyperelasticity and fragility, and hypermobility of joints (India-rubber man). Based upon clinical criteria, there are at least 10 variants of Ehlers–Danlos syndrome, but fewer than half of the patients can be accurately categorized.

The skin of affected patients is hyperextensible, returning to its normal position after stretching, and is

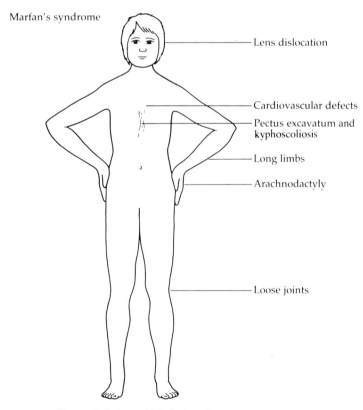

Fig. 1.14 *Features of Marfan's syndrome.*

Ehlers-Danlos syndrome

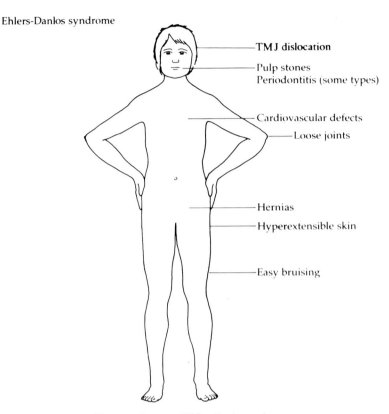

TMJ dislocation

Pulp stones
Periodontitis (some types)

Cardiovascular defects

Loose joints

Hernias

Hyperextensible skin

Easy bruising

Fig. 1.15 *Features of Ehlers-Danlos syndrome.*

thin and fragile, easily splitting to produce gaping wounds with relatively minor trauma. Healing is slow and may result in wrinkled 'cigarette-paper' scars that are thin, shiny and often hyperpigmented. The skin may easily bruise especially in the ecchymotic (type IV) form of Ehlers–Danlos syndrome. Other cutaneous manifestations of this syndrome include lumps (pseudo-tumours) that develop at pressure points and irregular subcutaneous calcified areas of organized haematomas (spherules).

Joint hypermobility is a classic feature but the degree depends upon the variant of Ehlers–Danlos syndrome. However, in the severe forms, all joints can be affected, with frequent joint dislocation and vertebral abnormalities such as kyphoscoliosis (Fig. 1.15).

There is an increased incidence of mitral valve prolapse (floppy valve syndrome) as well as arterial rupture following minor trauma, dissection of the aorta and spontaneous caroticocavernous fistulas.

Umbilical, inguinal and hiatus hernias are common in Ehlers–Danlos syndrome.

Dental aspects

Patients with severe Ehlers–Danlos syndrome may have an unusual 'parrot-like' facies with the ears pointing downwards and outwards. The patient may be able to touch the tip of his nose with his tongue—a diagnostic feature of the syndrome. Facial scarring, particularly about the chin and forehead, and recurrent dislocation of the temporomandibular joint are other common features.

The oral mucosa may be fragile, making difficult the effective closure of wounds with sutures. Gingival bleeding following minor trauma such as tooth-brushing and severe postextraction haemorrhage are common problems of the type IV variant. Patients with the type VIII syndrome characteristically suffer severe generalized early periodontitis.

Dental anomalies reported in some patients with Ehlers–Danlos syndrome include deeply fissured premolars and molars, dentinal abnormalities such as shortened deformed roots, and multiple large pulp stones (Fig. 1.15).

Patients with floppy mitral valve syndrome constitute a general anaesthetic risk and antibiotic cover is essential for all surgical procedures in order to prevent endocarditis (Volume 1).

FURTHER READING

Editorial (1984). Osteogenesis imperfecta. *Br. med. J.*, **289**: 394–395.

Leading Article (1980). Learning from Ehlers–Danlos syndrome. *Lancet*, **ii**: 1062–1063.

Pope F. M., Nicholls, A. C. (1987). Molecular abnormalities of collagen in human disease. *Arch. Dis. Child.*, **62**: 523–528.

Scully C., Flint S. (1988). *An atlas of stomatology.* London: Martin Dunitz (in press).

Metabolic bone disorders

BONE AND CALCIUM METABOLISM

Bone is continually being remodelled, resorption principally being carried out by osteoclasts (Fig. 2.1) and deposition mainly by osteoblasts—though it is now clear that bone resorption may also be effected by osteoblast-derived factors. These activities, along with maintenance of normal levels of serum calcium and phosphate, are controlled mainly by a metabolite of vitamin D (1,25-dihydroxycholecalciferol or dihydroxyvitamin D_3) synthesized in the kidneys from a precursor produced by the liver; by parathyroid hormone; and by calcitonin from the thyroid gland (Fig. 2.2). Bone metabolism is therefore dependent mainly on the parathyroid and thyroid glands, liver and kidneys.

Local factors such as pressure, prostaglandin secretion by cysts and neoplasms, or production of osteoclast-activating factor (OAF) in chronic inflammatory lesions may also cause resorption.

Vitamin D

The active metabolite of vitamin D—1,25-dihydroxycholecalciferol (1,25 $(OH)_2$ D_3)—acts as a hormone. Dihydroxycholecalciferol is generated as the end-product of a series of reactions in the skin, liver and kidneys (Fig. 2.3) and is the *major* control for calcium and phosphate absorption by the intestine. In addition it is indirectly involved in bone formation since it ensures the adequate availability of calcium and phosphate for the mineralization of osteoid, may increase the reabsorption of calcium and phosphate by the renal tubules, and may have wide-reaching effects on other cells and tissues.

The intermediate vitamin D metabolites—24,25-dihydroxycholecalciferol and 25,26-dihydroxycholecalciferol—may also possess some biological activity but their exact functions are unknown.

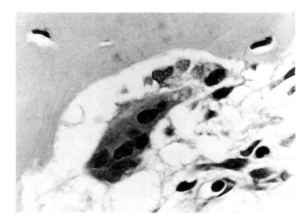

Fig. 2.1 *Osteoclastic resorption of bone. (Courtesy of Professor C. Scully.)*

Parathyroid hormone

Parathyroid hormone (PTH) is secreted by the parathyroid glands in response to a fall in serum calcium levels below normal limits. The PTH stimulates the enzyme 1α-hydroxylase in the kidney and thus increases production of 1,25-dihydroxycholecalciferol. Also, by activating existing osteoclasts and osteocytes in bone, and inducing new osteoclast formation, PTH mobilizes calcium and phosphate. In addition, PTH enhances the reabsorption of calcium from the glomerular filtrate in the kidney and increases the absorption of calcium in the small intestine. Secretion of PTH ceases when serum calcium returns to normal levels.

Calcitonin

Unlike PTH and 1,25-dihydroxycholecalciferol, calcitonin *reduces* serum calcium and phosphate levels. Calcitonin is a hormone secreted by C cells of the thyroid gland in response to high serum levels of calcium. It increases the

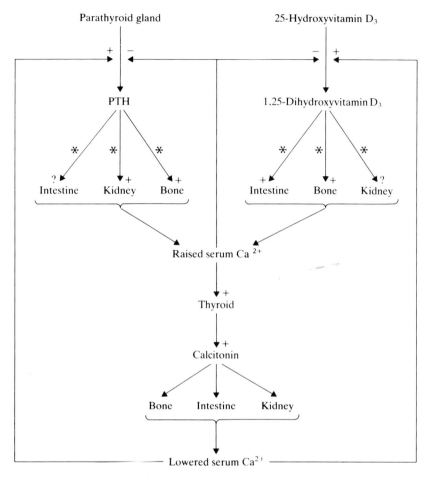

Fig. 2.2 *Hormonal control of calcium. (* Calcium absorption increased.)*

excretion of calcium and phosphate by the kidney, reduces osteoclastic bone resorption, and may have some effect upon intestinal absorption of calcium. Secretion of calcitonin ceases when serum calcium levels fall back to normal.

METABOLIC BONE DISORDERS

Metabolic disorders affecting bone may also, if they occur during early childhood, affect the developing teeth.

Hyperparathyroidism

Hyperparathyroidism is usually primary, but may occasionally be secondary to renal disease or malabsorption.

Primary hyperparathyroidism

Primary hyperparathyroidism is usually due to a parathyroid adenoma, but carcinoma or hyperplasia of parathyroid tissue or ectopic production of PTH (for example by tumours of lung or kidney) are other causes. Primary hyperparathyroidism may also rarely occur in association with adenomas of other endocrine glands—the multiple endocrine adenoma (MEA) syndromes.

The clinical features of hyperparathyroidism (Table 2.1) are the direct result of excess PTH or calcium, and particularly include renal stones, bone lesions (Figs. 2.4 and 2.5), polyuria and abdominal pain ('stones, bones and abdominal groans'). Anorexia and psychoses are not uncommon.

Serum calcium levels are raised, as, usually, is that of

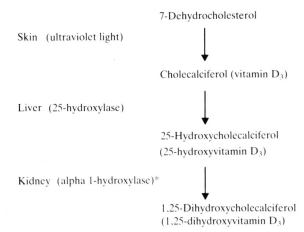

7-Dehydrocholesterol

Skin (ultraviolet light)

Cholecalciferol (vitamin D₃)

Liver (25-hydroxylase)

25-Hydroxycholecalciferol
(25-hydroxyvitamin D₃)

Kidney (alpha 1-hydroxylase)*

1,25-Dihydroxycholecalciferol
(1,25-dihydroxyvitamin D₃)

*This enzyme is controlled by calcium levels. Low calcium activates alpha 1-hydroxylase.

Fig. 2.3 *Synthesis of active vitamin D metabolites (mainly 1,25-dihydroxyvitamin D₃).*

Hyperparathyroidism

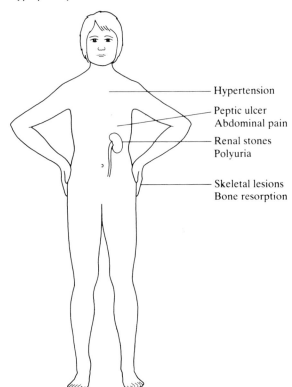

Hypertension

Peptic ulcer
Abdominal pain

Renal stones
Polyuria

Skeletal lesions
Bone resorption

Fig. 2.4 *Hyperparathyroidism—features.*

Table 2.1
Clinical features of primary hyperparathyroidism

Nephrocalcinosis
Peptic ulceration
Pancreatitis
Bone disease (osteitis fibrosa cystica, osteoporosis)
Muscle weakness, myalgia
Neurological and psychotic disorders
Polyuria and polydipsia
Constipation
Anorexia, nausea, vomiting
Hypertension
Arthralgia and arthritis

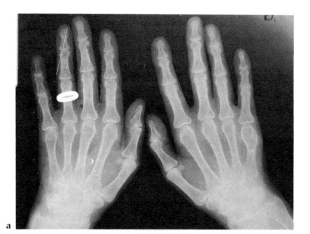

a

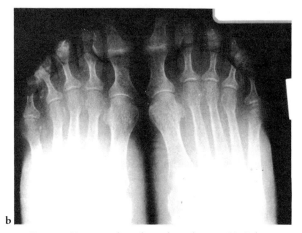

b

Fig. 2.5 *Hyperparathyroidism: bone lesions. (a) Subperiosteal erosions and tufting of terminal phalanges. (b) Bone lesions similar to those in (a). (Courtesy of Professor C. Scully.)*

Table 2.2
Biochemical findings in patients with disorders of calcium and bone metabolism

	Serum calcium (2.3–2.6 mmol/l)[a]	Serum phosphate (0.85–1.4 mmol/l)[a]	Serum alkaline phosphatase (3–13 KA units*)[a]	Serum urea (3.3–6.7 mmol/l)[a]
Osteoporosis	N	N	N	N
Hyperparathyroidism†	↑	N/↓	N/↑	N/↑
Hypoparathyroidism	↓	↑	N	N
Osteomalacia	N/↓	N/↓	↑	N

* King Armstrong units.
† The values vary according to the type of disease.
[a] Normal range.

alkaline phosphatase; phosphate levels are reduced (Table 2.2).

Secondary hyperparathyroidism

Secondary hyperparathyroidism is usually the consequence of renal disease in which low serum calcium as a consequence of impaired production of dihydroxycholecalciferol induces increased parathyroid activity, and eventually hyperplasia of the parathyroid glands. Secondary hyperparathyroidism may also follow malabsorption syndromes.

In contrast to the primary disorder, in which serum calcium levels are raised, calcium levels are usually normal or low in secondary hyperparathyroidism.

Tertiary hyperparathyroidism

Rarely chronic overstimulation of the gland in secondary hyperparathyroidism leads to neoplastic change in the parathyroids which then escape the normal control of serum calcium (tertiary hyperparathyroidism).

Management of hyperparathyroidism

In secondary and tertiary hyperparathyroidism, treatment of the underlying disorder (for example chronic renal disease) is required. Hyperparathyroidism is managed by excision of the neoplastic or hyperplastic parathyroid tissue.

Oral aspects of hyperparathyroidism

Oral manifestations of hyperparathyroidism, which are rare, include reduced bone density (the outlines of the maxillary antrum, inferior alveolar canal and inferior border of the mandible can become less distinct), loss of the lamina dura, root resorption, and radiolucencies (particularly of the mandible). The radiolucent lesions are either areas of high osteoclastic activity or giant-cell lesions. The giant-cell lesions can present intra-orally as gingival swellings (epulides) (Fig. 2.6). Patients with giant-cell lesions should be screened to exclude hyperparathyroidism.

Hypoparathyroidism

The most frequent cause of hypoparathyroidism is damage to, or loss of, parathyroid tissue during neck surgery (usually during thyroidectomy). It may also arise, rarely, as a familial disorder (idiopathic hypoparathyroidism) or very rarely as a consequence of *in utero* damage

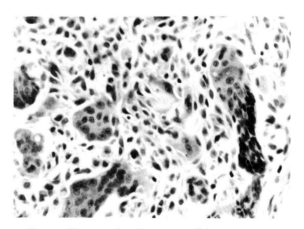

Fig. 2.6 *Hyperparathyroidism: giant-cell lesion. (Courtesy of Professor C. Scully.)*

Table 2.3
Clinical features of hypoparathyroidism

Tetany
Convulsions
Music cramps, twitching
Paraesthesia
Mental changes
Vomiting, constipation
Cardiac dysrhythmias
Loss of hair

when it is associated with cellular immunodeficiency (Di George syndrome). Hypoparathyroidism can be an accompanying feature of one of the polyendocrinopathy syndromes in which there is failure of several endocrine glands.

The major clinical features of hypoparathyroidism are related to the low serum calcium levels (Table 2.3). Tetany (hyperexcitability of muscles) is the most obvious and disturbing feature and can lead to facial twitching (Chvostek's sign) and laryngeal spasm.

Management

Patients with hypoparathyroidism are treated with α1-hydroxycholecalciferol.

Oral aspects

Hypoparathyroidism in childhood can give rise to enamel hypoplasia of developing teeth and delayed tooth eruption. Chronic mucocutaneous candidosis is often seen if there is an immune defect such as in the candidosis-endocrinopathy syndrome (Fig. 2.7).

Hypoparathyroidism frequently causes paraesthesia ('pins and needles') about the mouth. Tapping the skin over the facial nerve can elicit involuntary twitching of the muscles of the upper lip or ipsilateral side of the face (Chvostek's sign).

Tetany, convulsions, mental changes and cardiac problems may complicate the dental management of patients with this disorder.

Pseudohypoparathyroidism

Pseudohypoparathyroidism is a rare condition in which PTH is secreted normally but the tissue receptors are unresponsive. The features are similar to those of hypoparathyroidism, plus a tendency to short stature and small fingers but no dental manifestations.

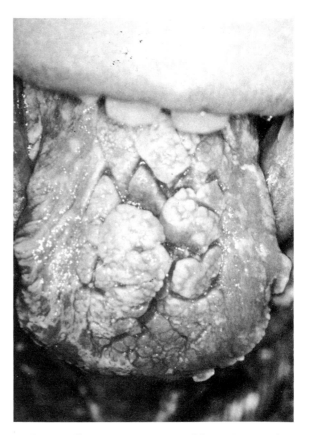

Fig. 2.7 *Chronic mucocutaneous candidosis. (Courtesy of Professor C. Scully.)*

Osteoporosis

Osteoporosis is a fairly common condition, characterized by the loss of both the organic matrix and the mineralized components of bone. Serum biochemistry is normal (Table 2.2). The most common cause of osteoporosis is ageing, especially in women (hormonal), but drugs and several other disorders can also increase the rate of bone loss (Table 2.4).

The main clinical problem of osteoporosis is either fracture of the neck of the femur, or collapse of vertebral bodies (which can lead to paraplegia).

Management

Osteoporosis is managed by treatment of the underlying disorder (where possible) and by use of stimulators of osteogenesis (fluoride, phosphate, sex hormones or PTH) or inhibitors of bone resorption (e.g. calcium, vitamin D

Table 2.4
Causes of osteoporosis

Sex-hormone deficiency
Hyperparathyroidism
Cushing's syndrome
Hyperthyroidism
Nutritional deficiencies (e.g. vitamin D or C)
Malabsorption
Chronic renal disease
Drugs
   corticosteroids
   chronic alcoholism
   long-term heparin therapy
Immobilization

Table 2.5
Causes of osteomalacia and rickets

Vitamin D deficiency
   Dietary deficiency
   Asian immigrants (high intake of phytates)
Malabsorption
   Post-gastrectomy
   Gluten-sensitive enteropathy (coeliac disease)
   Steatorrhoea
Disorders of vitamin D metabolism
   Chronic renal failure
   Impaired renal α-1-hydroxylase activity
   Renal tubular disorders
Hypophosphatasia
Drugs
   Diphosphonates
   Anticonvulsants (phenytoin)

or diphosphonates). Patients are encouraged to exercise and avoid long periods of inactivity.

Oral aspects

Osteoporosis has no notable oral manifestations but may affect the jaws and predispose to fracture. General anaesthesia may be difficult if vertebral or chest deformities are present.

Rickets and osteomalacia

These disorders are characterized by a decrease in the mineral but not organic content of bone. Unmineralized osteoid is present in large amounts but there is a deficiency of mature mineralized bone. The term rickets is used when the disorder affects children (when bones are still growing); the term osteomalacia when adults are affected.

The most common cause of rickets and osteomalacia in the Western world is a deficiency of vitamin D (Table 2.5) which can arise in dietary deficiency of vitamin D, gastrointestinal disease, or in disorders of vitamin D metabolism. Dietary deficiency of vitamin D is still seen in elderly patients, and in Asians living in Northern Europe with little exposure to sunlight, and on a poor diet which also contains phytates (such as in chapattis) since these inhibit calcium absorption from the gut. Renal disease impairs the conversion of vitamin D to di-hydroxycholecalciferol and consequently can lead to 'renal rickets'.

Rickets is clinically characterized by a spectrum of bony deformities which range from mild bowing of the long bones of the legs to gross skeletal deformity and dwarfism (Fig. 2.8). Osteomalacia causes generalized

Rickets

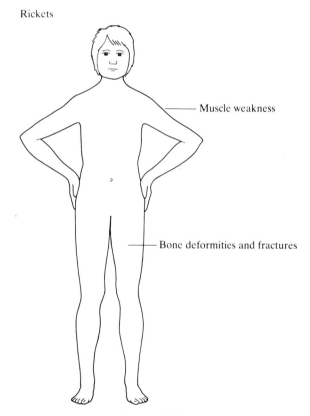

Muscle weakness

Bone deformities and fractures

Fig. 2.8 *Rickets.*

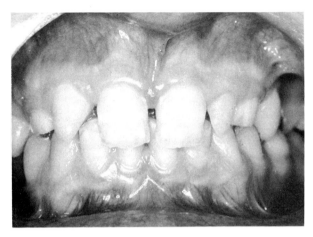

Fig. 2.9 *Dental hypoplasia in renal rickets. (Courtesy of Professor C. Scully.)*

bone pain and tenderness, vertebral collapse, pelvic deformities and myopathy.

Management

Correction of any underlying clinical disorder is required, and supplements of one of the metabolites of cholecalciferol are the usual lines of therapy for osteomalacia and rickets.

Oral aspects

Occasionally rickets may cause mild dental hypoplasia and delayed tooth eruption (Fig. 2.9). Osteomalacia can cause reduced bone density in the mandible and maxilla.

FURTHER READING

Avioli L. V., Krame S. M. (1978). *Metabolic bone disease. New York:* Academic Press.

Leading Article (1987). Vitamin D: New perspectives. *Lancet,* **i:** 1122–1123.

Scully C., Cawson R. A. (1988). *Colour aids to oral medicine.* Edinburgh and London: Churchill Livingstone.

Scully C., Flint S. (1988). *An atlas of stomatology.* London: Martin Dunitz.

Seow W. K., Latham S. C. (1986). The spectrum of dental manifestations in vitamin D resistant rickets and implications for management. *Pediatr. Dent.,* **8:** 245–250.

Sherwood L. M. (1987). Vitamin D, parathyroid hormone and renal failure. *N. Engl. J. Med.,* **316:** 1601–1602.

Fractures of the facial skeleton

Maxillofacial trauma is most commonly a consequence of road traffic accidents or assaults, but may also be due to sports injuries, civil disturbance and other causes. A severe maxillofacial injury is usually obvious, although quite extensive skeletal interruption can occur without marked displacement of bony fragments and uncomplicated by facial lacerations, and when the damage is trivial it is easily overlooked by those without dental knowledge. Medical staff dealing with accidents and emergencies need to be reminded that minimal degrees of malocclusion resulting from trauma can cause disproportionate discomfort to the patient, due to the rich nerve supply to the periodontal ligament and tongue, so that minor irregularities of tooth surface and of occlusion loom large in the patient's perception. In addition, secondary effects at the temporomandibular joint can result from minor tooth displacement.

The dental surgeon should in turn ensure a clear airway as a priority and seek to identify and record injuries in parts of the body outside the field of his or her specialty, particularly in the unconscious patient following a road accident or assault, where lesions may be overlooked (Fig. 3.1). Head injuries are particularly important.

This chapter will concentrate on injuries of the bony skeleton, with some mention of associated soft tissue injuries, but fracture of the cranial vault, the frontal bone and its sinus will be excluded. The management of trauma to individual teeth is described elsewhere (Volume 3).

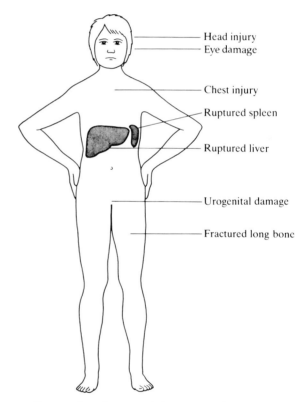

Fig. 3.1 *Sites that particularly require to be checked in patients with maxillofacial injuries.*

CLASSIFICATION OF FACIAL FRACTURES

Le Fort's classification is in general use for midface injuries, with additional descriptions of associated zygo-matic and orbital fractures. Mandibular fractures are classified by the region of the bone in which the fracture has occurred.

In general, fracture patterns are a result of the direction of the applied force and lines of weakness in the bone, but do not usually involve sutures, with the notable exceptions of the frontozygomatic suture and the midpalatal suture.

Middle third facial fractures

The Le Fort I fracture (Fig. 3.2a) passes immediately above the roots of the maxillary teeth to involve the floor of the antrum and the floor of the nose bilaterally. It is rarely impacted, more usually being somewhat mobile.

The Le Fort II fracture is at a higher level (Fig. 3.2b) and involves the lateral wall of the antrum, the infraorbital margin on both sides, and the nasal bones centrally. Impaction is common, due to overriding of the bony fragments at the fracture line under the influence of the original force, and may require considerable force to disimpact. The infraorbital foramen provides an area of weakness, and fracture through it results in numbness of the skin over the cheek. The cribriform plate of the ethmoid bone is frequently disrupted in the anterior cranial fossa, with consequent anosmia (Volume 1), cerebrospinal fluid rhinorrhoea (discharge of CSF from the nose) and risk of meningitis.

The Le Fort III fracture (Fig. 3.2c), at the highest level, produces complete craniofacial dysjunction involving the frontozygomatic suture, lateral wall of the bony orbit, and inferior orbital fissure bilaterally, and passing through the nasal bones and cribriform plate of the ethmoid bone medially. Craniofacial dysjunction, complicated by a downward and backward movement, can cause an unexpected respiratory obstruction by interposition of the soft palate between the tongue and the posterior wall of the pharynx (Fig. 3.3).

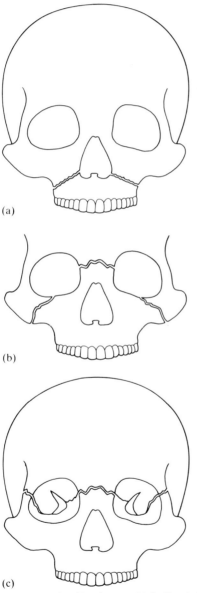

(a)

(b)

(c)

Fig. 3.2 *Patterns of midface fracture: (a) Le Fort I, (b) Le Fort II, (c) Le Fort III.*

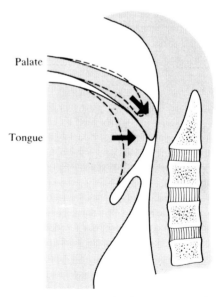

Fig. 3.3 *Impaction of soft palate between retroposed tongue and posterior pharyngeal wall, causing airway obstruction. The soft palate has moved backwards and downwards with the fragments constituting midface fracture.*

Zygomatic fractures

Zygomatic fractures are probably the most common facial fractures. They comprise the displacement of a single unitary fragment of bone, or they may be complicated by comminution, by adjacent orbital fractures, or by any of the Le Fort types of fracture. Occasionally the zygomatic arch alone is fractured, with resultant interference with the coronoid process of the mandible causing restricted mouth opening.

Where the orbital floor is fractured, interference with the movements of the inferior rectus and inferior oblique muscles may cause diplopia (double vision) when upward gaze is attempted (Fig. 3.4). The orbital floor can sometimes be fractured with the orbital rim remaining intact—the so-called blow-out fracture in allusion to its presumed aetiology from the transmission of hydraulic

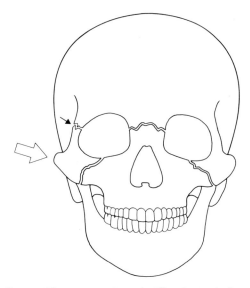

Fig. 3.5 *The common pattern of midface fracture is shown following a right-sided blow; the result is Le Fort II fracture with right zygoma fracture.*

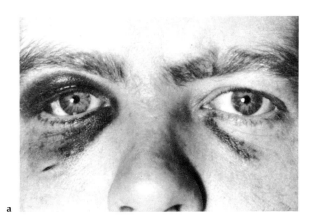

a

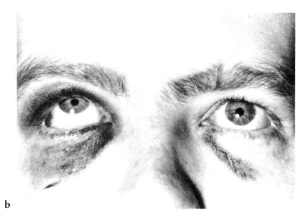

b

Fig. 3.4 *Fracture of the orbital floor, or 'blow-out' fracture, interferes with upward movement of the optic globe. In this patient, both orbital rims are intact, and the orbital floor is fractured on the left side.*

force through the optic globe within the inextensible bony orbit. Diplopia may also be caused by interference with the nerve supply to the ocular muscles, intraorbitally from trauma at the superior orbital fissure, or from haematoma or oedema, or alternatively at any point along the intracranial course of the motor nerves.

In the midface, a common fracture pattern is a Le Fort II fracture associated with a zygomatic fracture on the side of impact (Fig. 3.5).

Mandibular fractures

The lines of weakness in the mandible are at the neck of the condyle, the crypt of an unerupted third molar or other unerupted tooth, and below the canine, the tooth with the longest root (Fig. 3.6). The mandible fractures at any point in the body (Fig. 3.7), or the ascending ramus. The symphysis and the angle are commonly fractured.

Pathological fractures

A pathological fracture usually passes through a lesion such as a cyst, tumour, unerupted tooth or odontome which creates an area of weakness in the mandible. Although appropriate, the term pathological is not used regularly in connection with those fractures which result from osteoporosis. In addition, osteomyelitis and osteoradionecrosis also predispose to pathological fractures (Chapter 4).

Dentoalveolar fractures

Dentoalveolar fractures can complicate Le Fort and mandibular fractures, or occur alone. A tooth or teeth become displaced with a fragment of investing alveolar process. The fragment is usually mobile.

This account should also include the 'split palate', when the midpalatal suture gives way so that there is mobility of half the maxillary dental arch where one side is intact, or of both halves when a Le Fort fracture co-exists.

DIAGNOSIS OF FACIAL FRACTURES

History

An accurate history of the blow should be sought either from the patient, if he is able to communicate, or from a witness. The patient may remember the direction of the blow, and may have been conscious of the breaking of the jaw.

A common pattern of traumatic injury to the mandible is a fracture at the site of the blow, and an indirect fracture at a line of weakness on the opposite side, usually the condylar neck or angle of the jaw. The patient may remember a unilateral nose bleed (epistaxis) which, where the nose is undamaged, may indicate blood escaping from the antrum following a fracture of the zygomatic bone. The patient is often aware of an

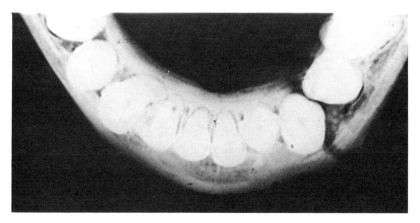

Fig. 3.6 Fracture of the lower left canine region. (Courtesy of Professor C. Scully.)

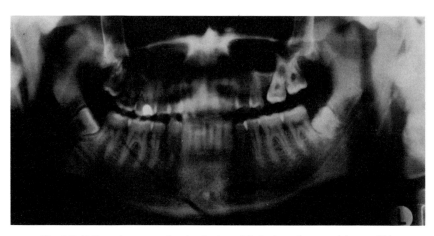

Fig. 3.7 Orthopantomogram showing fracture of the horizontal ramus of the mandible.

irregularity of the occlusion, which may be 'true', due to displacement of a tooth crown, or 'false', due to altered sensation or from an effusion in the temporomandibular joint. He will be aware of facial paraesthesia or hypoaesthesia, usually in the distribution of the infra-orbital or inferior alveolar nerve, but this may be due to pressure effects on terminal branches from trauma or oedema.

Inspection

Facial swelling and asymmetry or deformity are noted. The eyelids may be closed by oedema but, on parting them, it should be possible to confirm diplopia by asking the patient to follow a pointing finger or pencil through all the segments of usual gaze. The degree of diplopia may be recorded and illustrated by a Hess chart as a baseline record. A subconjunctival ecchymosis whose posterior limit cannot be defined (Fig. 3.8) is usually indicative of a fracture of the rim or wall of the orbit. The reaction of the eye to light assessed by shining a torch into the open eye is noted at 30-minute intervals for the first 24 hours, in order to detect failing function of the optic and oculomotor nerves, and intracranial haemorrhage.

Irregularity of bone contour may be identified immediately after the injury, but depression of the zygomatic bone or arch, or lengthening of the face in Le Fort injuries, is quickly masked by oedema (Fig. 3.9).

Where there is limitation of jaw opening, it may be due to spasm of the muscles or to displacement of the zygomatic arch, which impacts against the coronoid process on opening of the mouth. Deviation of the mandible towards the side of damage helps to identify fracture or contusion of the temporomandibular joint, and asymmetry will usually be obvious if the body of the mandible is fractured. Displacement and mobility of fragments is often obvious, but the presence of small discrepancies, as demonstrated by minor disorders of the occlusion and anterior open bite, should be excluded, particularly in the unconscious patient who is unable to report them.

The mouth and pharynx should be examined with a good light source and efficient suction to remove foreign bodies which might otherwise be inhaled. The foreign material may be extrinsic, for example metal or plastic from a road vehicle, or road grit; or it may be intrinsic,

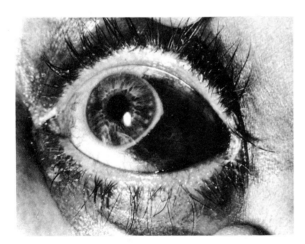

Fig. 3.8 *Subconjunctival ecchymosis whose posterior limit cannot be defined. The eye is directed towards the medial canthus; blood has extravasated from a lateral fracture of the left orbital margin.*

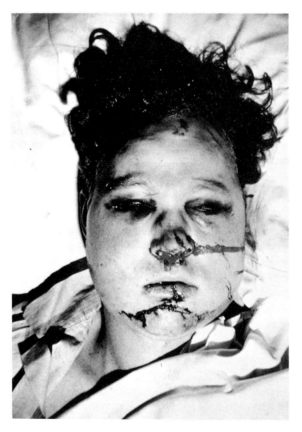

Fig. 3.9 *Facial oedema in a middle third fracture. (Courtesy of Professor C. Scully.)*

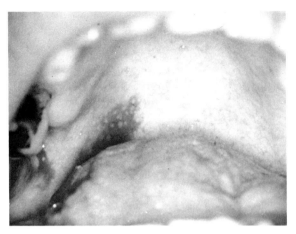

Fig. 3.10 Haematoma in a facial fracture (Guerin's sign). (Courtesy of Professor C. Scully.)

such as a tooth or teeth, blood clot, vomitus, restorations, or fragments of dentures. It should be remembered that methyl methacrylate is usually radiolucent, making the radiological identification of inhaled or ingested fragments of dentures very difficult.

Submucosal haematoma or ecchymosis (Fig. 3.10) is suggestive of an underlying fracture, and a sublingual haematoma is usually diagnostic of a fracture of the mandible. However, senile purpura in the elderly will exaggerate the amount of ecchymosis, and hence the significance of these signs.

The ears and nose should be inspected and any cerebrospinal fluid or haemorrhage noted. Inspection of the external auditory meatus with an auriscope may reveal a perforation of the tympanum if there is an underlying fracture of the skull base, and a discharge of cerebrospinal fluid and blood. A laceration of the anterior walls of the meatus is relatively common following posterior displacement of the major fragment in a condylar neck fracture, and disruption of the soft tissues may confuse the diagnosis. Basal skull fractures may cause bleeding into the middle ear, or haematoma over the mastoid process (Battle's sign).

Palpation

Accessible margins of the facial bones should be palpated for irregularity and tenderness. Particular attention should be paid to the orbital margins, the zygomatic arch, and the condyles and lower border of the mandible. Palpation within the oral vestibule will locate areas of tenderness and step deformities, which may identify sites of fracture. The sign of crepitus (grating together of the fracture margins) is painful to elicit, and is better not deliberately attempted but may sometimes be heard with a stethoscope, particularly at the temporomandibular joint when the mandible moves. Effusion in the joint can cause considerable tenderness and adjacent swelling, even in the absence of an underlying fracture.

Pressure in the palatal vault may elicit pain or mobility in the midface, indicative of Le Fort fracture. It is important to maintain counterpressure on the cranial vault or at the bridge of the nose, as it is easy to elicit a false positive sign because of movement of the head or of the scalp over the underlying bone. In addition, palpation of the nasal bridge while applying force in the palate may help to identify the level of the fracture.

Percussion

Tapping with a finger over the body of a facial bone is sometimes helpful in fracture diagnosis, as pain may be felt at the fracture site rather than at the point of percussion. Percussion of the maxillary incisors with the handle of a dental mirror may help to differentiate a fracture from a pre-existing congenital anterior open bite. If the bone is intact, the normal ringing tone will be heard, but an underlying fracture will give a dull note as of a cracked pot'.

Radiographs (see also Volume 1)

Some radiographic views require the cooperation of the patient and, in the severely injured or unconscious subject, good films may be unobtainable early on. Decisions may have to be deferred, or made on the basis of clinical examination, which sometimes must be carried out under a general anaesthetic.

Mandibular fractures

An orthopantomographic view is useful (see Fig. 3.7), and gives good information when the fracture is delineated. Oblique laterals are a good alternative. However, another film in a plane at right-angles is indicated, especially since the nature of tomography tends to obscure fractures which are running parallel with the tomographic 'slice'. A postero-anterior view should always be requested when clinical signs suggest a fracture. An occlusal view of the mandible is also useful in situations where the precise site of the fracture, or degree of displacement of fragments, is in doubt.

Zygomatic fractures

Two radiographic views at different angles are again essential, and it is usual to request 10° and 30° occipitomental radiographs. Where a fracture of the zygomatic arch is suspected, a submentovertex view is required. Further special techniques such as coronal tomography and computerized axial tomography will identify and locate fractures of the orbital floor and walls.

Midface fractures

Again, 10° and 30° occipitomental radiographs are required, supplemented by true lateral views. These radiographs can be difficult to interpret, and clinical findings should take precedence over radiographic appearances

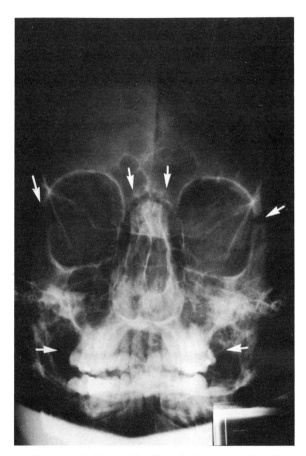

Fig. 3.11 *Occipitomental radiograph showing a Le Fort III fracture line (upper arrows). This patient also suffered a unilateral Le Fort I fracture with a midline split, causing separation of second molars (lower arrows).*

where there is doubt. In assessing the films, it is usual to inspect the supraorbital margins and zygomaticofrontal sutures, the lateral borders of the orbits, the infraorbital margins and nasal bones, and finally the maxillary antrum and its walls (Fig. 3.11). Radiographic signs of fracture are bony irregularity or displacement, opacity or a fluid level (blood) in the antrum, and displacement of orbital contents downwards into the antrum.

RESUSCITATION AND PRIMARY TREATMENT

The treatment of patients with maxillofacial injuries falls into three stages: resuscitation, primary treatment and definitive treatment. Where general injuries are minor, definitive treatment of a fracture may be initiated without delay, but it is appropriate here to give brief consideration to the earlier stages.

Resuscitation

The prime consideration is the integrity of the airway since asphyxia will kill the patient within minutes. The arrest of haemorrhage and the treatment of shock are also important.

Airway

Complex facial injuries, especially where there are fractures in both jaws, may compromise both nasal and oral airways. In fractures of the midface where the mandible is intact, the airway is usually easy to maintain—except in the rare instance where displacement of the midface results in obstruction of the nasopharynx by the soft palate (see Fig. 3.3). Unilateral fractures of the mandible seldom cause respiratory embarrassment, but where bilateral disruption of the mandible is sufficient to allow the anterior fragment to fall backwards, carrying the genioglossus and geniohyoid attachments and tongue with it, then the tongue will tend to obstruct the pharynx and the airway. The degree of tongue control is important for the patient to maintain his own airway, and bilateral fractures or the gross comminution observed in gun-shot injuries pose particular problems.

Until the airway is stable and controlled, patients must not be left unattended. In doubtful situations the patient is best cared for in the tonsillar position, semiprone with the upper leg flexed, and the head inclined in such a way that the sagittal plane is turned towards the pillow, but with the neck extended. A further pillow should be placed beneath the pelvis to aid postural drainage from the mouth (Fig. 3.12). The patient with a compromised airway should be supervised by a competent person throughout the initial phase of assessment and diagnosis, including the period in the radiology room.

If the tongue is uncontrolled, it may, in the unconscious patient, be grasped with tongue forceps or a towel clip, pulled forward and a traction suture inserted towards the posterior third. At the scene of the accident, the tongue may be grasped with a dry piece of linen material and the pharynx cleared of debris with a finger. Denture wearing is relatively common in the UK, and impaction of a denture or part of one into the respiratory passages may be the sole cause of airway obstruction. Fractures of the midface rarely cause obstruction of the airway, except by the occlusion of the nasal airway with blood clot and, as soon as suction is available, the nose, the pharynx and the mouth should be cleared. Where patency of the airway has not been maintained by posture or a tongue suture, an artificial airway may be successful, though the conscious or semiconscious patient may reject it. The oral airway functions by separating the tongue from the posterior pharyngeal wall but, where it is ineffective, a cuffed endotracheal tube should be passed below the laryngeal inlet. In extreme emergency a laryngotomy or tracheostomy may be necessary, but usually only where an endotracheal tube cannot be passed because of oedema or abnormal morphology preventing visualization of the laryngeal cords. The indications for *urgent* as distinct from *emergency* tracheostomy are loss of tongue control, respiratory inadequacy which may be pulmonary or central (due to brain damage) in origin, uncontrollable bleeding in the airway, glottic oedema, or an irreducible displacement of the midface with impaction of the soft palate in the pharynx (see Volume 1).

Brain damage may complicate an airway problem by decreasing gaseous exchange in lungs which are already impaired by pneumothorax, haemothorax, traumatic asphyxia or multiple fractures.

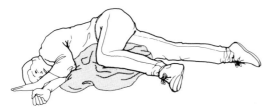

Fig. 3.12 *Tonsillar position. (Courtesy of Professor C. Scully.)*

Haemorrhage

Severe haemorrhage is not usually a feature of maxillofacial injuries despite the rich blood supply of the face. The facial artery may, however, on rare occasions, produce persistent bleeding and need to be clamped as a temporary measure. A torn inferior alveolar artery may suddenly bleed when a mandibular fracture is manipulated—particularly with a laryngoscope. Local pressure may suffice to stop the bleeding, but sometimes it may be desirable to approximate the fragments with a temporary wiring procedure (Fig. 3.13). Bleeding from oral wounds can usually be stopped by pressure with a swab or, when persistent, by oversewing the artery.

Bleeding into the nasal passages may be profuse at the time of injury, but persistent bleeding complicating midface fractures is not common, except where the fragments are very unstable. A notable example of this instability is provided by a gaping midline split in the palate, the fragments of which can be reduced and temporarily immobilized by simple wiring across the dental arch (Fig. 3.14). It may be necessary to insert a post-nasal gauze pack or inflatable balloon under general

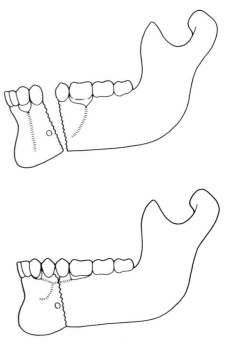

Fig. 3.13 *Wires twisted round firm teeth in the region of a displaced mandibular fracture, and then twisted together to provide temporary immobilization.*

anaesthesia to achieve final arrest of haemorrhage (Fig. 3.15). It is possible to ligate a bleeding maxillary artery by an approach through the maxillary antrum, but haemorrhage at this site is usually self-limiting. Persistent haemorrhage, which continues to well up from pharyngeal wounds even after insertion of post-nasal, pharyngeal and oral packs, and is accompanied by increasingly severe facial swelling, is indicative of a fracture of the base of the skull with disruption of the carotid arteries: it carries a grave prognosis.

Whereas all these methods of arresting haemorrhage need to be borne in mind, the need for fluid replacement must not be forgotten, and an intravenous infusion of fluid or sometimes whole blood, may be required.

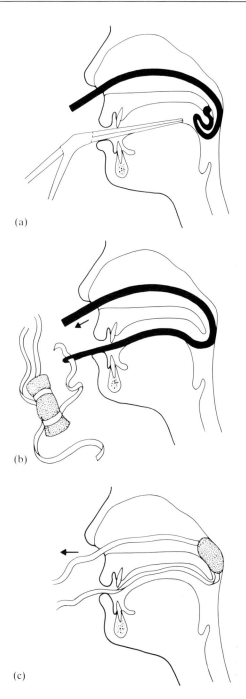

(a)

(b)

(c)

Fig. 3.15 *A method of insertion of a post-nasal pack to control nasal haemorrhage. (a) A catheter is passed through the nose. (b) A tape is attached to the end of the catheter. (c) The catheter is withdrawn, bringing the tape, and eventually the pack, to the nasopharynx.*

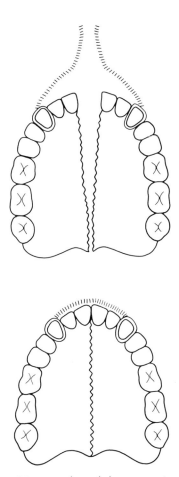

Fig. 3.14 *Wires passed round the upper canine teeth and twisted together will stabilize a gaping midline fracture of the maxilla.*

Shock

Maxillofacial injuries alone are rarely the cause of shock due to loss of blood volume (oligaemic shock). Therefore, if shock is present, obvious additional injuries causing substantial bleeding, such as fractured long bones (femur especially) or a hidden internal injury (such as a ruptured spleen) should be suspected (see Fig. 3.1).

The management of shock is not discussed here, but it is important to remember at this stage of care that morphine derivatives should be restricted in their use for the pharmacological control of pain and shock because they depress respiration and also cause pupil constriction, thereby complicating assessment of the pupil signs in the monitoring of intracranial injuries (see below).

Primary treatment of the jaw injury

Severely injured patients, fortunately, comprise a small but nevertheless important proportion of accident cases who have maxillofacial trauma. For the severely injured patient, primary care can begin only after resuscitation, but for most patients treatment begins with the primary care of their jaw injury. Primary treatment consists of control of pain, control of infection, and urgent simple measures to restore the injured tissues in order to reduce infection and improve comfort for the patient.

Control of pain

Pain is not a major feature of maxillofacial injury but when analgesia is needed for other injuries, account should be taken of an airway at risk. Reference should always be made to the local consultants' wishes, but a suitable analgesic for severe pain is 25 mg of pethidine intravenously. If the patient's conscious and pupil states have not deteriorated, this dose may be repeated, to a maximum of 100 mg in 4 hours. Where maxillofacial injury is not complicated by other injuries, 30–60 mg codeine phosphate by intramuscular injection or soluble paracetamol 500–1000 mg by mouth will usually suffice (Volume 1).

Control of infections

Contamination of facial injuries is the rule rather than the exception, particularly since mandibular fractures are compound into the mouth, zygomatic fractures may be compound into the antrum, and many maxillary fractures compound into the nasal air passages. A pre-existing dental apical granuloma (Volume 3) can readily infect a fracture, and damage to roots of teeth near to the fracture may predispose to infection. Systemic antibiotic cover should be instituted as soon as possible, except in condylar fractures (which are closed). The regimen of choice is 600 mg of benzylpenicillin 6-hourly for 5 days by intramuscular injection or via an intravenous drip, or phenoxymethyl penicillin 250 mg 6-hourly by mouth if feasible. Antitetanus prophylaxis may be required where facial lacerations are contaminated with dirt. Antibiotic prophylaxis against meningitis may be indicated when the cribriform plate of the ethmoid is fractured in Le Fort II and III injuries. In the past, immediate prophylaxis such as with sulphadiazine 2 g followed by 1 g 6-hourly was recommended, but many neurosurgeons now prefer to treat meningitis if and when it arises, withholding antibiotics from the start so as not to complicate the issue (Volume 1).

Soft tissue injury

Simple lacerations are usually sutured under local analgesia after cleaning away any debris. More complex lacerations are better repaired under general anaesthesia after underlying fractures have been reduced. The need for repair of such lacerations will often bring forward the timing of a general anaesthetic needed for treatment of a jaw fracture. Where there is tissue loss, it may be necessary to use plastic surgery techniques of tissue transfer in order to avoid the poor result inevitable if tissue is sutured across a gap. The extreme example of this is a gunshot wound, where it is always desirable to suture skin to mucosa around the edge of a large defect (Fig. 3.16).

The repair of intra-oral lacerations is not urgent if bleeding has stopped.

Skeletal injuries

Definitive treatment of skeletal injuries may have to be delayed for several days if the patient is not fit for a general anaesthetic and, in the interim, it may be desirable to apply some form of temporary fixation. A crepe bandage encircling the head as a barrel bandage provides support, but must be applied in such a way that it does not compromise the airway. Temporary support may also be provided by the use of strapping attached to a 'scrum cap'.

A delay of 10 days will not usually prejudice the efficient treatment of jaw injuries, but union may already have begun by then in midface fractures and, in children, even in mandibular fractures. Where the prognosis for

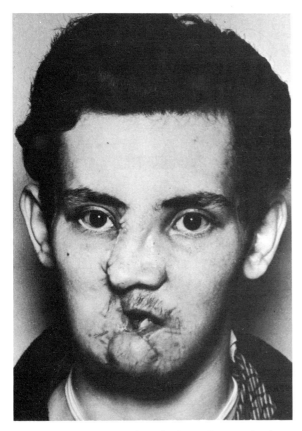

Fig. 3.16 *This patient, who suffered a gunshot wound of the face, has received inappropriate treatment. The wound has been closed restricting the oral aperture and distorting the face. The correct approach would have been to suture skin to mucous membrane, leaving a wide defect for reconstruction by tissue transfer. This is an old photograph: modern treatment would consider tissue transfer by microvascular surgery as an immediate procedure.*

loose teeth appears hopeless, they should be removed under local analgesia, particularly where they are broken down or so loose that they may be inhaled or ingested. However, the decision to remove teeth should not be taken lightly and, for example, localized alveolar fractures may be encouraged to unite by immobilization of the teeth, even if they subsequently need to be removed.

It is always useful to make record models at an early stage, from impressions recorded in the ward or if the patient is anaesthetized for some other purpose. Plaster models give information about the expected occlusion, and may be cut and repositioned in imitation of

reduction. They are of course essential for the fabrication of splints when these are indicated for definitive treatment.

Dislocation and subluxation of the mandible (see Chapter 9)

Records of the injuries

Careful recording of clinical data is always important, but it is doubly so in assaults or in accident cases, particularly where injury has resulted from a road traffic accident. The position and size of facial lacerations should be recorded, and the site and complexity of fractures of the facial skeleton should be set down visually in addition to the use of radiographs. It is most important to record, *at the time of injury,* loss of, and damage to, teeth which can be attributed to the assault or accident.

Definitive treatment of jaw fractures

Fortunately for the patient, bony union in jaw fractures is almost inevitable. Where the fragments are correctly reduced and immobilized, and infection is controlled, non-union is rare. However, there should be no laxity in applying the orthodox orthopaedic principles of accurate reduction and rigid fixation. The occlusion of the teeth provides an accurate record of the correct anatomical position; the dental occlusion should be accurately restored by reducing and immobilizing the skeletal elements, since even minor degrees of malocclusion and facial deformity can be difficult for the patient to accept. In most patients with facial fractures the normal dental occlusion can be readily identified but, where there is a pre-existing malocclusion or an underlying skeletal deformity, it may be necessary to study records very carefully, and assess the teeth and the plaster casts for cuspal arrangement and tooth wear, in order to define the correct occlusion.

Mandibular fractures

The usual form of fixation for simple mandibular fractures is by eyelet wires and intermaxillary tie wires. Eyelet wires are fabricated from stainless steel wire 0.35 mm in diameter, which is usually supplied in soft form and work hardened by stretching it so that its length is increased by 10% before it is made into eyelets (Fig. 3.17). Though local irregularities and the location of fractures will determine the precise placement of eyelet wires, it is

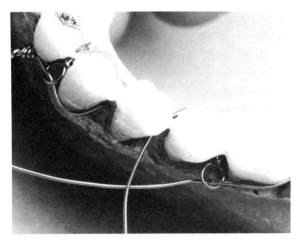

Fig. 3.17 *Eyelet wires placed on a model skull.*

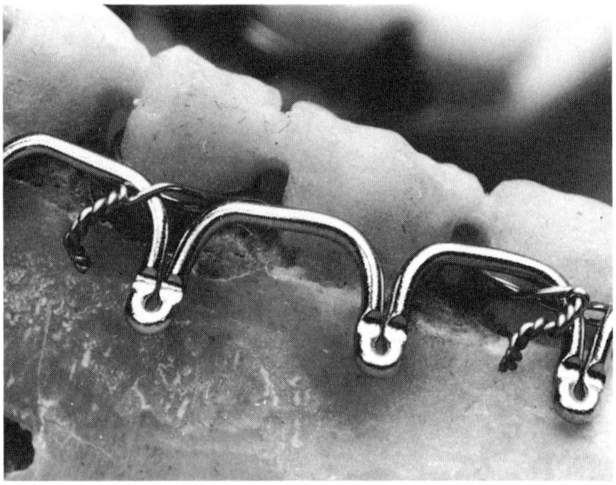

usual to place a minimum of five wires in each jaw, distributed more or less equally between the second molars. The wires should be placed such that the distance between eyelets when the tie wires are tightened with the teeth in occlusion is not less than 5.0 mm nor more than 15.0 mm. Oblique placement of the wires is helpful both in reducing the fracture and in controlling deviation of the jaw (Fig. 3.18). A reinforcing wire can be placed across the fracture site to approximate fragments by exerting tension between eyelets in the same arch and it may be necessary to place an intra-osseous wire to control a mandibular fragment which remains displaced even after interdental wiring (see below).

An alternative method of providing anchorage for intermaxillary fixation is by the use of an arch-bar wired to the teeth. The usual types of preformed material available are the Jelenko (Fig. 3.19) and Erich arch-bars (Fig. 3.20). Custom-made arch-bars can be fabricated on plaster casts, either by bending oval section heavy German silver wire (similar to lingual bar material for a partial denture), or by casting silver or chrome cobalt into an appropriate shape (Fig. 3.21). Metal buttons have also been designed for wiring to the teeth and these combine the advantages of both eyelets and arch-bars.

Eyelets are usually used where the teeth are stable in their sockets with satisfactory contact points, and there is

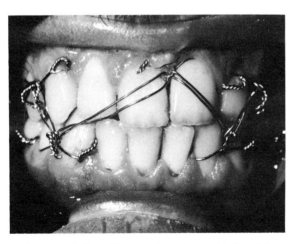

Fig. 3.18 *Eyelet and intermaxillary wires used to immobilize a fractured mandible to an intact maxilla.*

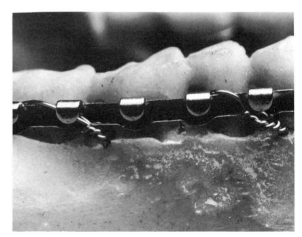

Fig. 3.19 *Jelenko arch-bar applied to a model skull.*

Fig. 3.20 *Erich arch-bar applied to a model skull.*

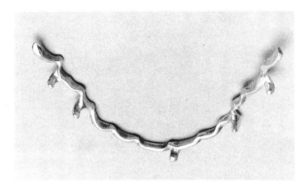

Fig. 3.21 *Cast silver bar suitable for wiring to the teeth. Stability is enhanced by the accurate contouring to the buccal and labial surfaces of the teeth.*

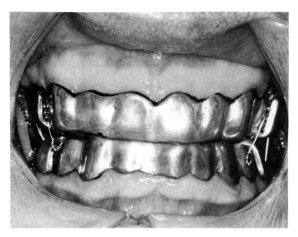

Fig. 3.22 *Cast silver cap splints. (Courtesy of Professor C. Scully.)*

no requirement for elastics. Elastic bands are useful where it is desirable to have instant release of the fixation, and when early function is desirable, for example in the case of a fractured condyle—where the elastics can be removed for meals to allow function and discourage ankylosis. Arch-bars are indicated where contact points are deficient, or where teeth are loose from periodontal disease or the trauma of the accident. Additionally, arch-bars are more convenient when their hooks can be used for elastic bands to provide intermaxillary fixation.

Interdental eyelet wiring is the treatment of choice for most simple fractures, and when it has been completed the patient will be returned to the ward with a pair of suitable wire cutters and an indication of the position of the tie wires, should it be necessary for a non-expert person to release the fixation in the event of respiratory obstruction. If the patient is to be transported by air or sea, intermaxillary fixation with elastic bands is the most satisfactory method.

Cast silver cap splints are occasionally indicated for immobilization of mandibular fractures (Fig. 3.22). Their main advantage is their ability to carry locking plates appropriate for the control of adjacent fractures via the teeth, or to carry external rods which may be connected to other skeletal fixation. However, there is always a delay due to the preoperative fabrication of the splints. Furthermore, their thickness over the occlusal surface can lead to minor occlusal irregularity when the splints are removed. A description of cap splints follows in the section on midface fractures.

Intermaxillary fixation alone may be sufficient to achieve reduction of mandibular fractures but, in a significant number of patients, displacement of a major fragment or fragments will remain, even though the

occlusion is correct. In such cases, it may be necessary to place an intra-osseous wire or a bone plate. An intra-oral or extra-oral approach is made to explore the fracture site and, after holes have been drilled adjacent to the fracture, 0.35 mm stainless steel wire is placed to reduce and immobilize the fragment (Fig. 3.23). The holes for the wire are placed in the bone with care to avoid the underlying inferior alveolar nerve and roots of teeth.

An alternative treatment is to use bone plates placed across fracture sites through an extra-oral or intra-oral approach. Orthopaedic finger plates and small compression plates have been used in the past, but both of these suffer from the disadvantage that they have been designed to treat fractures in straight long bones, whereas the mandible is curved in two directions. Although anatomical reduction apparently may be achieved, small discrepancies at the occlusal plane are difficult to eliminate. A recent development has been the introduction of malleable mini plates (Champy) which are

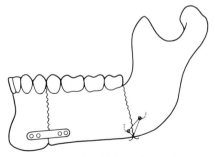

Fig. 3.23 *Diagram of small bone plate and intra-osseous wires in appropriate sites of the mandible.*

carefully contoured to any discrepancy before the screws are driven home. The great advantage of plating fractures is the partial or complete avoidance of a period of immobilization, to the obvious benefit of the patient's comfort, airway and nutrition. However, it is desirable to remove the plate after bony union has occurred, and for this a second operation is needed.

If the maxilla is intact, the mandible will be immobilized correctly by these means, and intermaxillary fixation is maintained for 4 or 5 weeks, during which time the patient eats a soft diet.

Minimally displaced fractures of the edentulous mandible do not require surgical intervention, since new complete dentures can compensate for the minor changes in mandibular shape. However, where the displacement is unacceptable, a fractured edentulous mandible can usually be successfully treated by the insertion of intra-osseous wires or the use of bone plates. Immobilization of the mandible by means of splints may not be necessary but it is still essential to define the occlusal plane by the provision of Gunning splints, which are simple acrylic bite blocks mounted on acrylic base plates. The anterior part of the splint is cut away for access for suction, for an airway and for nutrition. The most satisfactory way to construct the splint is to modify the existing dentures by removing the anterior teeth and providing hooks and attachments for intermaxillary and retaining wires. The mandibular splint is secured to the lower jaw by a circumferential wire passed around the splint and mandible using an awl (Fig. 3.24). The maxillary splint is secured to the upper jaw by one or more of several methods. Transalveolar wires can be passed through the cancellous bone of the alveolar process, through holes prepared in the base plate of the splint, and then tied over the occlusal surface. Screws may be passed into the maxillary bone, usually of the hard palate. A wire may be passed around the hard palate in an anteroposterior direction. Suspension wires may be attached to holes drilled in the pyriform margin of the anterior nares, the infraorbital margin, or malar buttress (Fig. 3.25). All these methods are carried out by means of an intra-oral approach.

The frontozygomatic suture region may be used as a suspension point for a maxillary splint (Fig. 3.25). The zygomatic process of the frontal bone is approached by a skin incision, and a hole is drilled obliquely. An awl is then used to pass the wire down the anterior border of the temporalis muscle into the mouth. An awl can be used in a similar fashion to pass circumferential wires around the zygomatic arches where these are intact and can be incorporated in the fixation. Whatever method is

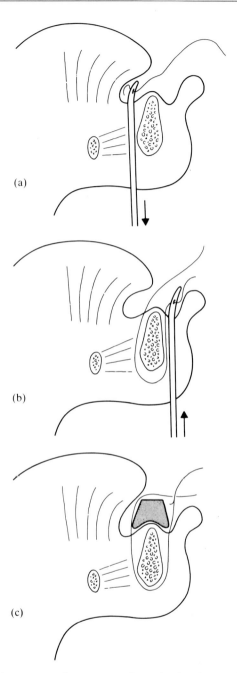

(a)

(b)

(c)

Fig. 3.24 *In order to secure a splint to the edentulous mandible, an awl is passed medial to the horizontal ramus. (a) A strand of 0.35 mm stainless steel wire is passed through the eye of the instrument and partially withdrawn. (b) The awl is subsequently passed to the vestibule of the mouth, and the wire removed from the eye. (c) The wire can be twisted over the splint to secure it.*

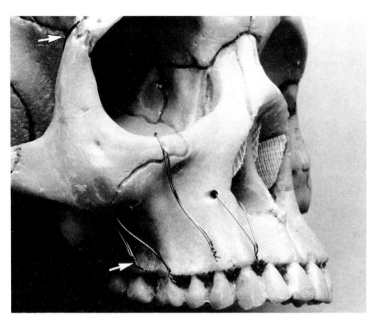

Fig. 3.25 *Suspension wires attached to fixed points on a model of the skull. From left to right: frontal suspension wire (arrow), malar buttress wire, infraorbital wire, pyriform margin wire. Clinically, one or more of these wires would be attached to a splint on the upper teeth on each side to resist downward displacement.*

selected for retaining the splint, it is important that intraosseous fixation in the mandible, whether using a wire or a plate, is secured with the occlusal plane defined as accurately as possible, and with intermaxillary fixation in place.

Unilateral fractures of the neck of the mandibular condyle do not usually produce permanent occlusal derangement but, in bilateral condylar fractures, the mandible may move posteriorly and produce an anterior open bite. A direct surgical approach to the fracture is possible but is difficult because it lies medial to the facial nerve, and intra-osseous fixation is problematical. Where occlusal disturbance results from condylar fracture or fractures alone, it usually resolves. However, if derangement persists for 10 days or more after injury, it is desirable to fit cast silver cap splints with provision for elastic traction so that the open bite may be reduced and, after a period of immobilization, alternating function and immobilization may be allowed until satisfactory union with good occlusion is obtained.

Midface fractures

Displaced Le Fort I, II and III level fractures can be accurately reduced in the anteroposterior plane by fixing the teeth in occlusion. The mandible will, of course, still be able to move following the application of the intermaxillary fixation, and could pull the mobile fractured maxillary complex with it. Craniomaxillary fixation to prevent this undesirable movement is usually achieved by means of rods extending from a cast upper cap splint cemented on the teeth to a skull halo (Figs. 3.26 and 3.27) or to supra-orbital pins (Fig. 3.28). The correct vertical dimension of the face has to be assessed by the operator. Alternatively, cranial suspension may be applied by wires suspending the maxilla from the zygomatic process of the frontal bone, or the frontal process of the zygomatic bone, or the zygomatic arches (see Fig. 3.25). These wires pull in a posterior direction, and their use is therefore contraindicated in the presence of unstable mandibular fractures. For example, the presence of bilateral condylar neck fractures destroys the continuity of the mandible and is not readily restored. A further disadvantage of suspension wires is that upward forces are not resisted, except by impaction of the fracture, and there can be movement at the cribriform plate of the ethmoid bone, with an increased risk of intracranial infection. Cranio*maxillary* fixation is preferred to cranio*mandibular* fixation as the former facilitates quick release of the mandible with

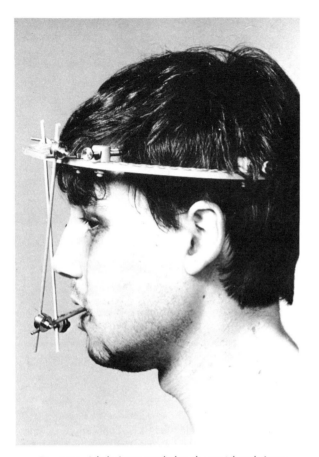

Fig. 3.26 *A halo frame attached to the cranial vault forms the upper component of craniomaxillary fixation—lateral view.*

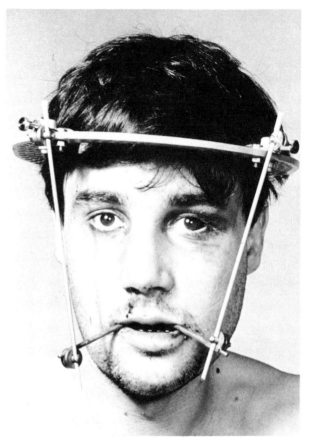

Fig. 3.27 *Anterior view of halo frame showing rods attached to bars projecting from a cap splint.*

minimal disturbance of the maxillary fracture, should airway impairment demand jaw opening and forward traction of the tongue. In most patients, once the correct occlusion and reduction of the maxillary component have been achieved and craniomaxillary fixation applied at operation, the mandible can be temporarily released in order to ensure a satisfactory oral airway in the immediate postoperative period. Recent modifications of the Champy system may, in the absence of comminution, permit plating of maxillary fractures—thereby dispensing with these external methods of fixation. Reapplication of the intermaxillary wires is desirable within 48 hours, since otherwise movements of the mandible may gradually displace the fractured maxilla, and malunion and malocclusion could result. Even after 24 hours, strong elastics may be necessary to restore the

normal occlusion achieved at operation. Although these methods usually produce good reduction of the fractured maxilla, complete reduction of the naso-ethmoidal region can be difficult and subsequent recession of the central region of the midface may result. It may be possible to place interosseous wires between nasal and frontal bones in order to minimize this recession and to avoid traumatic hypertelorism (increased intercanthal distance). The best access to the naso-ethmoid region is through a bicoronal skin incision.

Most fractures of the midface are multiple and relatively mobile, but in those few cases where the impaction resulting from overriding of the fragments proves resistant to manual pressure, reduction cannot be achieved without the use of disimpaction forceps (Fig. 3.29).

ing plates machined to precise limits are interchangeable, but electrolytic ulcers are easily caused unless both brass plates and silver splints are gold-plated. Some are individually made in cast silver with the advantage of eliminating electrolytic effects due to the presence of dissimilar metals. The localizing plates are used to carry rods connecting with external fixation, or localizing bars which pass across a fracture from one fragment to another. This may be appropriate in the maxilla, most commonly at the midline (Fig. 3.31), or in the mandible. In those patients whose severe injuries render them unfit for general anaesthesia, it is sometimes possible to reduce displaced fractures by the use of elastics over suitably placed hooks on the splints. Slow movement of the fragments takes place and, when complete reduction has been affected by elastic traction, a localizing bar is made. The precise relationship of the localizing plates is recorded in the mouth using plaster of Paris as a rigid matrix poured over the ends of extension wires so that when the plates have been removed it is possible for the laboratory to invest them and solder a rigid bar across the gap.

Combined mandibular and maxillary fractures

Where both mandibular and maxillary fractures are present, the mandible should first be reconstituted, where possible, by means of intra-osseous wires or bone plates, or cap splints. The fractured maxilla can then be located and controlled by the mandible. Where a fracture of the maxilla is complicated by bilateral fractures of mandibular condyles, the latter cannot be rendered intact, so that craniomaxillary fixation must have an anterior component which is necessary to restore normal facial contour. It may also be necessary to insert bone pins at the angles of the mandible in order to distract the mandible from the base of the skull, and allow the condyles to take up a satisfactory position.

Zygomatic and orbital fractures

Simple displaced fractures of the zygomatic bone may be elevated with a Kilner or Rowe elevator through a Gillies' incision in the temporal fascia (Fig. 3.32). It is sometimes possible to elevate through an intra-oral incision, and certain depressed zygomas can be elevated using a hook via a stab incision in the cheek. Most zygomatic fractures which are single fragments will remain stable after elevation because of the interdigitation of the bony edges at the fracture sites. However, it is important that they are not re-depressed by minor pressure in the immediate

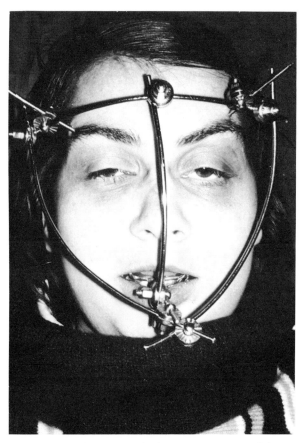

Fig. 3.28 *This patient suffered a Le Fort II fracture with left zygomatic fracture, and bilateral fracture of the mandible. Supra-orbital pins have been screwed into the frontal bone, and three rods are attached to a projecting bar from a cap splint to exert forward traction.*

Cap splints

Cast silver cap splints are fabricated on plaster models of the standing teeth. Once immobilized in the correct position, adequate control of the underlying dento-alveolar or body fracture may be obtained, but the splints are falling out of favour with the advent of intra-osseous wires and bone plates. Cap splints still have a place, particularly in midface fractures, complex maxillomandibular fractures, and bilateral fractures of the condylar neck. The splints bear hooks which have their openings facing away from the occlusal plane for intermaxillary fixation and facing towards the occlusal plane where suspension wires are to be used (Fig. 3.30).

Localizing plates are of two main types. Brass localiz-

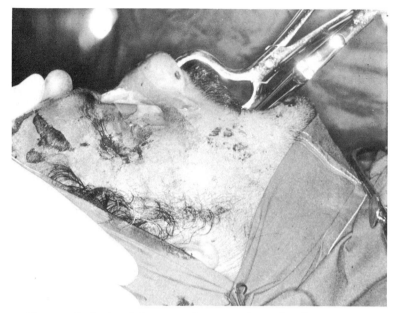

Fig. 3.29 *Application of disimpaction forceps to a fractured midface in an anaes-thetized patient. Note the assistant's hands restraining the cranial vault.*

post-operative period before the patient regains control. Unstable fractures are stabilized by the insertion of 0.35 mm stainless steel wires at the frontozygomatic suture, and often at the infra-orbital margin after elevation (Fig. 3.33). Complementary methods of stabilizing the main fragment are to use a pack of Whitehead's varnish on gauze to fill the antrum via a Caldwell–Luc procedure (Chapter 10), or to attach a pin to the zygoma, stabilizing it with another pin at the supra-orbital margin.

Comminuted fractures involving the orbital rim may extend along the floor of the orbit allowing herniation of

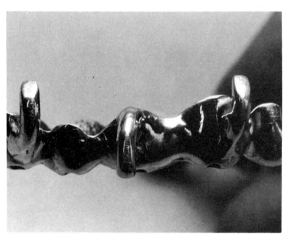

Fig. 3.30 *Part of a maxillary silver cap splint. Hooks for intermaxillary fixation are placed buccal to the lower right first molar and the lower right canine and a hook for a suspension wire at the lower right first premolar.*

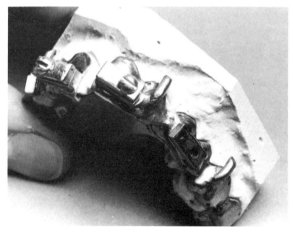

Fig. 3.31 *A maxillary silver cap splint in two parts, with localizing plates in situ adjacent to the midline. A localizing plate for an external rod has been removed from the canine region.*

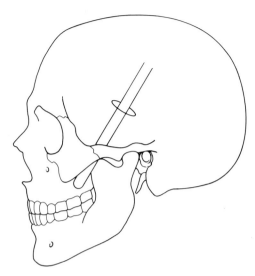

Fig. 3.32 *Gillies' approach, via a temporal incision, enables a Kilner zygomatic elevator to be passed beneath the temporalis fascia to the displaced zygomatic bone or arch in order to elevate the fragments.*

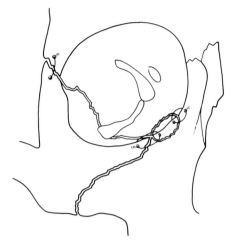

Fig. 3.33 *Unstable zygomatic and infra-orbital rim fractures can be stabilized by the insertion of interosseous wires, as shown.*

the orbital contents into the maxillary antrum. The orbital floor should be explored in these cases via an infra-orbital incision, the trapped orbital tissue freed, and possibly an implant inserted to separate the soft tissue from the fracture site. The implant may be a thin sheet of synthetic material such as silastic, cartilage or bone. True 'blowout' fractures, where the orbital rim is intact but the floor fractured, should be similarly treated. Where a zygomatic fracture complicates a Le Fort fracture, it is essential to elevate the zygomatic bone at the beginning of the operative procedures to release any latent impaction.

Nasal fractures

Nasal fractures complicating Le Fort II and III level injuries should receive attention immediately after the maxillary complex has been reduced and immobilized. It is necessary to manipulate displaced fragments using nasal forceps (Asche's and Walsham's) around the nasal endotracheal tube. The fragments are stabilized between a plaster splint externally and internally a carefully inserted gauze pack soaked in an antiseptic such as flavine emulsion.

Facial fractures in children

The principles of treatment of facial fracture are the same in children as in adults, but there are differences of emphasis. The presence of unerupted permanent teeth influences the selection of sites for the insertion of wires or of screws for plates. The plastic nature of the bones renders them less liable to fracture with mild to moderate trauma, and the remodelling processes of growth will usually smooth out minor discrepancies of contour. The developing occlusion will adapt to small disturbances of cuspal contact and, in many situations, simple treatment measures are sufficient.

Two aspects of injuries specific to children deserve attention. The first is the need to monitor condylar growth where a fracture is thought to have disturbed the condylar cartilage, so that any facial asymmetry may be corrected at an early stage. Secondly, it is important to remember the possibility of parental assault or other child abuse when a child is brought in with facial injuries which are not easily explained as the result of an accident (Volume 1).

FURTHER READING

Lewis A. F. (1983). *The management of acute head injury.* London: HMSO.

Rowe N. L., Williams J. L. (Eds.) (1985). *Maxillofacial injuries.* London: Churchill Livingstone.

Schultz R. C., de Camera D. L. (1984). Athletic facial injuries. *JAMA,* **252**: 3395.

Zook E. G. (1980). *The primary care of facial injuries.* Littleton, Mass.: PSG.

Chapter
4   *Infection of bone*

Surgical infections of the orofacial region and principles of treatment are discussed in Volume 1. This chapter deals with infection of bone.

Dental extractions, jaw fractures and many oral surgical procedures expose the cancellous bone of the jaw to saliva and the oral flora and yet, despite this contaminated environment, the bones almost invariably heal well because of their excellent blood supply from the alveolar arteries and periosteum. The maxilla is even more resistant to infection than the thicker mandible whose form and vascularity more closely resemble those of a long bone.

Severe bone infections of the jaws are therefore rare, especially in Western and other societies where the level of nutrition ensures a high resistance.

DRY SOCKET

A dry socket is a localized osteitis of the alveolar bone, which occurs as a postoperative complication in up to 3% of tooth extractions. The prevalence is highest following the removal of wisdom teeth and where various predisposing factors are operative.

Predisposing factors

The condition is most common:

1. in the mandible,
2. in the molar region,
3. following difficult extractions,
4. after operation under local analgesia rather than general anaesthesia,
5. in women—there is an increased incidence in patients taking oral contraceptives,
6. in smokers,
7. where there are local bone diseases, e.g. Paget's disease and osteopetrosis,
8. where there is an immune defect,
9. where there is a previous history of dry socket.

Aetiology

Dry socket appears to be caused by dissolution of the postextraction clot; both infection and fibrinolysis by enzymes such as plasmin have been implicated.

Features

The clinical feature of dry socket is postextraction pain which is often severe, throbbing and deep seated and frequently worse than any original toothache that necessitated the extraction. The pain usually begins 2–4 days after the extraction and the socket is devoid of clot but may contain food debris, and has a swollen erythematous mucosal margin. Exposed bone is often visible in the socket and is exquisitely tender to touch. A foul halitosis and bad taste may be complained of by the patient.

Prophylaxis

Antimicrobials given before extractions have a prophylactic effect. The particular efficacy of metronidazole has shown the important part played in this condition by anaerobic bacteria.

Treatment

Treatment consists of local measures and analgesics. The socket should be gently irrigated with warm normal saline or warm aqueous 0.2% chlorhexidine in order to remove debris, and lightly packed with a resorbable proprietary paste containing an antiseptic and local analgesic. The treatment is repeated every few days until granulation of the socket occurs. The patient is instructed in the use of hot (50°C) salt-water mouthwashes to be used at least four times daily. Systemic antibiotic therapy is rarely necessary and although some have advocated topical antibiotic pastes for use in the socket both for prophylaxis and treatment, they are rarely needed and might, at least in theory, lead to sensitization to the drug.

OSTEOMYELITIS

Osteomyelitis literally means inflammation of the bone marrow, although sometimes the subperiosteal bone is mainly affected. Osteomyelitis usually occurs in adults, and the affected bone responds either by osteoclastic resorption or by osteoblastic bone formation. Classic acute osteomyelitis .is essentially an osteolytic, destructive process, but an osteoblastic response is typical of chronic sclerosing osteomyelitis. In children, proliferative periostitis may occur with the production of large quantities of subperiosteal new bone.

Microbiology

Staphylococcus aureus is the commonest organism causing osteomyelitis in the jaws, but streptococci (both alpha and beta haemolytic) and anaerobic organisms (e.g. bacteroides, peptostreptococci and anaerobic streptococci) are increasingly recognized. The appreciation of the important role of anaerobes is due not only to better techniques of culture and transport, but also to the realization that these organisms show syngergism with aerobic bacteria and that they are not mere contaminants in a mixed infection. Mixed aerobic and anaerobic bony infections are particularly difficult to treat.

Rarely, osteomyelitis of the jaws may be caused by more specific organisms, e.g. salmonellae, mycobacteria or *Treponema pallidum.*

Predisposing factors

There are three possible sources from which bacteria can spread to bone.

1. From local infection, the commonest causes being compound fractures where foreign bodies are present, or odontogenic infection.

2. Spread from other adjacent structures, e.g. from middle-ear infection (otitis media), tonsillitis, or salivary gland infection.

3. Haematogenous spread of organisms: this is rare in relation to the jaws.

When osteomyelitis of the mandible does occur, it may be a sign of an underlying debilitating disease, such as diabetes mellitus, an immune defect, or the effects of alcoholism; alternatively, it may be related to reduced vascularity such as occurs after irradiation (see below and Volume 1) or in rare conditions such as osteopetrosis (Chapter 1).

Pathology

In acute osteomyelitis the organisms excite an acute inflammatory response in the medullary bone and the consequent oedema and exudation within the rigidly enclosed bone marrow causes pus to be forced under pressure through the medullary bone. The pressure causes thrombosis of the intrabony blood vessels, i.e. the inferior alveolar artery, reducing the vascular supply to the bone, which then necroses (Fig. 4.1). Eventually the pus bursts through the cortical plate to drain via sinuses in the skin or mucosa. Where pus penetrates the cortex it may spread subperiosteally, stripping the periosteum from the bone and thus further reducing the blood supply. Necrotic areas of bone become sequestra surrounded by pus, and either spontaneously discharge or remain and perpetuate the infection. The periosteum which has been lifted from the underlying bone lays down new bone to form an involucrum encasing the infected and sequestrated bone. The involucrum, though perforated by sinuses which drain pus, may prevent sequestra from being shed. Finally, if little new bone is formed, a pathological fracture may occur.

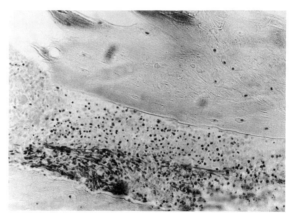

Fig. 4.1 *Osteomyelitis of the jaws, showing necrotic bone and inflammatory infiltrate. (Courtesy of Professor C. Scully.)*

Treatment

Treatment of bone infections may be medical, surgical or a combination of the two (Table 4.1).

The principles of antibiotic use are discussed in Volume 1. A high bone penetrance of antibiotic is essential to treat osteomyelitis, since bone vascularity is reduced. Penicillin is still the drug of choice, but many staphylococci are now penicillin resistant, and for these infections flucloxacillin or fusidic acid may be used. Fusidic acid should always be used in combination with another antibiotic to discourage the development of drug resistance. Lincomycin and clindamycin also give high bone levels but, because of a high incidence of colonic inflammation due to *Clostridium difficile* (pseudomembranous colitis), are now rarely used. Metronidazole gives good bone levels and is indicated where anaerobic infection is suspected. Tetracycline penetrates bone well, but is bacteriostatic and is less effective than bacteriocidal antibiotics.

Drainage of established pus follows the same guidelines used for other infections. When dead bone is exposed in the mouth, it can often be left to sequestrate without surgical interference, but sequestrectomy should be undertaken if the separated dead bone fails to discharge, and decortication of the mandible may be needed in order to allow this and drainage. Infected endosteal bone should be curetted. Occasionally radical resection of the infected bone may be required.

High-pressure oxygen therapy (hyperbaric oxygen) is

an effective adjunct for recalcitrant osteomyelitis, especially where anaerobic organisms are involved.

Acute osteomyelitis

Acute osteomyelitis primarily affects the mandible (Fig. 4.1) but, in very young children, may affect the maxilla (Figs. 4.2 and 4.3), presumably because the lack of development of the antrum at this age makes the maxilla a dense bone.

Mandibular osteomyelitis presents with a deep-seated, boring pain and swelling (Fig. 4.4). Teeth in the affected segment are mobile and tender to percussion, and pus oozes from the gingival crevices. Once pus penetrates the cortical plate the pain improves and pus discharges intra- or extra-orally, often through several sinuses (Figs. 4.5 and 4.6). Labial anaesthesia is a characteristic feature because of pressure on the inferior alveolar nerve. The patient is often febrile and toxic with enlarged cervical lymph nodes.

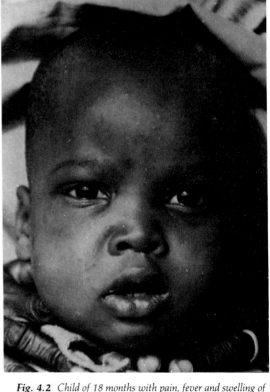

Fig. 4.2 *Child of 18 months with pain, fever and swelling of right maxilla from osteomyelitis (patient of Professor A. O. Adekeye, Nigeria).*

Table 4.1
Treatment of osteomyelitis

Treatment	Comments
Medical	
Antibiotics	Specific for causative organism
Analgesics	Pain relief
Hyperbaric oxygen	Improves vascularity and healing, especially in anaerobic infection
Surgical	
Drainage	For release of pus
Sequestrectomy	For removal of dead bone
Decortication	To allow drainage of endosteal infection
Removal of infective source	Tooth extraction
Resection	Where entire sections of mandible are dead and destroyed
Reconstruction	After resection, e.g. hip graft, vascularized flap

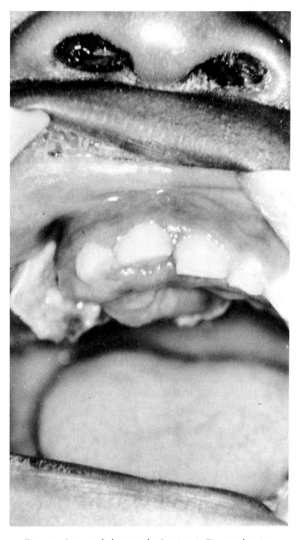

Fig. 4.3 *Intra-oral photograph of patient in Fig. 4.2 showing large bone sequestrum in upper deciduous molar region.*

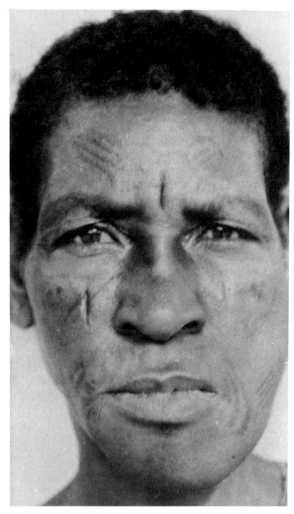

Fig. 4.4 *40-year-old woman with facial pain, numb left lower lip and swelling of the left face (patient of Professor A. O. Adekeye, Nigeria).*

Radiographs in established cases show marked bony destruction and sequestration (Figs. 4.7 and 4.8), but since the radiographic changes are seen only after there has been significant demineralization of bone, early cases may not be detected and, in these, isotope bone scanning using technetium diphosphonate may show increased uptake (Fig. 4.9). Blood tests show a leucocytosis with neutrophilia, and a raised erythrocyte sedimentation rate (or plasma viscosity). Treatment is by antibiotic therapy and usually drainage.

Chronic osteomyelitis

Chronic osteomyelitis presents with intermittent pain and swelling, relieved by the discharge of pus through longstanding sinuses. Bone destruction is localized and often a single sequestrum may be the source of chronic infection (Fig. 4.10). Removal of the sequestrum and curettage of the associated granulation tissue usually produces complete resolution.

Focal sclerosing osteomyelitis

Focal sclerosing osteomyelitis is usually asymptomatic

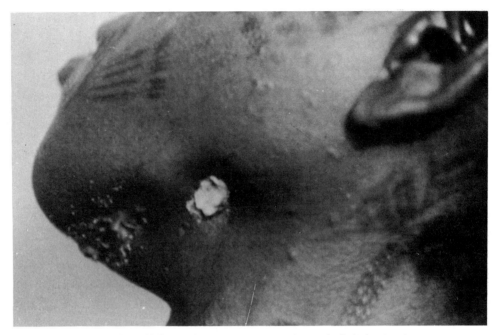

Fig. 4.5 *Submandibular view of patient in Fig. 4.4 to show multiple discharging sinuses.*

and revealed as an incidental radiographic finding (Fig. 4.11). Most common in young adults, it is usually associated with apical infection of a mandibular molar. Radiographically there is a dense, radio-opaque area of sclerotic bone related to the apical area, caused by formation of endosteal bone. This appears to be a response to low-grade infection in a highly immune host. Following tooth extraction the infection usually resolves (but the area of sclerotic bone often remains).

Diffuse sclerosing osteomyelitis

Diffuse sclerosing osteomyelitis is a sclerotic endosteal reaction which, like focal sclerosing osteomyelitis, appears to be a response to low-grade infection. However, the area of bone affected is widespread and sometimes involves most of the mandible or occasionally the maxilla (Fig. 4.12). Sometimes the infection arises in an abnormally osteosclerotic mandible such as in Paget's disease, osteopetrosis or fibrous dysplasia. Intermittent swelling, pain and discharge of pus may go on for years.

Management is difficult because of the extensive nature of the disease process. Long-term antibiotics, curettage and limited sequestrectomy all have their place.

Proliferative periostitis (Garre's osteomyelitis)

Garre's osteomyelitis is more common in children than adults. The cellular osteogenic periosteum of the child responds to low-grade infection such as apical infection of a lower first molar tooth by proliferation and deposition of subperiosteal new bone.

The subperiosteal bone may be deposited in layers, producing an onion-skin appearance radiologically, which can simulate a sarcoma. The endosteal bone, however, may appear to be completely normal, but in severe cases also appears 'moth-eaten' radiologically (Fig. 4.13). Removal of the infective source is usually followed by complete resolution, although subsequent bone remodelling can take a considerable time.

Pulse granuloma (Lewar's disease)

Pulse granuloma is a variety of periostitis and osteitis. The typical presentation is of an edentulous patient with a bony hard, subperiosteal mass in the lower buccal sulcus, indented or ulcerated by a denture flange. Hyaline bodies seen on histology seem to be vegetable leguminous pulse fragments, which have provoked a foreign body reaction. Vegetable matter may become embed-

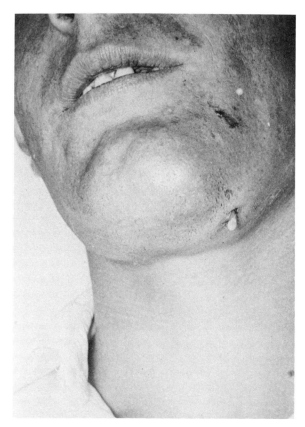

Fig. 4.6 *Sinus discharging pus in acute osteomyelitis. (Courtesy of Professor C. Scully.)*

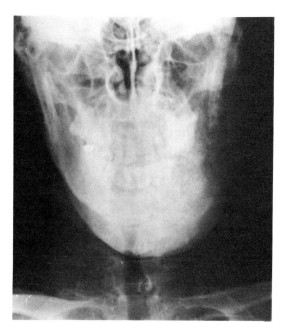

Fig. 4.7 *Radiograph of acute osteomyelitis of the jaws: postero-anterior (PA) radiograph showing extensive destruction of left angle of mandible.*

ded under the mucosa following tooth extraction or by pressure from the denture. Treatment is by curettage.

Osteoradionecrosis

Osteoradionecrosis used to be a common complication of radiotherapy for head and neck cancers (Volume 1). Modern techniques of radiotherapy have significantly reduced this risk, but osteoradionecrosis may still occur. The initiating factor is often trauma, such as tooth extraction or infection. Presentation is of exposed bone in an irradiated mouth, with or without external sinuses, pain and pathological fracture (Fig. 4.14 and 4.15). Once established, the process may spread to involve the whole jaw, usually the mandible.

Treatment is by long-term antimicrobials, especially tetracycline (which has high bone penetrance), and local cleansing of debris with aqueous 0.2% chlorhexidine

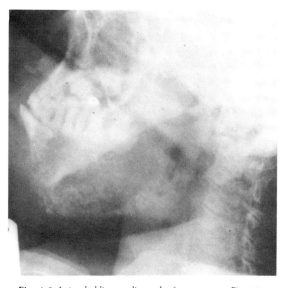

Fig. 4.8 *Lateral oblique radiograph of same case as Fig. 4.7, showing virtual destruction of the left hemimandible. Note moth-eaten appearance.*

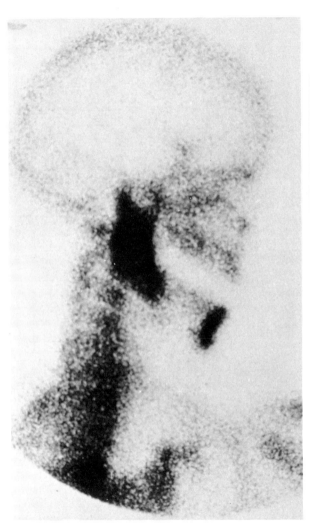

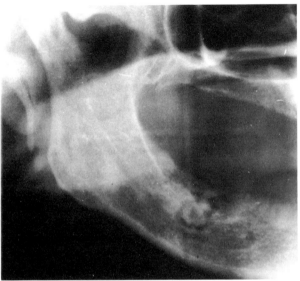

Fig. 4.10 *Radiograph of patient with an 8-year history of recurrent swelling and discharge in the lower first molar region. Radiograph demonstrates a well-demarcated chronic sequestrum.*

Fig. 4.9 *Isotope scan of patient with early osteomyelitis showing hot spots in the vertical ramus and angle and also the anterior mandible.*

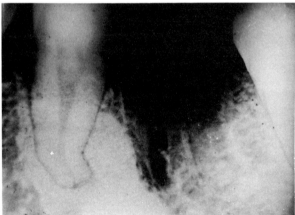

Fig. 4.11 *Focal sclerosing osteomyelitis. (Courtesy of Professor C. Scully.)*

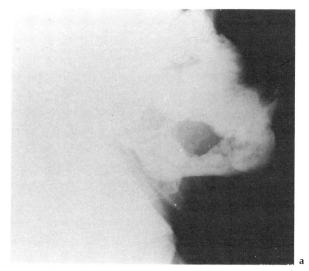

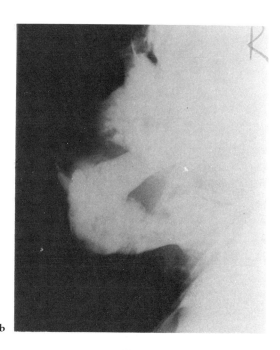

Fig. 4.12 (a) Right and (b) left lateral–oblique radiographs of a patient with fibrous dysplasia of maxilla and mandible, with superimposed diffuse sclerosing osteomyelitis of the mandible with a 6-year history of draining submandibular sinuses.

b

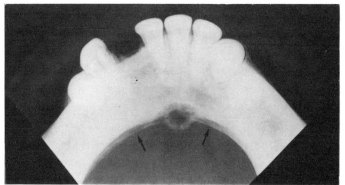

Fig. 4.13 Garre's osteomyelitis related to apical infection of the mandibular incisors. Note new subperiosteal bone formation.

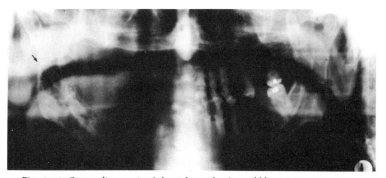

Fig. 4.14 Osteoradionecrosis of the right angle of mandible postextraction. Arrow demonstrates a pathological fracture. Note the extensive cervical caries affecting teeth in the left jaws (patient of Mr R. P. Ward-Booth).

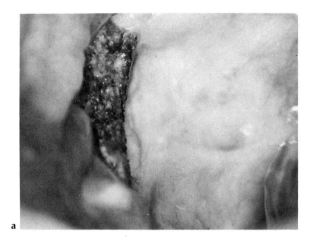

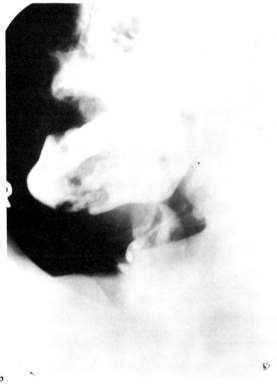

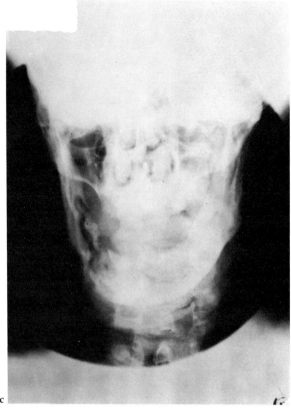

Fig. 4.15 *Osteoradionecrosis. (a) Clinical appearance of sequestrum. (b) and (c) Radiographic moth-eaten appearance. (Courtesy of Professor C. Scully.)*

mouthbaths. Sequestrectomy and surgical intervention should be minimal. Hyperbaric oxygen has proved useful in the USA for both initial treatment and during reconstruction. As a last resort, resection may become necessary because of chronic pain and destruction. Since there is reduced tissue vascularity, later reconstruction is complex.

FURTHER READING

Adherhold L., Knothe H., Frenkel G. (1981). The bacteriology of dentogenous pyrogenic infections. *Oral Surg.,* **52**: 583–587.

Heimdahl A., Nord C. E. (1983). Orofacial infections of odontogenic origin. *Scand. J. Infect. Dis.,* (Suppl.) **39**: 86–91.

McCracken A. W., Cawson R. A. (1983). *Clinical and oral microbiology.* Washington: Hemisphere.

Chapter

5   *Cysts in the jaws*

Definition

A cyst is a pathological cavity having liquid, semi-liquid or gaseous contents. It is frequently, but not always, lined with epithelium.

Classification

Table 5.1 shows a simplification of a classification of jaw cysts established by the World Health Organisation (WHO) in 1971.

This chapter discusses cysts based on the WHO classification; antral cysts are discussed in Chapter 10.

Table 5.1
Classification of jaw cysts

Developmental
Odontogenic
   Odontogenic keratocyst (primordial cyst)
   Follicular (dentigerous) cyst
   Eruption cyst
   Other developmental odontogenic cysts
Non-odontogenic
   Nasopalatine (incisive canal) cyst
   Nasolabial cyst
   Cysts of debatable origin

Inflammatory
Radicular (apical, dental) cyst
Lateral periodontal cyst
Residual cyst

Non-epithelial
Simple (traumatic, haemorrhagic) bone cyst
Aneurysmal bone cyst

Mechanisms of cyst growth

The mechanisms of cyst development are not fully understood, but the main factors are as follows.

1. Epithelial proliferation, either stimulated by inflammation (in the case of radicular cysts) or occurring without apparent stimulation (in the case of keratocysts).
2. Hydrostatic or osmotic factors may play a part in cyst growth since the cyst wall acts as a semipermeable membrane. Keratin formation may be prominent in keratocysts.
3. Bone-resorbing factors such as prostaglandins have been demonstrated in tissue cultures from cysts, and collagenase may be present in the walls of keratocysts.

The significance of each of these three factors in cyst formation and growth is speculative; all may well act to varying degrees.

Clinical features

Cysts of the jaws are relatively common. Inflammatory cysts are the most frequent, accounting for about 55% of all jaw cysts. Jaw cysts are generally slow growing and expansive, rather than invasive. Individual cysts often reach a large size before they give rise to symptoms, such as noticeable swelling (Fig. 5.1), discharge into the mouth, or pain due to secondary infection. Many cystic lesions appear as symptomless coincidental radiographic findings (Fig. 5.2).

Cysts in bone initially become apparent as a smooth, bony hard lump with normal overlying mucosa but, as the bone thins, it may crackle on palpation rather like an egg shell. When the overlying bone is resorbed, the cyst may show through as a bluish fluctuant swelling.

The diagnosis of jaw cysts, as in other conditions, is

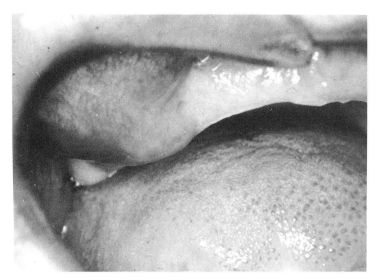

Fig. 5.1 *Cyst in right maxillary alveolus. (Courtesy of Professor C. Scully.)*

based on the combination of an adequate history, clinical examination and selected investigations (Volume 1).

Investigations

The appropriate tests include: pulp testing of associated teeth, preferably with a carbon-dioxide pencil; radiographs (both intra-oral and extra-oral); aspiration and analysis of cyst fluids; and biopsy. Aspiration through a large-bore needle may confirm that a lesion is cystic (though it may be a generally solid lesion with cystic areas) and may help in the differentiation of keratocysts from other odontogenic cysts (page 54).

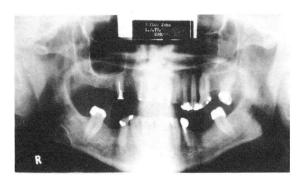

Fig. 5.2 *Asymptomatic cystic radiolucency at the angle of the right mandible: a Stafne bone cavity. (Courtesy of Professor C. Scully.)*

Management

Cysts are generally managed either by enucleation or by marsupialization. Enucleation is the complete removal of the cyst, and has the advantages of leaving behind no pathological tissue and of permitting histopathological examination of the complete cyst (Fig. 5.3). In marsupialization, only part of the cyst can be histologically examined; some pathological tissue is left in situ and healing is slower (Fig. 5.4). Marsupialization is sometimes preferable, however, if there is a large cyst close to structures that could be damaged by enucleation (see page 58).

DEVELOPMENTAL CYSTS

Odontogenic developmental cysts

Odontogenic keratocysts (primordial cysts)

These cysts have generally been thought to arise from the dental lamina or its derivatives, but there is some suggestion that they may also arise from basal cells of the oral mucosa.

Clinical features

Keratocysts may be seen over a wide age range. Most involve the mandibular angle and may expand to occupy the major part of the mandibular ramus. They are often

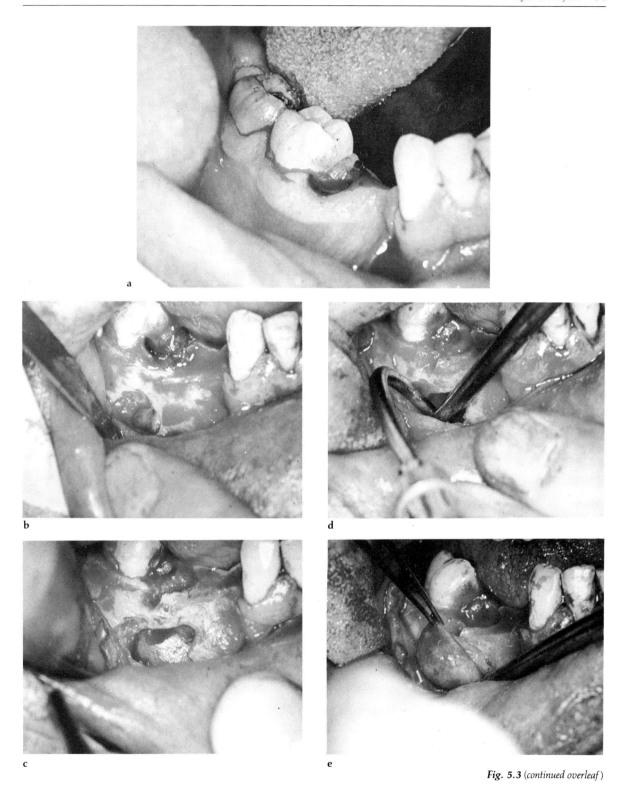

Fig. 5.3 (*continued overleaf*)

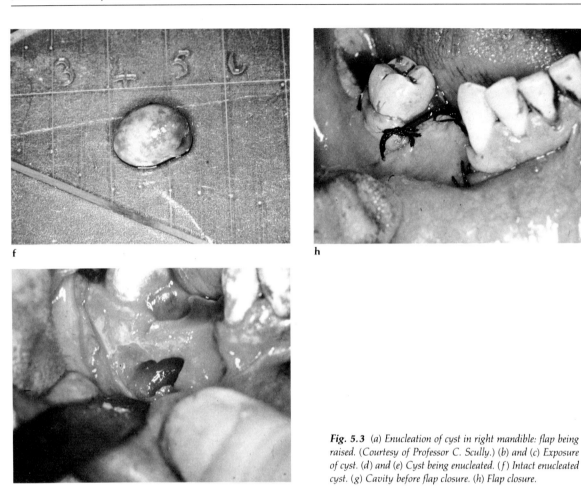

Fig. 5.3 (a) Enucleation of cyst in right mandible: flap being raised. (Courtesy of Professor C. Scully.) (b) and (c) Exposure of cyst. (d) and (e) Cyst being enucleated. (f) Intact enucleated cyst. (g) Cavity before flap closure. (h) Flap closure.

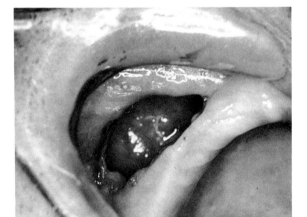

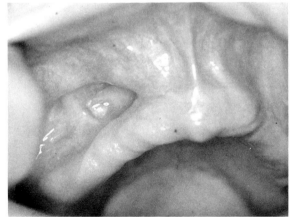

Fig. 5.4 (a) Marsupialized cyst of right maxilla (cyst in Fig. 5.1). (Courtesy of Professor C. Scully.) (b) Healing marsupialized cyst after 6 months.

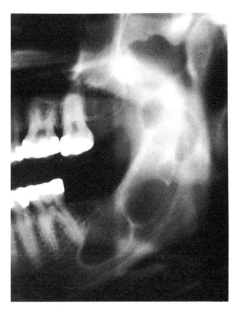

Fig. 5.5 *Orthopantomogram demonstrating a multilocular keratocyst in the mandibular ramus extending towards the coronoid process.* (*Courtesy of Mr R. M. Cook.*)

multilocular (Fig. 5.5). They may resorb the cortical plates and expand into the soft tissues, may envelop unerupted teeth giving a dentigerous appearance, or they may displace teeth. Odontogenic keratocysts are generally painless, unless they become secondarily infected, and often grow to a large size before giving rise to symptoms.

The most important feature of keratocysts is their tendency to recur following removal: recurrence rates as high as 60% have been recorded. There are many reasons for this high rate of recurrence, with surgical aspects being significant. Growth of the cyst wall seems to be more prominent than expansion of the cyst cavity, and the lesions tend to extend through cancellous spaces, forming finger-like projections permeating throughout the bone before there is any bony expansion. Invagination of the epithelium may also give rise to the formation of 'daughter cysts' within the cyst wall which are difficult to remove surgically. Hence recurrence is likely.

Pathology

The cyst lining usually has a characteristic appearance of a regular keratinized stratified squamous epithelium, commonly five to eight cell layers thick and without rete pegs (Fig. 5.6). There is a well-defined basal layer

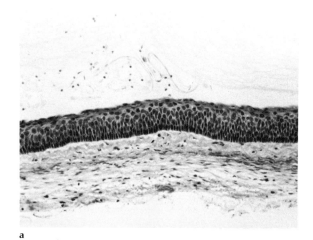

a

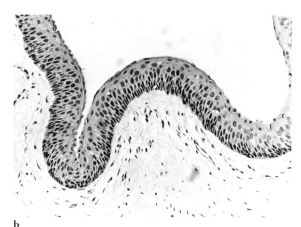

b

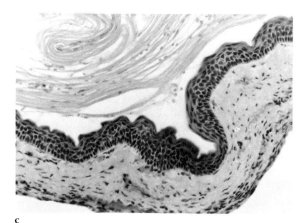

c

Fig. 5.6 *Photomicrographs of a keratocyst.* (a) *Histological appearance of keratocyst wall* (*medium power: courtesy of Dr B. G. Radden*); (b) *higher power* (*courtesy of Professor C. Scully*). (c) *Keratin contents.* (*Courtesy of Professor C. Scully.*)

predominantly of columnar, but occasionally cuboidal, cells. Desquamated keratin is often present within the cyst lumen and the fibrous wall is usually thin.

Biochemistry

The estimation of the soluble protein level in aspirated cyst fluid is an aid to the diagnosis of keratocysts since a protein level of less than 4.0 g per 100 ml suggests a keratocyst, whereas a value over 5 g per 100 ml suggests a radicular or follicular cyst or, rarely, a cystic ameloblastoma. The demonstration of keratin squames in a cyst aspirate is virtually diagnostic of a keratocyst.

Management

Although there is some dispute over the most appropriate treatment for keratocysts, all agree that the cyst lining should be meticulously removed. Small unilocular lesions should be thoroughly *enucleated*. When the cysts are large or multiloculated, excision with a margin of surrounding bone may be more appropriate. When the cysts have perforated the cortical plate and extend into the soft tissue, a supraperiosteal approach is indicated.

There are advocates of marsupialization for large keratocysts. This technique involves making a large opening into the cyst cavity which is then made confluent with the oral mucosa (see Fig. 5.4). The opening is maintained and in many cases the cyst may shrink in size, allowing for a more conservative secondary removal (see pp. 50 and 58).

Long-term clinical and radiographic follow-up of all keratocysts is mandatory as they can recur many years after initial treatment.

Gorlin's syndrome

Multiple naevoid basal cell carcinoma and jaw cyst syndrome is inherited as an autosomal dominant trait. The features include multiple odontogenic keratocysts of the jaws (Fig. 5.7; see also Fig. 32.16), multiple basal cell carcinomas of the skin (Fig. 5.8), skeletal anomalies such as bifid ribs and vertebral abnormalities (Fig. 5.9), frontal and temporoparietal bossing with a broad root of the nose, calcification of the falx cerebri and an abnormally shaped sella turcica (Fig. 5.10).

The jaw cysts in these patients are indistinguishable from other odontogenic keratocysts and are treated in a similar manner.

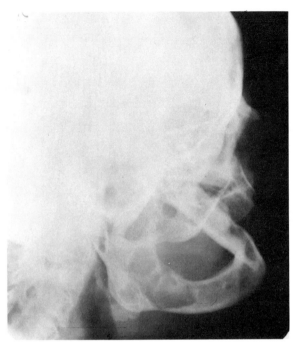

Fig. 5.7 *Odontogenic keratocysts in Gorlin's syndrome. (Courtesy of Professor C. Scully.)*

Follicular (dentigerous) cysts

Follicular cysts arise by separation of the dental follicle from around the anatomical crown of an unerupted tooth (Fig. 5.11). They may also form due to degeneration of the stellate reticulum, or an accumulation of fluid between the layers of the reduced enamel epithelium.

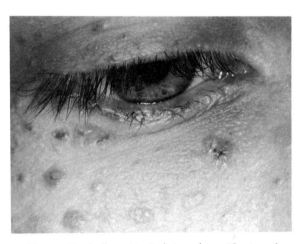

Fig. 5.8 *Basal cell naevi in Gorlin's syndrome. (Courtesy of Professor C. Scully.)*

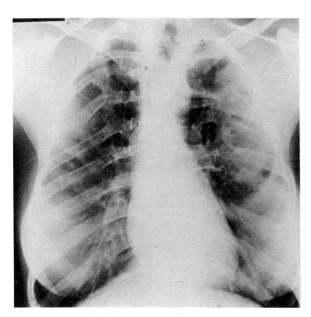

Fig. 5.9 *Bifid ribs in Gorlin's syndrome. (Courtesy of Professor C. Scully.)*

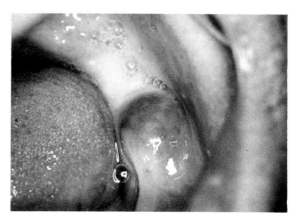

Fig. 5.11 *Intra-oral swelling caused by a dentigerous cyst in the left mandible. (Courtesy of Professor C. Scully.)*

Clinical features

Follicular cysts may grow to a large size, displace the tooth with which they are associated (Fig. 5.12) or, rarely, cause resorption of adjacent teeth. They are most common in association with mandibular third molars and maxillary canines (Figs. 5.12 and 5.13).

Pathology

The lining of follicular cysts typically consists of thin and non-keratinized, flattened stratified epithelium (Figs. 5.14 5.15).

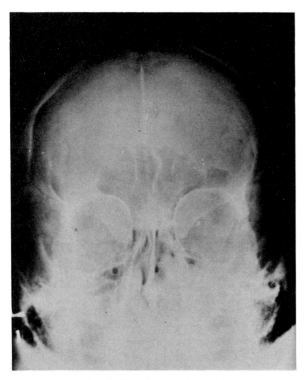

Fig. 5.10 *Calcified falx cerebri in Gorlin's syndrome. (Courtesy of Professor C. Scully.)*

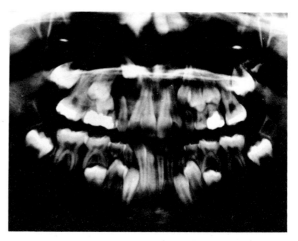

Fig. 5.12 *Orthopantomogram demonstrating a dentigerous cyst involving the upper canine which has been superiorly displaced.*

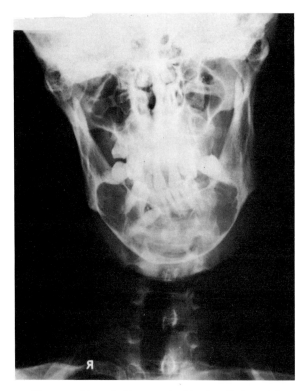

Fig. 5.13 *A large dentigerous cyst arising from the impacted mandibular canine. (Courtesy of Professor C. Scully.)*

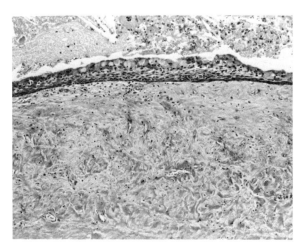

Fig. 5.15 *Photomicrograph demonstrating the histological appearance of a dentigerous cyst (medium power). (Courtesy of Dr B. G. Radden.)*

Management

Diagnosis is usually made by clinical and radiographic assessment—when the follicular space exceeds 5 mm from the crown it is likely that a cyst is present. However, odontogenic keratocysts and ameloblastomas may occasionally mimic the radiological appearances of follicular cysts. Aspiration may assist the diagnosis.

Treatment may be either marsupialization, allowing the tooth to erupt, or enucleation, with removal of the associated tooth.

Eruption cysts

Eruption cysts are considered as minor soft tissue forms of follicular cysts. They often burst spontaneously before eruption of the associated tooth, and only require excision if impeding normal eruption (Fig. 5.16).

Other odontogenic developmental cysts

These cysts are uncommon. They can be subdivided into three groups: gingival cysts of adults and infants, and lateral periodontal cysts. The pathogenesis of these cysts is far from clear: gingival cysts of adults arise from epithelial rests in the gingiva, those in infants arise from remnants of the dental lamina. Lateral periodontal cysts of developmental type arise in the periodontal membrane alongside a vital tooth. Treatment of these cysts is generally by enucleation.

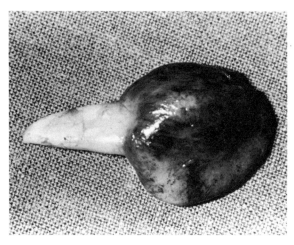

Fig. 5.14 *Surgical specimen showing a dentigerous cyst enveloping the crown of a canine.*

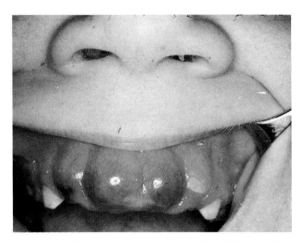

Fig. 5.16 *Eruption cysts on the central incisors. (Courtesy of Professor C. Scully.)*

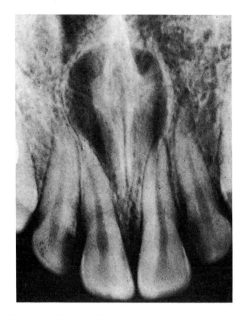

Fig. 5.17 *Radiograph demonstrating a nasopalatine cyst.*

Non-odontogenic developmental cysts

Originally these cysts were said to form from entrapped epithelium during the fusion of embryological processes, but this embryological concept has now been discarded. The lining of these cysts is either stratified squamous epithelium or pseudostratified ciliated columnar (respiratory) epithelium.

Nasopalatine or incisive canal cysts

These rare cysts are derived from the vestigial oronasal ducts. They may occur either within the nasopalatine canal or in the soft tissue of the palate at the opening of the canal, they grow slowly, and may discharge into the mouth giving a salty taste. Radiological examination shows a well-defined, rounded ovoid or occasionally heart-shaped defect in the anterior maxilla (Figs. 5.17 and 5.18). Nasopalatine cysts must be distinguished from a normal large anterior palatine fossa which may be up to 7 mm in diameter, and from radicular cysts associated with the maxillary incisor teeth. These cysts should be enucleated and seldom recur.

Nasolabial cysts

The nasolabial cyst is a soft tissue cyst found within the nasolabial fold. It is lined by respiratory epithelium and if allowed to grow may distort the upper lip and alar base. Treatment is by simple excision.

Others

Other cysts described include the globulomaxillary cyst, median mandibular cyst, and median palatal cyst, but there are few case reports of these cysts which fulfil the criteria of non-odontogenic developmental cysts; most are probably odontogenic cysts that have been misdiagnosed.

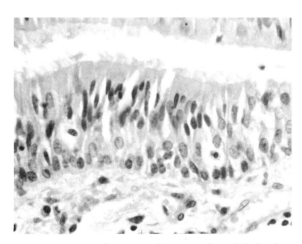

Fig. 5.18 *Nasopalatine cyst—showing pseudostratified ciliated epithelium. (Courtesy of Professor C. Scully.)*

INFLAMMATORY CYSTS

By far the most common of all jaw cysts are inflammatory cysts arising in association with a non-vital tooth.

There are three closely related varieties of inflammatory cysts.

1. Radicular cyst (dental cyst)—where the cyst is associated with the apex of a non-vital tooth (Figs. 5.19 and 5.20).
2. Lateral periodontal cyst—where the cyst is found to lie on the lateral aspect of a non-vital tooth, usually associated with a lateral pulp canal and foramen. From time to time periodontal cysts may be found in association with a vital tooth (see also developmental cysts), due to periodontal inflammation or pericoronitis (particularly with a mandibular third molar tooth).
3. Residual cysts—where one of the above inflammatory cysts (usually a radicular cyst) remains after removal of the non-vital tooth from which it arose (Fig. 5.21).

Pathology

The epithelial lining is derived from the epithelial rests of Malassez which proliferate to produce thick, irregular squamous epithelium (Figs. 5.22–5.25). The epithelial lining is often non-keratinized and incomplete, with granulation tissue forming the cyst wall in the denuded areas. Depending on the nature of the inflammatory response, there may be areas of chronic inflammation, or acute inflammation with abscess formation. Cholesterol crystal clefts are often present and mucous cells may be found. The cyst capsule consists of collagenous fibrous connective tissue. The cyst fluid is usually watery but may be thick and viscid with cholesterol crystals giving it a shimmering appearance. These cysts cause resorption of bone and may erode the cortical plates and can become quite large (see Fig. 5.20).

Management

The treatment of inflammatory cysts depends on whether the involved non-vital tooth is to be retained. Conventional intracanal endodontic treatment will often lead to the resolution of very small radicular cysts, but regular radiographic review is necessary until there has been complete resolution of the cyst. If, when the tooth has been root-filled the cyst does not resolve, or if the cyst is of such a size that it is unlikely to resolve with endodontic treatment alone, surgery is indicated. The benefit of enucleation is that all of the cyst tissue is available for histological examination and the cyst cavity will usually heal uneventfully with minimal aftercare. Enucleation is potentially problematic when the cyst involves the apices of adjacent vital teeth, as the surgery may deprive the teeth of their blood supply and render them non-vital. Marsupialization of the cyst may be an

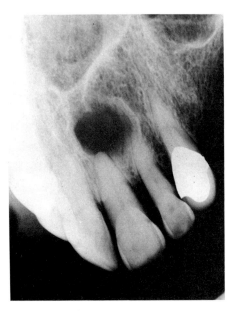

Fig. 5.19 *Radiograph demonstrating a radicular cyst associated with the non-vital central incisor. (Courtesy of Mr R. M. Cook.)*

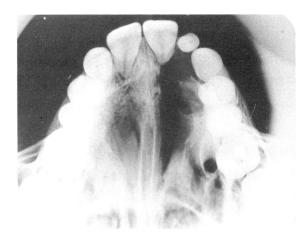

Fig. 5.20 *Large radicular cyst associated with maxillary lateral incisor. (Courtesy of Professor C. Scully.)*

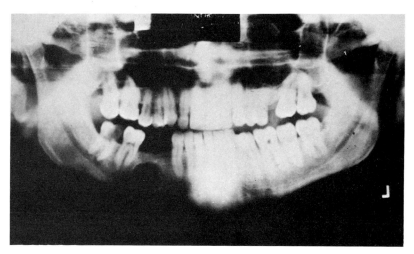

Fig. 5.21 *Residual cyst in lower first molar region. (Courtesy of Professor C. Scully.)*

option in these cases, but this treatment requires considerable aftercare and good patient co-operation in keeping the cavity clean whilst it resolves. Marsupialization consists of removing a window of cyst lining to decompress the cyst, which will then gradually reduce in size provided that the cavity is kept open with a 'bung', or acrylic plug, often attached to a denture or acrylic splint. The bung stops food collecting in the cavity but the cavity must still be syringed by the patient after each meal. Marsupialized cyst cavities may take up to 6

months to close down to the extent of becoming 'self-cleansing'. The other disadvantage of marsupialization is that all of the cyst lining is not available to histopathological examination, and this may lead to misdiagnosis.

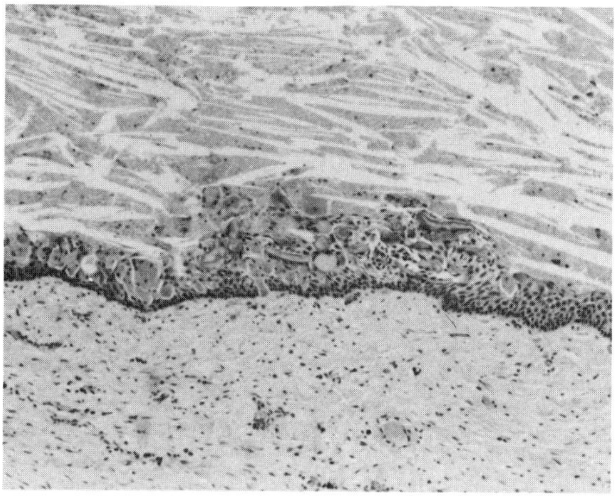

NON-EPITHELIAL CYSTS

Solitary (traumatic, haemorrhagic) bone cysts

These lesions occur most commonly in the long bones but may also be found occasionally in the jaws. Their cause is speculative but they may arise after trauma to the

Fig. 5.22 *Photomicrograph demonstrating the histological appearance of a radicular cyst of long standing, with few inflammatory cells and cholesterol crystal clefts in the lumen. (Courtesy of Dr B. G. Radden.)*

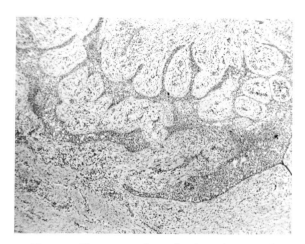

Fig. 5.23 *Photomicrograph of a dental cyst showing proliferating epithelium. (Courtesy of Professor C. Scully.)*

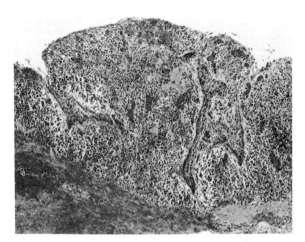

Fig. 5.24 *Photomicrograph demonstrating the histological appearance of a radicular cyst, with acute inflammation, epithelial disruption and proliferation of granulation tissue (medium power). (Courtesy of Dr B. G. Radden.)*

bone when an intramedullary haematoma forms and then degenerates rather than progressing to normal healing.

Clinical features

Haemorrhagic bone cysts are generally painless and expansion is uncommon, the lesions usually being coincidentally discovered during radiographic examination. They are seen most often in the posterior body of the mandible in young persons. Radiologically there is a well-defined translucency with a scalloped appearance around the apices of the teeth, *which are vital* (Fig. 5.26).

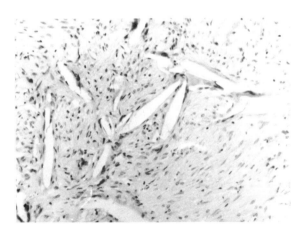

Fig. 5.25 *Cholesterol clefts in the wall of a dental radicular cyst. (Courtesy of Professor C. Scully.)*

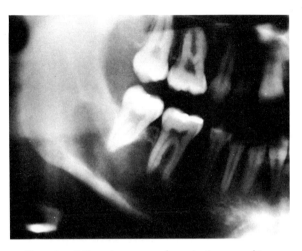

Fig. 5.26 *Orthopantomogram demonstrating a solitary bone cyst, with a scalloped appearance around the roots of the teeth.*

Management

Surgery is undertaken in order to make a definitive diagnosis. Clear or blood-stained fluid may be found within the bony cavity, but preoperative aspiration may at times not yield any product. There is no detectable cyst lining and sometimes only a thin fibrous membrane. Curettage produces bone fragments and connective tissue, sometimes with granulation tissue. However, such surgical opening of the cavity usually leads to spontaneous resolution.

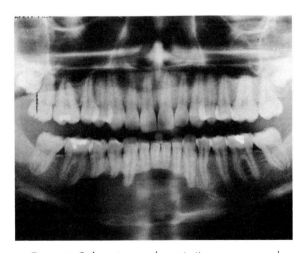

Fig. 5.27 *Orthopantogram demonstrating an aneurysmal bone cyst in the anterior mandible. (Courtesy of Mr M. K. Ruljancich.)*

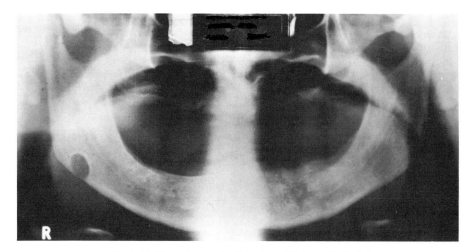

Fig. 5.28 *Stafne bone cavity. (Courtesy of Professor C. Scully.)*

Aneurysmal bone cyst

This lesion is quite rare, and in fact is not a cyst at all. It may occur in any part of the skeleton (see also Chapter 8). A significant number of these lesions may be associated with other bony pathology such a fibrous dysplasia,

ossifying fibroma and giant-cell granuloma. The aetiology of the aneurysmal bone cyst remains obscure.

Clinical features

An aneurysmal bone cyst usually presents as a firm,

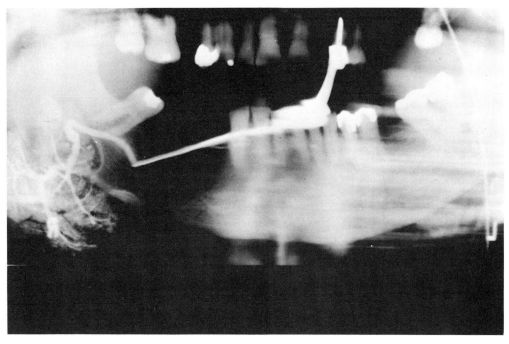

Fig. 5.29 *Following the injection of Conray 420 into the submandibular duct, this radiolucent lesion is shown to be an ectopic salivary gland inclusion, confirming the diagnosis of a Stafne cavity.*

painless swelling of the mandible, which expands and subsequently perforates the cortex. Radiographs show a unilocular or multilocular translucency with a honeycomb or soap-bubble appearance (Fig. 5.27).

Pathology

Preoperative aspiration shows bloody fluid. An haematocrit should be performed on the aspirate, which will often be low, differentiating it from undiluted blood in a vascular anomaly such as an haemangioma.

The 'cyst' cavity contains blood and reddish-brown tissue. Histology reveals numerous capillaries and blood-filled spaces with old and new haemorrhage in the connective tissue. Irregular areas of osteoid and multinucleated giant cells are often present.

Management

Treatment is by thorough curettage or excision as these lesions have a propensity to recur.

Stafne bone cavity

This is not a cyst of the jaws but an ectopic inclusion of salivary tissue, often from the submandibular gland, which on radiography shows a radiolucency just above the lower border of the mandible in the posterior body, resembling a cyst. No treatment is indicated but exploratory surgery is necessary when a diagnosis cannot be made by non-invasive means such as sialography (Figs. 5.28 and 5.29), or when serial radiographs show an increase in cavity size.

FURTHER READING

Cowan C. G. (1980). Traumatic bone cysts of the jaws and their presentation. *Int. J. Oral Surg.*, **9**: 287–291.

El Deeb M., Sedano H. O., Waite D. E. (1980). Aneurysmal bone cysts of the jaws. *Int. J. Oral Surg.*, **9**: 301–311.

Hollinshead M. B., Schneider L. C. (1980). A histologic and embryologic analysis of so-called globulomaxillary cysts. *Int. J. Oral Surg.*, **9**: 281–286.

Shear M. (1983). *Cysts of the oral regions*, 2nd edn. Bristol: Wright.

Wysocki G. P. *et al.* (1980). Histogenesis of the lateral periodontal cyst and the gingival cyst of the adult. *Oral Surg.*, **50**: 327–334.

Chapter
6

Tumours of the dental tissues

Tumours in the mandible and maxilla may arise from the dental tissues (odontogenic tumours), from bone and related tissues, or may invade as metastases from elsewhere. This chapter deals with odontogenic tumours, both neoplasms (autonomous growths) and hamartomas (developmental anomalies consisting of tissues indigenous to the area).

Tumours of the dental tissues are classified according to the tissues of origin and histopathological features (Table 6.1).

Tumours consisting predominantly of epithelium originate from odontogenic epithelium but it is uncertain whether this epithelium is derived from the enamel organ itself, the remnants of the dental lamina (cell rests of Serres) or Hertwig's root sheath (cell rests of Malassez),

the epithelium of odontogenic cysts (particularly the dentigerous cyst) or from the oral mucosa.

Tumours composed of odontogenic connective tissue originate from the mesenchymal portion of the tooth germ—either from the dental papilla or the dental follicle.

Tumours of mixed origin consist of both odontogenic epithelium and mesenchyme and during the period of active growth contain both ameloblastic epithelium and odontoblastic tissue but, when completely developed, consist principally of enamel, dentine, cementum or combinations thereof.

Enamel, dentine and their precursors are also present in a number of other lesions and their presence is usually indicated by inclusion of the suffix 'odonto' (e.g. ameloblastic fibro-odontoma, odontoameloblastoma, ameloblastic odontosarcoma).

TUMOURS OF EPITHELIAL ORIGIN

Ameloblastoma

The ameloblastoma is an odontogenic neoplasm that rarely metastasizes but does invade locally.

Clinical features and diagnosis

Ameloblastomas are more frequent in males, usually after the age of 40 years. Some 80% are found in the posterior mandible. The tumour is not uncommon in Blacks compared to the low incidence in Caucasians.

The initial detection of an ameloblastoma is likely to be a 'chance finding', but when the tumour is evident clinically there is a slow-growing, painless, expansile swelling of bone. The lesion expands to produce progressive facial deformity and there may be evidence of malocclusion and mobile teeth. Eventually the bone is perforated and soft tissues are involved. Radiographi-

Table 6.1
Classification of tumours of the dental tissues

Epithelial
    Ameloblastoma (adanantinoma)
    Adenomatoid odontogenic tumour (adenoameloblastoma)
    Calcifying epithelial odontogenic tumour
    Calcifying odontogenic cyst

Mesenchymal
    Myxoma
    Odontogenic fibroma

Epithelial and mesenchymal
    Ameloblastic fibroma (and ameloblastic sarcoma)

Odontogenic hard tissues without epithelium
    Odontome
    Enameloma
    Dentinoma
    Cementoma
    Dens invaginatus (dilated odontome)

Odontogenic hard tissues with epithelium
    Odontoameloblastoma

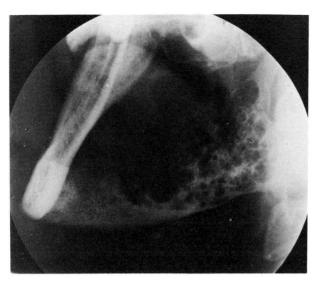

Fig. 6.1 *Ameloblastoma showing a 'soap bubble' appearance. (Courtesy of Professor C. Scully.)*

cally, a monocystic or polycystic ('soap bubble') radiolucency is evident (Figs. 6.1 and 6.2).

There is a tenuous association with dentigerous cysts but it remains unresolved whether such cases represent cystic ameloblastomas or an ameloblastoma arising from the cyst lining.

Diagnosis is confirmed by histological examination of a biopsy specimen.

Pathology

Ameloblastomas are composed of epithelial cells arranged as a peripheral layer of ameloblast-like cells around a central area of cells resembling stellate reticulum (Fig. 6.3). Two main histological types are seen—follicular and plexiform. In the follicular type, discrete islands (follicles) of epithelial cells are evident (Fig. 6.4), whereas in the plexiform type the epithelium forms continuous anastomosing strands (Fig. 6.5). Enamel formation is not evident, presumably because no odontogenic mesenchyme is present to give the inductive forces critical in the formation of dentine.

Histological variations occasionally seen in ameloblastomas include the presence of granular cells, squamous metaplasia and keratinization, areas of calcification and variable degrees of vascularity. However, there appears to be little correlation between these histological patterns and the clinical course of the tumour. Features such as increased cellular pleomorphism and mitotic activity do, however, suggest that the lesions will behave more aggressively.

Treatment and behaviour

Despite the ameloblastoma expanding rather than de-

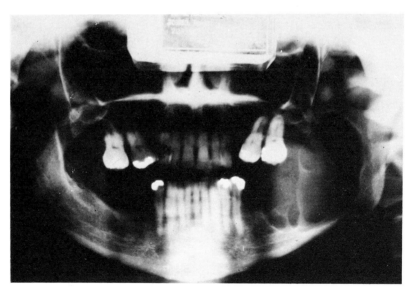

Fig. 6.2 *Ameloblastoma showing a multilocular appearance. (Courtesy of Professor C. Scully.)*

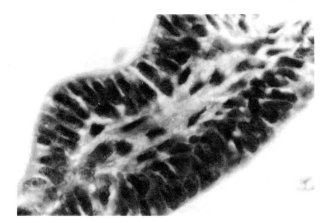

Fig. 6.3 *Ameloblastoma showing ameloblast-like cells surrounding a central area resembling stellate reticulum.*

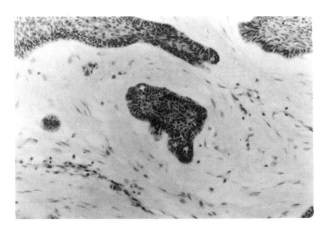

Fig. 6.4 *Follicular ameloblastoma.*

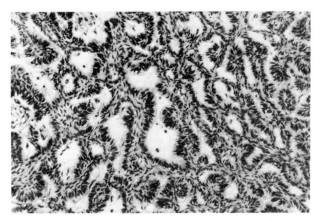

Fig. 6.5 *Plexiform ameloblastoma. (Courtesy of Professor C. Scully.)*

stroying bone, there is some local invasion of the surrounding bone. The treatment of choice, therefore, is surgical excision of the tumour together with removal of a margin of normal bone and retention of the lower border of the mandible if at all possible. Extension of the tumour into the adjacent soft tissues makes treatment difficult as the tumour is radioresistant. Metastatic dissemination of the ameloblastoma is rare and usually occurs by aspiration to the lungs following long-standing local disease or recurrence after previous surgical intervention.

Adenomatoid odontogenic tumour (adenoameloblastoma)

Clinical features and diagnosis

This tumour typically presents in the second and third decades, is more common in females than males, and affects the maxilla more than the mandible. There is a

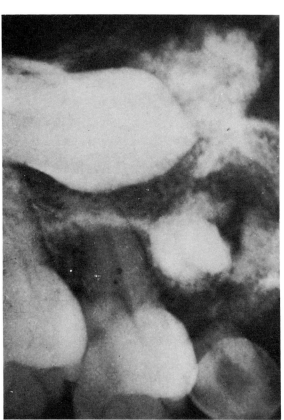

Fig. 6.6 *Adenomatoid odontogenic tumour showing radio-opacities.*

propensity for the lateral incisor, canine and premolar regions.

Clinically, the lesion presents as a gradually increasing intrabony swelling which is occasionally painful. On radiographs, the tumour appears as a unilocular radiolucency and in some lesions there are radio-opaque foci (Fig. 6.6). A clinical provisional diagnosis should include either a lateral periodontal cyst or a dentigerous cyst, particularly as, in the latter case, the tumour is sometimes associated with an unerupted tooth (Chapter 5).

On histological examination, the tumour is encapsulated and consists of sheets and strands of epithelial cells arranged as convoluted bands and tubular structures (Fig. 6.7). In the tubular structures, ameloblast-like cells are

arranged radially around spaces containing an homogeneous eosinophilic material. The nature of this material is unknown, although suggestions have included pre-enamel, predentine, amyloid and basement membrane material. Separate from the homogeneous material, foci of calcification frequently are evident throughout the lesion. The tumour contains little intervening mesenchymal stroma, although cystic degeneration of this tissue is common.

Treatment

Unlike the ameloblastoma, the adenomatoid odontogenic tumour is not locally invasive and shows no tendency to recur following conservative surgical excision.

Calcifying epithelial odontogenic tumour (Pindborg tumour)

Clinical features and diagnosis

This rare tumour has been reported in all age groups (10–90 years), but manifests most commonly at approximately 40 years of age. It is found equally in males and females and is most frequent in the mandibular premolar/molar region. Rarely, it is extra-osseous in more anterior parts of the mouth.

Clinically, there is a progressive painless swelling of the jaws. Radiographically, the tumour usually appears as a radiolucency containing focal opacities. Approximately 50% of the lesions are associated with an unerupted tooth.

Histological examination shows three distinct features (Fig. 6.8).

1. The lesion consists of sheets of epithelial cells (containing tonofilaments, desmosomes and hemidesmosomes) which frequently are pleomorphic and which contain abnormal nuclei. In places, these cells are characterized by a clear cytoplasm, and hence have been termed 'clear cells'. Mitoses are rare.

2. Amyloid, with its characteristic staining reactions (green birefringence with congo red stain; positive fluorescence with thioflavine T), is evident throughout the tumour and is considered to be a product of the epithelial cells.

3. Concentric masses of calcified tissues are present, often closely associated with the epithelial cells. It has been suggested that these may be a feature of the age of a tumour. Older lesions are characterized by more confluent calcified areas and by less prominent cellular features than are young lesions.

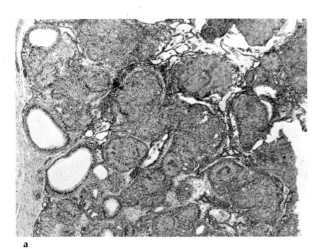

a

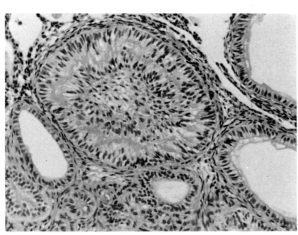

b

Fig. 6.7 *Adenomatoid odontogenic tumour: (a) tubular arrangements of epithelial cells; (b) high power.*

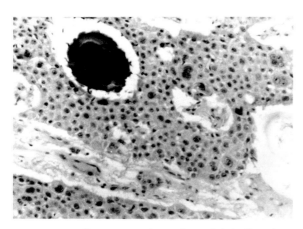

Fig. 6.8 *Pindborg tumour: pleomorphic epithelial cells with abnormal nuclei and concentric masses of calcified tissue.*

Treatment

The calcifying epithelial odontogenic tumour is locally invasive and, therefore, treated similarly to the ameloblastoma—that is, with surgical excision of the lesion plus a margin of normal bone.

Calcifying odontogenic cyst

The calcifying epithelial odontogenic cyst is an extremely rare lesion, now recognized as an entity distinct from the ameloblastoma and Pindborg tumour. It is sometimes termed the calcifying epithelial odontogenic cyst.

Clinical features and diagnosis

Calcifying odontogenic cyst can occur at any age but most commonly presents in adults younger than 40 years. Either jaw of either sex may be affected but the general site predilection is anterior to the first molar.

Clinically, there is a slowly enlarging, painless swelling of the jaws which, on radiographic examination, commonly appears as a well-defined unilocular or multilocular radiolucency containing flecks of opacity. Embedded teeth and/or denticle-like structures are not infrequent findings (see Fig. 10.21).

Microscopically, the tumour may be solid or cystic. In cystic lesions, the cyst wall is lined by odontogenic epithelium resembling that in an ameloblastoma, with peripheral ameloblast-like cells in close association with more central cells comparable to the stratum intermedium and the stellate reticulum. In places, the epithelial cells undergo aberrant keratinization to form large eosinophi-lic cells without a nucleus, termed 'ghost cells'. With further development, large masses of keratin accumulate and a foreign body giant cell reaction may be evoked if there is breakdown of the epithelial cyst lining. Foci of calcification and dentine-like material frequently are present throughout the specimen.

Treatment

Conservative enucleation of the lesion is rarely followed by recurrence.

TUMOURS OF MESENCHYMAL ORIGIN

Myxoma

Myxomas have been reported in the soft tissues and as intra-osseous lesions of the jaws.

Myxomas of the soft tissues

The origin of these lesions is uncertain but they may arise from:

    (i) primitive mesenchyme;
    (ii) myxomatous lesions following degeneration in fibromas;
    (iii) oral lesions analogous to cutaneous focal mucinosis or the cutaneous myxoid cyst;
    (iv) nerve sheath.

Myxomas of the jaws

Myxomas in the jaws are distinct pathological entities, derived from odontogenic mesenchyme.

Clinical features and diagnosis

Myxoma of the jaws usually occurs in adolescents and young adults (10–40 years), manifests more frequently in females than males, and presents in the posterior region of the mandible. The maxillary lesions that have been reported are characterized frequently by extensive involvement of the alveolar bone, the maxillary antrum and the zygomatic process.

Clinically, the myxoma is an intrabony lesion which slowly expands the bony cortex and only perforates later. The lesion is rarely painful but there may be loosening and displacement of the teeth. Radiographic examination shows a well-defined unilocular or multi-locular ('soap-bubble') radiolucency which may extend between the roots of the teeth and thus form a scalloped margin. Root resorption is sometimes seen.

On microscopic examination of the biopsy specimen, spindle/stellate-shaped cells are present in an intercellular mucoid stroma sometimes containing nests of epithelial cells. Fibrous tissue and collagen are frequently evident throughout the lesion (fibromyxoma). There is widespread infiltration of the surrounding bone.

Treatment

Myxomas infiltrate and therefore should be treated similarly to ameloblastomas, with surgical excision of the tumour and removal of a margin of normal bone.

Odontogenic fibroma

The rarity of this tumour has resulted in an incomplete understanding of its incidence, clinical features and long-term behaviour. The tumour, however, generally presents in close relation to the root of a tooth, the crown of an unerupted tooth, or in the site of a tooth which is congenitally missing from the area. Histologically, the lesion consists of fibrous tissue which has a similar appearance to the dental pulp but contains small nests of odontogenic epithelium. Conservative enucleation is the treatment of choice.

TUMOURS OF EPITHELIAL AND MESENCHYMAL ORIGIN

Ameloblastic fibroma

Clinical features and diagnosis

The ameloblastic fibroma is a tumour that occurs in young adults (15–25 years), shows no sex predilection, and is found most commonly in the molar region of the mandible.

There is a slow, painless expansion of the jaws and the lesion appears as a unilocular radiolucency on radiographic examination. Infrequently, the tumour may be associated with an unerupted tooth.

Histologically, epithelium of odontogenic origin is present as small islands or terminal buds of peripheral ameloblast-like cells and central stellate reticulum cells. The odontogenic mesenchyme resembles the dental papilla. Surrounding the epithelial component there is frequently a cellular hyaline material thought to be the product of epithelial–mesenchymal interaction. Uncom-

monly, dentine may be present and has led to the term ameloblastic fibro-odontoma being used.

Treatment

Conservative enucleation of the tumour is the treatment of choice.

Ameloblastic sarcoma

Malignant counterparts of the ameloblastic fibroma are very rare. The lesions are associated with pain and are characterized by a rapid enlargement of the jaw. A biopsy shows an odontogenic epithelial component similar to that found in an ameloblastic fibroma, whereas the mesenchymal tissues resemble a fibrosarcoma with cellular pleomorphism, tumour giant cells and numerous, atypical mitotic figures. Treatment involves radical surgery combined with radiotherapy.

TUMOURS OF ODONTOGENIC HARD TISSUES NOT CONTAINING EPITHELIUM

Odontomes

Odontomes are hamartomatous malformations of the dental hard tissues rather than neoplasms and consist of dental tissues in normal relationship one to another. They are calcified and have been classified according to the type and spatial arrangement of the dental tissues.

Composite odontomes

Compound odontomes consist of multiple small simple teeth embedded in fibrous connective tissue within a fibrous capsule (Fig. 6.9). *Complex* odontomes consist of an irregular mass of all the dental tissues (Fig. 6.10).

The classification, however, has little practical value because different areas of the same lesion can show 'compound' or 'complex' patterns, and furthermore, the classification bears no relationship to the prognosis.

Clinical features and diagnosis

Odontomes typically present in children and adolescents, are more common in females than males, and show a distinct predilection for the premolar/molar region of the mandible.

Typically, they behave like teeth: they grow to a

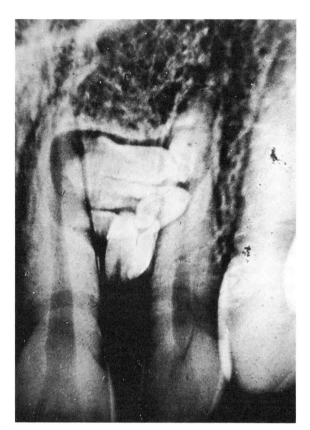

Fig. 6.9 *Compound odontome. (Courtesy of Professor C. Scully.)*

certain size and then tend to erupt with ulceration of the overlying oral mucosa. Alternatively, they may go unnoticed or, if located over the crown of an unerupted tooth, may prevent eruption. Radiographically, the lesions appear as well-defined radio-opacities (Figs. 6.9 and 6.10).

Treatment

The lesions are excised if producing symptoms, but considerable mechanical difficulty may be encountered in this procedure.

Enameloma

Rarely, disturbances in odontogenesis cause small deposits of enamel, termed enamelomas, between the roots of the first permanent molars.

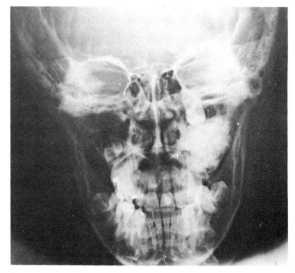

a

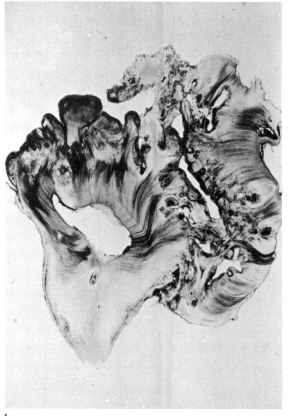

b

Fig. 6.10 *Complex odontome. (Courtesy of Professor C. Scully.)*

Dentinoma

Focal deposits of dentine or osteodentine have been found overlying the crowns of unerupted mandibular molar teeth in young adults and have been termed dentinomas. The lesions are usually asymptomatic and appear as chance findings, as opacities on radiographic examination.

The pathogenesis of this lesion, as with the enameloma, is an enigma because the development of the dental hard tissues in the absence of odontogenic epithelium confounds the current concept that odontogenesis is reliant on an epithelial–mesenchymal interaction.

Cementoma

Cementum is normally deposited on the root of a tooth throughout life to compensate for occlusal wear; an excess of such physiological deposition is termed hypercementosis. Alternatively, cementum may be deposited neoplastically, when the lesion is termed a cementoma.

Hypercementosis

The common causes of hypercementosis are chronic periapical infection, a functionless tooth, a reaction to increased stress and Paget's disease (Fig. 6.11). Hypercementosis is often symptomless and causes complications only during exodontia.

Cementomas

Cementomas are uncommon but include the cementoblastoma, the gigantiform cementoma, periapical cemental dysplasia, and the cementifying fibroma. The characteristics of these lesions are summarized in Table 6.2 (see also Figs. 6.12–6.15).

Dens invaginatus (dens in dente; dilated odontome)

Dens invaginatus is a distorted tooth which contains an invagination of dentine and enamel and radiographically resembles a tooth within a tooth (dens in dente).

During odontogenesis, a portion of the enamel organ may protrude, or invaginate, into the dental papilla (Fig. 6.16). Thus, when development has been completed, the affected tooth contains a cavity that is completely or partially lined by enamel. The cause of this defect is unknown. Theories of its pathogenesis have included the

Table 6.2
Classification of cementomas

	Cementoblastoma	Gigantiform cementoma	Periapical cemental dysplasia	Cementifying fibroma
Occurrence	<25 years ♂>♀ Mandible—premolar/ molar region Solitary	Middle age (more common in Blacks ♀>♂) Mandible Multiple and symmetrical	Middle age and over ♀>♂ Mandible—incisor region Multiple	Middle age and over ♀=♂ Mandible—premolar/ molar region Solitary
Clinical features	±Localized swelling and sometimes expansion of jaws Vital teeth Well-defined apical opacity surrounded by lucent zone	±Localized swelling and sometimes expansion of jaws Vital teeth Lobulated apical opacity without lucent zone	Lesions very small—no expansion of jaws Vital teeth Circumscribed radiolucency becoming opaque with age	Lesions very small—no expansion of jaws Vital teeth Circumscribed radiolucency becoming opaque with age
Histology	Cementum-like tissue fused to tooth Numerous cementoblasts and reversal lines Zone of uncalcified tissue at periphery	Acellular cementum continuous with the normal cementum of the root	Replacement of a localized area of bone with fibrous tissue Deposition of trabeculae of cementum-like tissue Fusion of cementum mass	
Treatment	Enucleation	Excision	Enucleation	Enucleation

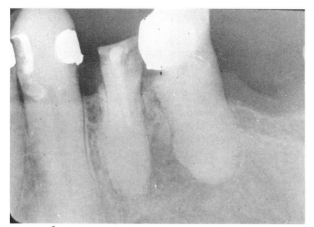

Fig. 6.11 *Hypercementosis.* (*Courtesy of Professor C. Scully.*)

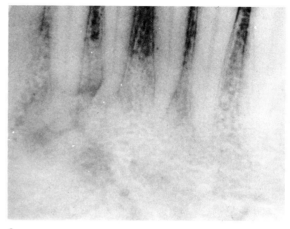

a

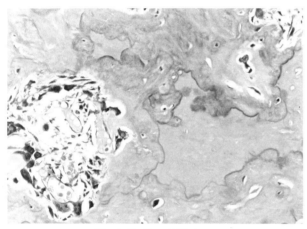

Fig. 6.12 *Cementoblastoma.*

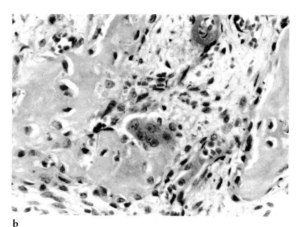

b

Fig. 6.14 *Periapical cemental dysplasia.* (*Courtesy of Professor C. Scully.*)

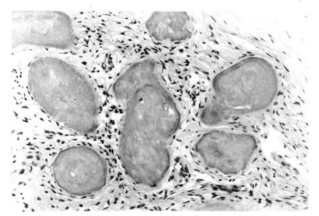

Fig. 6.13 *Gigantiform cementoma.* (*Courtesy of Professor C. Scully.*)

suggestion that there may be an area of active proliferation of the enamel organ with ingrowth into the dental papilla, such that there is a relative retardation in the growth of a portion of the enamel organ with the result that the remaining tissues envelop this area. Alternatively, local causes, such as infection, trauma, or disproportionate maxillary pressures, may be the initiators of the invagination.

Clinical features

Dens invaginatus occurs in children and adolescents, shows no sex predilection, commonly affects the permanent dentition, usually the upper lateral incisor or an upper anterior tooth, and not infrequently is bilateral.

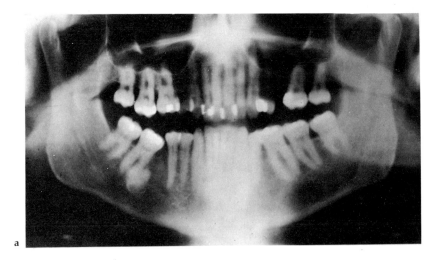

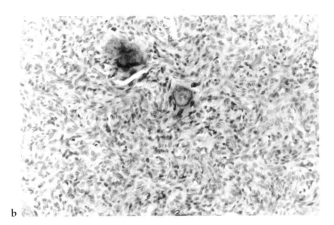

Fig. 6.15 *Cementifying fibroma.*

The degree of invagination may be mild to severe, and the lesion presents as a small pit on the palatal surface of the affected tooth (Fig. 6.16). The actual defect collects plaque and food debris, as a result of which there is often caries and consequently pulpitis and periapical infection.

Treatment

Routine conservation is adequate for mild defects, but in more severe cases, particularly where there is pulpitis or periapical infection, endodontics or extraction are needed.

Dens evaginatus

In this instance, an evagination causes a nodule on the occlusal surface. It is most common in mongoloid races (Fig. 6.17).

Geminated odontome

A geminated odontome is a large abnormal tooth that is actually composed of two joined teeth, resulting either from partial division of a tooth germ or from the fusion of

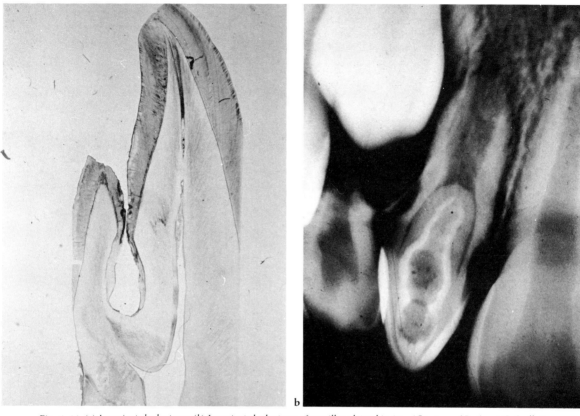

a   b

Fig. 6.16 (a) *Invaginated odontome.* (b) *Invaginated odontome of maxillary lateral incisor. (Courtesy of Professor C. Scully.)*

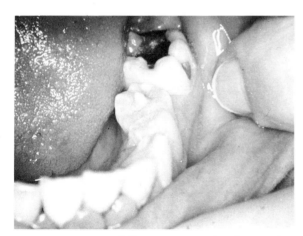

Fig. 6.17 *Evaginated odontome on a premolar. (Courtesy of Professor C. Scully.)*

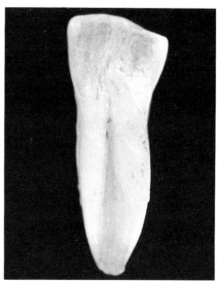

Fig. 6.18 *Gemination of a lower incisor. (Courtesy of Professor C. Scully.)*

adjacent tooth germs. Gemination is seen mainly anteriorly; the crowns may be separate or divided by a groove. Similarly, the roots may be fused or separate (Fig. 6.18).

TUMOURS OF ODONTOGENIC HARD TISSUES WITH EPITHELIUM

Odontoameloblastoma

This extremely rare lesion is identical clinically and in its behaviour to the ameloblastoma. Histologically, however, in addition to the epithelial component resembling the ameloblastoma, there are also enamel and dentine.

FURTHER READING

Gardner D. G., Pecack A. M. (1980). The treatment of ameloblastoma based on pathologic and anatomic principles. *Cancer*, **46**: 2514–2519.

Lucas R. B. (1984). *Pathology of tumours of the oral tissues*, 4th edn. Edinburgh: Churchill Livingstone.

Pindborg J. J., Kramer I. R. H., Torloni H. (1971). Histological typing of odontogenic tumours, jaw cysts and allied lesions. *International histological classification of tumours, No 5*. Geneva: World Health Organisation.

Reichart P. A., Ries P. (1983). Consideration on the classification of odontogenic tumours. *Int. J. Oral Surg.*, **13**: 323–333.

Smith R. R. L. *et al.* (1979). Adenomatoid odontogenic tumour. Ultrastructural demonstration of two cell types and amyloid. *Cancer*, **13**: 505–511.

Chapter
7   *Tumours of bone and cartilage*

The skeleton consists mainly of bone and cartilage together with fibrous tissue, neural and haemopoietic elements. Any of these tissues may undergo neoplastic change but most neoplasms in bone are metastases from lung or breast carcinomas and are seen in middle-aged or elderly persons. In contrast, primary malignant tumours of bone affect mainly younger patients.

Torus palatinus and torus mandibularis are discussed in Chapter 1. This chapter discusses mainly primary neoplasms of bone and cartilage; metastatic neoplasms are covered mainly in Chapter 15.

BENIGN NEOPLASMS OF BONE

Osteoma

Osteomas are benign neoplasms of cancellous or compact bone. They are painless, slow-growing lesions which often present as a lump on the jaw (Fig. 7.1). The mandible is particularly involved. Osteomas tend to become apparent in the fourth decade. Histologically, they are composed of essentially normal bone (Fig. 7.2).

Gardner's syndrome

Multiple osteomas are rare except in Gardner's syndrome, a familial condition in which multiple osteomas are seen, especially in the mandible, in association with multiple fibromas and desmoid tumours of the skin, sebaceous cysts, and multiple polyps of the colon which have a strong propensity to undergo malignant change (Figs. 7.3 and 7.4).

Osteoid osteoma and osteoblastoma

These benign neoplasms of bone are uncommon in the skeleton generally and are very rare in the jaws.

Microscopically these tumours are similar but they have distinctive clinical and radiological features. Osteoid osteoma is usually seen in adolescents and young adults, most frequently in the femur and tibia. It is often painful, particularly at night. Osteoid osteoma has a characteristic radiographic appearance with a central radiolucent area (nidus) surrounded by a rim of densely sclerotic bone of variable thickness. The nidus rarely exceeds 1 cm in diameter. Osteoblastoma, on the other hand, shows progressive growth without the osteosclerotic rim and is rarely painful. Microscopically both lesions consist of a vascular stroma in which there are trabeculae of osteoid surrounded by numerous darkly staining osteoblasts.

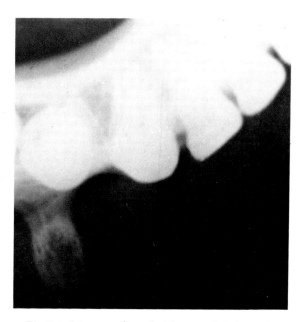

Fig. 7.1 *Osteoma: radiograph. (Courtesy of Professor C. Scully.)*

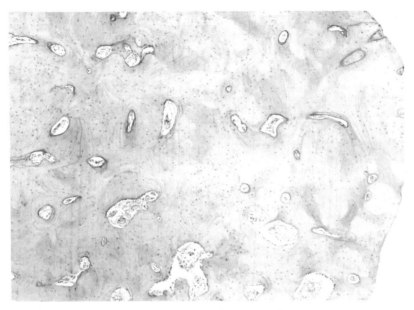

Fig. 7.2 *Osteoma: photomicrograph.*

MALIGNANT NEOPLASMS OF BONE

Osteosarcoma

Osteosarcoma is an aggressive malignant neoplasm which typically affects young patients. Males are affected twice as frequently as females. The long bones, particularly the lower end of the femur, are typical sites and only rarely is the mandible or maxilla affected. The aetiology

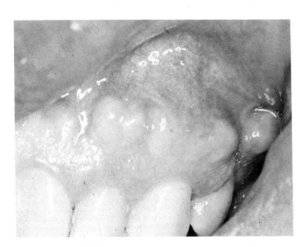

Fig. 7.3 *Multiple osteomas in Gardner's syndrome. (Courtesy of Professor C. Scully.)*

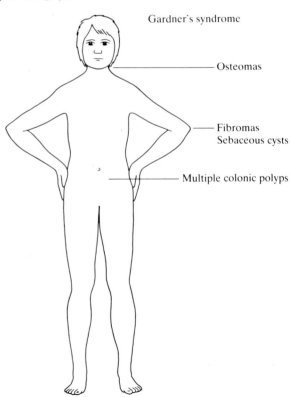

Gardner's syndrome

Osteomas

Fibromas
Sebaceous cysts

Multiple colonic polyps

Fig. 7.4 *Features of Gardner's syndrome. (Courtesy of Professor C. Scully.)*

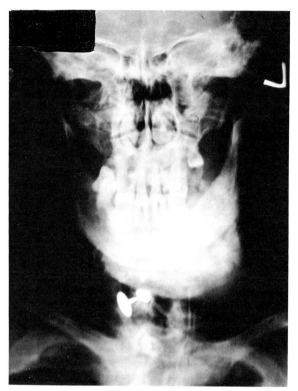

Fig. 7.5 *Osteosarcoma of the mandible. (Courtesy of Professor C. Scully.)*

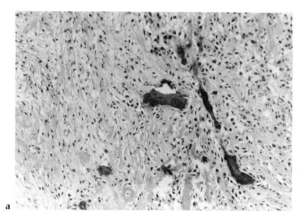

a

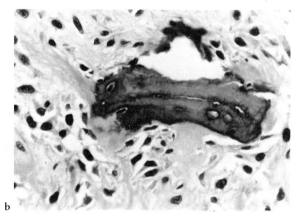

b

Fig. 7.6 *(a) Photomicrograph of osteosarcoma; (b) high power. (Courtesy of Professor C. Scully.)*

is largely unknown although about 3% of patients with osteosarcomas have a history of irradiation for other lesions. It should be noted that there is another peak incidence of osteosarcoma in the over-fifties which probably represents the small but significant malignant change in patients with pre-existing Paget's disease (Chapter 8).

Osteosarcomas are classified as either sclerosing or osteolytic depending on the degree of bone formation or destruction, and may be predominantly medullary or subperiosteal. There is a rare subtype called a parosteal or juxtacortical osteosarcoma which grows from the superficial surface of the bone and is relatively well differentiated. This variant grows much more slowly than the conventional osteosarcoma and metastasizes late.

A characteristic feature of osteosarcoma is the so-called sunray appearance on radiography (Fig. 7.5). In the jaws, symmetrical widening of the periodontal ligament in associated teeth may be an early sign. Microscopy shows a stroma of sarcomatous cells in which abnormal osteoid is being directly deposited (Fig. 7.6). In some

tumours there is abundant formation of cartilage (chondroblastic variant) and it may be difficult to distinguish them from chondrosarcomas.

Although the prognosis for osteosarcomas of the jaws is marginally better than that for the long bones, the outlook for most patients is still poor. Local recurrence and its consequences tend to be the major problems in the head and neck.

Ewing's tumour

Ewing's tumour is a primary malignant neoplasm of undifferentiated mesenchymal cells of bone, of uncertain origin. It characteristically affects children and young adults, particularly males, and is rare in the jaws.

The tumour is extremely aggressive, expands rapidly

and invades the soft tissues, and metastasizes early via both the lymphatics and bloodstream. Radiographically it has either a sunray appearance or an onion-peel appearance due to deposition of new bone in layers. Microscopy shows sheets of uniform small, round cells with scanty, indistinct cytoplasm containing glycogen.

Until recently the prognosis for patients was very poor. Current treatment, which is usually a combination of chemotherapy and radiotherapy, has led to a 5-year survival rate of over 50% in some series.

BENIGN NEOPLASMS OF CARTILAGE

Chondroma

This benign neoplasm is rare in the jaws. The anterior maxilla, mandibular symphysis and the coronoid and condylar processes are the most common sites. Chrondomas are typically found in the elderly and form slow-growing, painless masses. Microscopy shows well-defined lobulated masses of hyaline cartilage separated by fibrous septa. Providing surgical excision of these masses is complete, recurrence is unlikely.

There have been cases described where there was apparent malignant transformation of chondromas to chondrosarcomas, but the microscopical distinction between these lesions can be extremely difficult so there is some doubt as to whether the diagnosis was correct.

Multiple enchondromas constitute the rare Ollier's syndrome, but oral tumours are not a feature of this condition.

Osteochondroma (osteocartilaginous exostosis)

This arises from the epiphyseal region of bone as cartilage-capped bony outgrowths, usually in children. Lesions may be solitary, or multiple in the syndrome of hereditary multiple exostoses (diaphyseal aclasia). In the jaws the most common site is the coronoid process. The solitary lesions are entirely benign but in patients with multiple osteochondromas there is a significant risk of malignant change.

MALIGNANT NEOPLASMS OF CARTILAGE

Chondrosarcomas tend to affect the elderly and, although isolated cases might possibly arise from chondromas, most arise *de novo*. The behaviour of chondrosarcomas of the jaws is very unpredictable but many grow rapidly and produce extensive local destruction.

Radical surgery, the only means of eradicating the tumour, can be difficult as the edges may not be apparent clinically or radiographically. Multiple local recurrence is common and the prognosis is worse than for osteosarcoma.

Other tumours of cartilage, such as mesenchymal chondrosarcoma, chondroblastoma and chondromyxoid-fibroma, are extremely rare and predominantly affect bones other than the jaws.

METASTATIC TUMOURS OF THE JAWS
(see Chapter 15)

Although the jaws are not a common site for clinically obvious metastases, it is probable that subclinical secondary deposits are not rare. The mandible is involved four times as frequently as the maxilla, especially in the premolar and molar regions.

Typical symptoms are pain and swelling, anaesthesia or paraesthesia, loosening of teeth and occasionally pathological fracture. In up to one-third of patients, the jaw lesions are the first manifestation of the tumour.

The most common sites of the primary neoplasm are the bronchus, breast, kidney and thyroid gland, and metastases from these sites usually form destructive, osteolytic lesions (see Fig. 32.17). Metastases from the prostate tend to be osteoblastic and may be confused radiographically with chronic forms of osteomyelitis, Paget's disease and cemental lesions.

OTHER NEOPLASMS

Myeloma (multiple myeloma; myelomatosis)

Myeloma is a malignant neoplasm of plasma cells (Fig. 7.7). It usually forms multiple endosteal deposits, though occasionally there may be solitary lesions (plasmacytomas) in either bone or soft tissue. Nevertheless, most plasmacytomas usually progress to multiple myeloma.

Multiple myeloma is seen mainly in the middle aged and elderly, with a 4:1 male:female predominance. Multiple myeloma is characterized by osteolytic lesions which cause severe bone pain and tenderness. The jaws are involved in 30% of patients and the skull is affected in over 70%. The lesions form discrete, punched-out radiolucent areas in the affected bones (e.g. the 'pepper-pot' skull).

When the jaws are involved there may be paraesthesia or anaesthesia, loosening of teeth and pathological fracture.

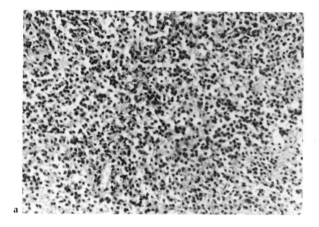

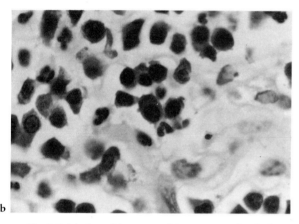

Fig. 7.7 *Myeloma: (a) monomorphic appearance of multiple plasma cells; (b) high power. (Courtesy of Professor C. Scully.)*

Myelomatosis

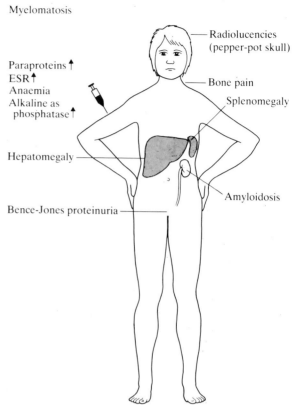

Fig. 7.8 *Features of myelomatosis. (Courtesy of Professor C. Scully.)*

Anaemia, weakness and weight loss are manifestations of advanced disease. About 10% of patients also develop amyloidosis—a rare cause of macroglossia and intra-oral purpura.

Serum electrophoresis shows a monoclonal gammopathy due to the production of fragments of immunoglobulin, typically light chains, by the neoplastic plasma cells. These may also be detected in the urine (Bence–Jones proteinuria). In addition, the erythrocyte sedimentation rate (ESR) or plasma viscosity is greatly raised (Fig. 7.8).

The prognosis for multiple myeloma is poor and, despite frequent early responses to chemotherapeutic agents such as melphalan, less than 20% of patients survive more than 5 years.

Histiocytosis

Eosinophilic granuloma

Eosinophilic granuloma is a non-neoplastic destructive lesion of bone which may be solitary or multifocal. The aetiology is unknown but lesions consist of cells of the mononuclear phagocyte system and eosinophils. It is probably a lesion of Langerhan's cells. Many regard eosinophilic granuloma as a manifestation of a group of diseases called histiocytosis X or Langerhan's cell histiocytosis. This is a spectrum of lesions which includes solitary eosinophilic granuloma, multifocal eosinophilic granuloma (including Hand–Schuller–Christian disease) and Letterer–Siwe disease. However, some regard Letterer–Siwe disease as a type of lymphoma, fundamentally different from eosinophilic granuloma.

In eosinophilic granuloma of the jaws, lesions develop within the cancellous bone and cause such extensive destruction that the cortex is often perforated and the lesion extends into soft tissues. Swelling and gingival ulceration, particularly in the molar region, are common manifestations and the teeth may loosen and exfoliate. Failure of healing of a socket or appearance of a pathological fracture may be the presenting feature. Multifocal lesions are most common in infants and young children, particularly in the calvarium and facial bones.

Hand–Schuller–Christian syndrome

About 25% of patients with multifocal eosinophilic granuloma have the triad of exophthalmos, multifocal cystic lesions, particularly of the skull, and diabetes insipidus (Hand–Schuller–Christian syndrome).

Radiographs in the histiocytoses may show extensive destruction of bone with no new bone formation within the lesion (Fig. 7.9). The punched-out radiolucent areas in the skull in multifocal lesions closely resemble the radiographic appearances of multiple myeloma. Microscopy shows replacement of bone by sheets of histiocytes and focal aggregates of eosinophils which may form microabscesses. Electron microscopy shows that the histiocytes contain the rod-shaped Birbeck granules typical of Langerhan's cells. Monoclonal antibodies can be used to stain these cells.

Letterer–Siwe disease

This condition is usually seen in children in the first two years of life. There is generalized lymphadenopathy, hepatosplenomegaly and destructive lesions in the lungs and bones and the condition is rapidly fatal. The affected tissues are infiltrated by sheets of large, pale-staining histiocytes and occasional multinucleated giant cells.

CENTRAL GIANT-CELL GRANULOMA
(see also Chapter 21)

This uncommon lesion is only seen in the tooth-bearing regions of the jaws, most commonly in the mandible, and typically in the second and third decades. The true nature of these lesions is unknown but, as they are invariably destructive, the term 'reparative' giant-cell granuloma would appear to be inappropriate.

Lesions may be symptomless or simulate a malignant neoplasm clinically and radiographically. Occasionally, the lesion erodes through the cortical bone where it presents as a domed, purplish submucosal swelling (Fig. 7.10).

Radiography shows an ill-defined area of radiolucency and there may be resorption of the roots of related teeth. Microscopy shows multinucleated giant cells irregularly distributed in a cellular stroma of plump, spindle-shaped cells which is often highly vascular (Fig. 7.11). There may be areas of new and old haemorrhage with haemosiderin pigment deposition. These microscopical features are indistinguishable from the focal lesions of hyperparathyr-

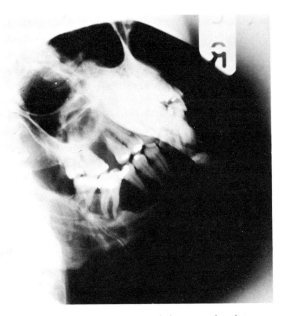

Fig. 7.9 *Histiocytosis showing a radiolucent osteolytic lesion in lower premolar/molar region. (Courtesy of Professor C. Scully.)*

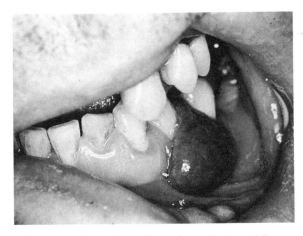

Fig. 7.10 *Central giant-cell granuloma. (Courtesy of Professor C. Scully.)*

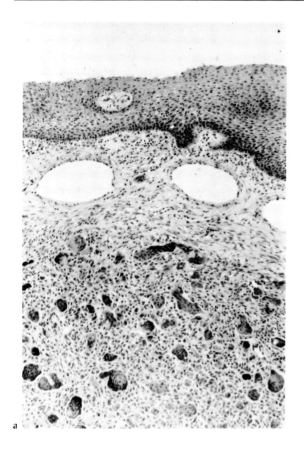

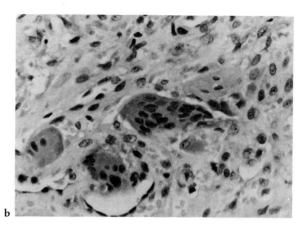

Fig. 7.11 (*a*) *Photomicrograph of a giant-cell granuloma;* (*b*) *high power.* (*Courtesy of Professor C. Scully.*)

oidism, which can only be excluded by the appropriate serological tests (calcium and phosphate levels and alkaline phosphatase: Chapter 2).

Although central giant-cell granulomas may recur following curettage, they virtually never metastasize.

OSSIFYING FIBROMA (see Chapter 8)

FURTHER READING

Beckstead J. H., Wood G. S., Turner R. R. (1984). Histiocytosis X and Langerhans cells: enzyme, histochemical and immunologic similarities. *Human Pathol.*, **15**: 826–833.

Beeching B. W. (1980). Neoplasms and tumour-like lesions of the jaws—part 2. *Dental Update*, March/April: 97–111.

Clark J. L., Unni K. K., Dahlin C. C., Devine K. D. (1983). Osteosarcoma of the jaw. *Cancer*, **51**: 2311–2316.

Fitzpatrick R., Rapaport M. J., Silva D. G. (1981). Histiocytosis X. *Arch. Dermatol.*, **117**: 253–257.

Groopman J. E., Golde D. W. (1981). The histiocytic disorders: a pathophysiologic analysis. *Ann. Int. Med.*, **94**: 95–107.

Hartman K. S. (1980). Histiocytosis X: a review of 114 cases with oral involvement. *Oral Surg.*, **49**: 38–54.

Harvei S., Solheim O. (1981). The prognosis in osteosarcoma: Norwegian national data. *Cancer*, **48**: 1719–1723.

Jones R. O., Pillsbury H. C., Hill C. (1984). Histiocytosis X of the head and neck. *Laryngoscope*, **94**: 1031–1035.

Chapter
8

Fibro-osseous lesions

Fibro-osseous lesions comprise a group of disorders of unknown aetiology, composed of fibrous and ossified tissue (Table 8.1). The main disorders include Paget's disease of bone; fibrous dysplasia and cherubism; and the ossifying fibroma.

PAGET'S DISEASE OF BONE

Paget's disease is a fairly common disorder in the UK. It is found predominantly in elderly males and may affect up to 5% of those over 55 years of age. The aetiology is unclear, but recently infection with measles or respiratory syncytial virus has been implicated.

Clinical features

Paget's disease is characterized by the total disorganization of the normally orderly remodelling of bone and an anarchic alternation of bone resorption and apposition. In early lesions, bone destruction predominates (osteolytic stage) and there is bowing of the long bones, especially

Table 8.1

Fibro-osseous lesions

	Age (years)	Sex	Site General	Oral	Dental
Paget's disease	>40	♂>♀	Vertebral column, pelvis, skull, long bones (tibia and femur)	Maxilla > mandible	Hypercementosis, loss of lamina dura
Fibrous dysplasia	0–20	♀>♂		Maxilla > mandible	
Monostotic			Single lesion—long bones, rib, jaw, skull	Frequent involvement	—
Polyostotic			Multiple lesions—head of femur, vertebrae, skull, pelvis	25% of patients with fibrous dysplasia	—
Albright's syndrome			Polyostotic fibrous dysplasia, cutaneous pigmentation, endocrine disorders	Rare	—
Cherubism	2–4	♂>♀	—	Mandible always Mandible and maxilla in severe cases	—
Ossifying fibroma	Chidren and young adults		—	Mandible > maxilla	—

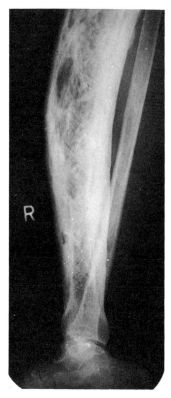

Fig. 8.1 *Paget's disease producing bowing of the legs. (Courtesy of Professor C. Scully.)*

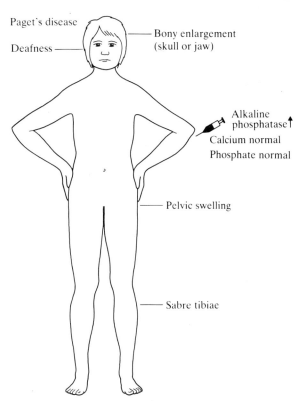

Fig. 8.2 *Features of Paget's disease. (Courtesy of Professor C. Scully.)*

the tibia (Fig. 8.1), pathological fractures of bone, broadening/flattening of the chest and spinal deformity. There may also be severe bone pain and headaches and, if the disease is widespread, the increased vascularity of the bones can lead to cardiac failure (Fig. 8.2).

Orofacial manifestations

As the disease activity declines, bone apposition becomes more evident (osteosclerotic stage) and the bones enlarge. If the skull is affected, the patient who wears a hat may notice that it becomes tight. Constriction of skull foramina may cause cranial neuropathies. The maxilla often enlarges (Figs. 8.3 and 32.18), particularly in the molar region, with widening of the alveolar ridge. Classically patients are said to present with dentures that appear to become too tight, but in fact this is rare. Hypercementosis and loss of the lamina dura may be evident (Figs. 8.4 and 8.5). Extractions can be difficult both because of the hypercementosis and the dense bone,

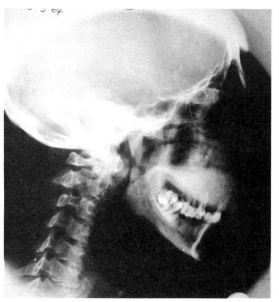

Fig. 8.3 *Paget's disease of the maxilla. (Courtesy of Professor C. Scully.)*

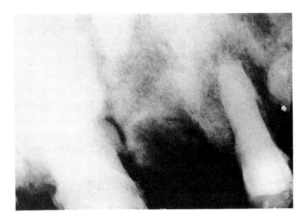

Fig. 8.4 *Hypercementosis, loss of lamina dura and cotton-wool appearance of bone in Paget's disease. (Courtesy of Professor C. Scully.)*

and there is a liability to haemorrhage and infection of bone in Paget's disease.

Other complications in Paget's disease, together with the appropriate precautions in dental treatment, are summarized in Table 8.2.

Diagnosis

Diagnosis of Paget's disease is based on the history and examination supported by radiography, biochemistry and histopathology.

In early lesions, radiographs show large, irregular areas of relative radiolucency (osteoporosis circumscripta), but later there is increased radio-opacity, with the loss of the normal radiographic landmarks, and appearance of an irregular 'cotton-wool' pattern. There is progressive thickening of the diploë and base of the skull as well as of the sphenoid, orbital and frontal bones (Fig. 8.6). Isotope bone scanning shows localized areas of very high uptake. Patients present with a considerable increase in plasma alkaline phosphatase and urine hydroxyproline levels which reflect the accelerated bone turnover. However, there are little or no changes in plasma calcium or phosphate levels.

Histopathological examination shows evidence of bony trabeculae being resorbed and deposited as a continuous process, as shown by numerous prominent 'reversal lines' producing a mosaic pattern in the bone (Fig. 8.7). The marrow is fibrous and very vascular in early lesions, but these features are less evident later.

The differential diagnosis includes other fibro-osseous lesions such as fibrous dysplasia, and conditions with a raised alkaline phosphatase, e.g. osteomalacia, hyperparathyroidism, and osteoblastic metastatic deposits (e.g. carcinoma of the prostate).

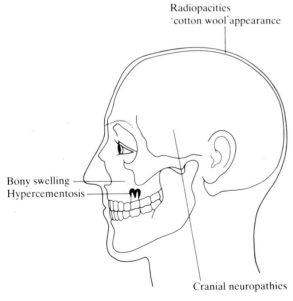

Fig. 8.5 *Orofacial complications of Paget's disease. (Courtesy of Professor C. Scully.)*

Table 8.2
Paget's disease and preventive measures during dental care

	Prevention
General	
Congestive cardiac failure	Avoid general anaesthesia
Bone deformities	—
vertebral column	Avoid general anaesthesia
thoracic cage (bronchitis, bronchopneumonia)	
fractures	
Malignant change to osteosarcoma (very rare in jaws)	Frequent assessment of clinical behaviour; biopsy as required
Dental	
Hypercementosed teeth	Surgical dento-alveolar approach to extractions
Haemorrhage	Ensure haemostasis before discharging patient
Infection (chronic suppurative osteomyelitis)	Antibiotic cover for surgery
Expansion of dento-alveolar ridge	Frequent replacement of dentures

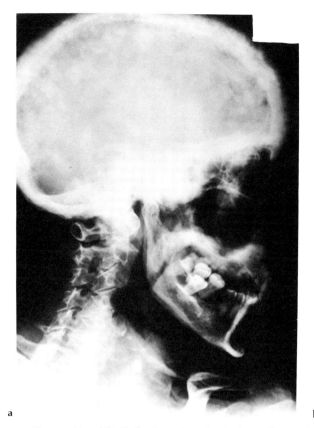

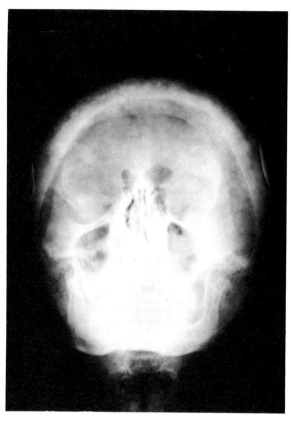

a   b

Fig. 8.6 (a) and (b) Skull radiographs in Paget's disease showing thic ?ning of the skull and cotton-wool appearance. (Courtesy of Professor C. Scully.)

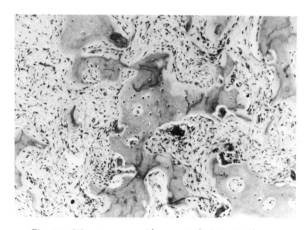

Fig. 8.7 Mosaic pattern of bone typical of Paget's disease. (Courtesy of Professor C. Scully.)

Management

Treatment of Paget's disease is medical, reducing bone turnover with diphosphonates or calcitonin, and, as far as possible, preventing complications (Table 8.2).

FIBROUS DYSPLASIA

Fibrous dysplasia is a disorder characterized by the replacement of an area of bone with fibrous tissue. The process typically starts in childhood and, as the skeleton matures, the lesions progressively ossify. As skeletal growth ceases, the lesion stabilizes.

Three types of fibrous dysplasia are recognized.

1. Monostotic—in which there is a single lesion in only one bone.

2. Polyostotic—in which several lesions are present in one or more bones.

3. Albright's syndrome—where polyostotic fibrous dysplasia is associated with cutaneous pigmentation (café-au-lait type) on the same side as the bony lesion; precocious puberty; and, rarely, overactivity of other endocrine glands such as the thyroid, adrenal cortex or pituitary.

Clinical features

Fibrous dysplasia usually presents as a painless, bony hard swelling. The maxillary sinus is often involved, when there may be encroachment on the orbit—causing protrusion of the eye (proptosis)—and nasal cavity—causing obstruction. Expansion of the alveolar bone leads to disruption of occlusion, displacement of teeth and possibly failure of eruption of teeth (see Fig. 10.20).

In Albright's syndrome, polyostotic fibrous dysplasia is accompanied by areas of skin and sometimes oral pigmentation overlying the bone lesions.

Diagnosis

Radiographically, there is either a translucent cystic appearance in the affected bone, or mottled opaque areas likened to ground glass (Fig. 8.8). The lesions are often ill-defined and may extend to, but not cross, suture lines.

Serum calcium and phosphate levels are normal, but in many the serum alkaline phosphatase level is high and

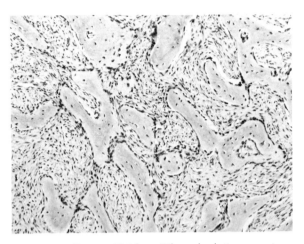

Fig. 8.9 *Histology of fibrous dysplasia.*

urinary hydroxyproline is increased—findings similar to those in Paget's disease.

Microscopically, the lesion consists of fibrous tissue that replaces the normal bone and gives rise to osseous trabeculae by metaplasia. The osseous tissue is composed of irregular ('Chinese characters') trabeculae of woven bone lined by osteoblasts (Fig. 8.9). Focal degeneration of fibrous tissue accounts for the cystic spaces seen macroscopically.

A differential diagnosis includes the other fibro-osseous lesions and, where cutaneous pigmentation is present, Addison's disease and neurofibromatosis should also be excluded.

Management

The treatment of choice to correct any cosmetic defect is conservative surgery, preferably after the cessation of normal skeletal growth. The lesion is not radiosensitive; indeed, irradiation may cause sarcomatous change.

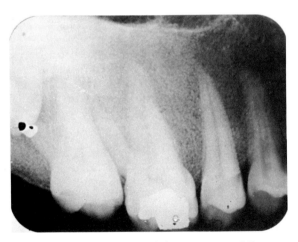

Fig. 8.8 *Radiographic 'ground-glass' appearance of fibrous dysplasia. (Courtesy of Professor C. Scully.)*

CHERUBISM

Cherubism is a genetically determined disease of the jaws which in many ways closely resembles fibrous dysplasia, except that there is an autosomal dominant mode of inheritance (but variable expression) and it presents at 2–4 years of age. The lesions grow progressively until puberty, when they usually arrest or regress.

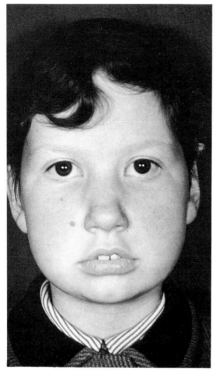

Fig. 8.10 Facial appearance in cherubism. (Courtesy of Professor C. Scully.)

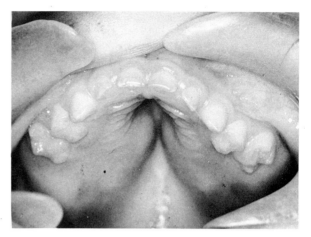

Fig. 8.11 Maxillary swelling in cherubism. (Courtesy of Professor C. Scully.)

Clinical features

Painless symmetrical enlargement at the angles of the mandible and often in the maxilla leads to the typical 'cherubic' facial appearance (Fig. 8.10). Expansion of the alveolar bone results in irregular spacing and premature loss of teeth and possibly disturbances to the developing dentition (Fig. 8.11).

Diagnosis

Radiography shows well-defined multilocular radiolucencies in the mandible but maxillary lesions are less clearly defined. Blood chemistry is essentially normal, although there may be a raised alkaline phosphatase during the periods of most active growth. Histologically, the lesion consists of loose vascular connective tissue with numerous multinucleated giant cells and, as in fibrous dysplasia, there is replacement of bone by the fibrous tissue. However, metaplastic bone formation is an infrequent finding.

Other fibro-osseous lesions and giant-cell lesions of bone (giant-cell granuloma, hyperparathyroidism, giant-cell tumours) should be excluded.

Management

Treatment of cherubism is as for fibrous dysplasia.

OSSIFYING FIBROMA

The nature of the ossifying fibroma is obscure because it has features both of a developmental anomaly and a neoplasm (Table 8.3). Nevertheless, it is a distinct entity which presents as a painless, localized, slow-growing, hard swelling of the jaw which radiographically is a well-defined radiolucent area with a thin sclerotic margin containing irregular opaque masses.

Table 8.3
Features of ossifying fibroma

Developmental	Neoplastic
Occurs in children and young adults	Clearly demarcated from normal bone
Shows occasional multiplicity	Can grow to large dimensions
Lesions in children may cease to grow with skeletal maturity	Recurrence if inadequate removal

Histological examination shows little or no distinction between ossifying fibroma and fibrous dysplasia, except perhaps that a cellular, homogeneous calcified material is usually more obvious in the former. Distinction between ossifying fibroma and fibrous dysplasia, therefore, relies heavily on the localized nature and slow growth pattern of the ossifying fibroma. Surgical enucleation is usually curative.

Juvenile ossifying fibroma

Juvenile ossifying fibromas appear to behave more aggressively in children than in adults. They present as rapidly enlarging swellings of the jaw but are entirely benign, and growth often ceases with skeletal maturation. Cosmetic surgery may then be needed.

ANEURYSMAL BONE CYST (see also Chapter 5)

Approximately one-third of aneurysmal bone cysts appear to be associated with other disorders such as a giant-cell lesion, fibrous dysplasia and fibromas.

This rare lesion presents as an asymptomatic hard swelling of the jaw, sometimes following a history of previous trauma. The lesion generally expands the cortex and may go on to perforate it.

Radiologically, there is a well-defined unilocular or multilocular radiolucency.

Diagnosis is confirmed by histology which shows numerous capillaries and blood-filled spaces, areas of haemorrhage associated with multinucleated giant cells and irregular areas of osteoid.

Treatment is by surgical curettage.

FURTHER READING

Hosking D. J. (1982). *Paget's disease of bone.* London: Update Publications.

Scully C., Flint S. (1988). *An atlas of stomatology.* London: Martin Dunitz (in press).

Smith B. J., Eveson J. W. (1981). Paget's disease of bone with particular reference to dentistry. *J. oral Pathol.,* **10**: 233–247.

Waldron C. A. (1985). Fibro-osseous lesions of the jaws. *J. oral max-fac. Surg.,* **43**: 249–262.

Chapter
9
Temporomandibular joint disorders

The temporomandibular joint (TMJ) should not be viewed in isolation but considered with its opposite joint, as part of the stomatognathic system, even though many disorders which affect the joint appear to be unilateral.

DEVELOPMENT OF TMJ

The joint itself develops from two groups of prototype cells (blastemas) at 6–8 weeks of fetal life. The condylar blastema and the glenoid blastema are widely separated until they meet at the twelfth week. The articular disc develops from a mesenchymal condensation between these two blastemas. The condylar blastema contributes the anterior portion and the glenoid blastema contributes the lesser posterior portion. Cavitation to produce the lower and upper joint compartments occurs at 12 and 14 weeks respectively.

The traditional view of postnatal condylar development considers the condyle as a primary growth centre. Its upward and backward growth was said to push the mandible down and forward. The more recent view is that the condyle is a secondary growth site capable of remodelling in response to functional requirements. Condylar growth maintains contact with the articular fossa while the mandible is carried down by soft tissue forces. This latter view is partly supported by morphological differences between the condylar cartilage and endochondral growth plates, and by recent studies of monkeys involving artificial occlusal interferences to stimulate condylar adaptation in various directions.

During childhood the condylar cartilage is hypertrophic in form. Cessation of growth is accompanied by maturation of the cartilage to a non-hypertrophic form which has a reduced potential for adaptive remodelling.

Nevertheless remodelling continues throughout life as part of normal ageing, and this is sometimes difficult to distinguish from alteration due to disease.

HISTORY AND EXAMINATION

A history must include date(s) of onset of symptoms; pain details such as duration, daily timing, character, spread, aggravating factors, relieving factors and associated phenomena; details of any joint noises such as clicking or grating; details of any restriction to mouth opening, any facial asymmetry or mandibular disproportion and any personal or family history of arthritis.

The area should be inspected and then the TMJ should be palpated over both condyles to detect abnormal movements or clicking within the joint. Palpation of the condyle via the external auditory meatus may detect tenderness posteriorly. The interincisal distance should be measured at maximum mouth opening. The mandibular muscles should be palpated: the lateral pterygoid (lower head) by placing a finger up behind the maxillary tuberosity; the masseter by intra-oral–extra-oral compression between finger and thumb; and the temporalis by direct palpation in the temporal region. The dentition and occlusion are also thoroughly examined.

INVESTIGATIONS

The following radiographs show the articular surface (Volume 1).

1. Transpharyngeal (Toller view).
2. Orthopantomogram.
3. Transcranioblique (TMJ view).

Additional views which display the condylar *neck* rather than the articular surface include:

4. Reverse Townes view.
5. Zimmer's transorbital view.

Three-dimensional information may be gained from:

6. Tomography in both the coronal and sagittal planes.
7. Computerized tomography (CT scan). This multi-plexed horizontal image can be reconstructed by computer to display the condyle in different planes (e.g. the sagittal plane). The image density can also be altered to help separate and identify different tissues.

The position of the meniscus can be deduced by arthrography following injection of radio-opaque dye into, preferably, the lower joint compartment. This is viewed on a transcranioblique radiograph or a sagittal tomogram. If an image intensifier is used, a dynamic arthrogram during opening and closing of the mandible can be recorded on videotape.

Direct visualization of the meniscus can be obtained using a fibre-optic arthroscope. Recently, nuclear magnetic resonance imaging of the joint has been accomplished. Both latter techniques avoid irradiating the patient.

Detailed examination of the occlusion may require monitoring of study models on a semi- or fully adjustable articulator. Special haematological investigations might be required for rheumatoid arthritis of the TMJ (e.g. rheumatoid factor; raised plasma viscosity or ESR). Electromyography can be helpful in the diagnosis of condylar hyperplasia by showing whether increased jaw muscle activity is on the same side as the apparent deformity.

TMJ DYSFUNCTION PAIN

(Myofascial pain dysfunction, mandibular dysfunction, or mandibular stress syndrome)

This refers to a triad of symptoms—clicking, jaw locking (or limitation of opening) and pain. TMJ dysfunction is neither new nor confined to Western 'civilized' communities.

Clinical features

The main features are locking (or limitation of opening) and pain.

Pain may occur at an early stage or sometimes after the onset of clicking or stiffness of the jaw. It may range from a vague dull ache to an acute pain. The site is usually pre-auricular but can radiate to the back of the mouth, down the neck or up to the head. Sometimes discomfort is more clearly sited in a jaw muscle, e.g. the masseter.

Clicking occurs either on attempted opening or closing. Often the click allows the completion of that phase of mandibular movement. Sometimes clicking ceases and the jaw locks either open or closed. There may be reduced mouth opening and deviation of the jaw to one side on attempted opening. A grating noise (crepitus) often signifies intra-articular arthritic change.

Symptoms can be quantified by the indices of Helkimo, based on both patient information (the anamnestic dysfunction index Ai) and on clinical findings (the clinical dysfunction index Di).

In the anamnestic index:

Ai O denotes complete absence of subjective symptoms of dysfunction,

Ai I denotes mild symptoms such as TMJ sounds, feelings of stiffness of the jaws,

Ai II denotes more severe symptoms, e.g. difficulty in opening the mouth wide, locking, fixations, pain on movement, facial and jaw pain.

The clinical dysfunction index grades five common signs according to severity to classify patients as:

Di 0   clinically symptom free,
Di I   mild dysfunction,
Di II   moderate dysfunction,
Di III   severe dysfunction.

These indices include a numerical scoring system.

Many patients presenting for treatment can be graded as Ai II, Di II/Di III.

Epidemiology

TMJ symptoms have been reported by up to 88% of the UK general population, with as many as 25% reporting severe symptoms. However, patient populations are much smaller and most patients are females between 20 and 30 years of age.

Aetiology

This is multifactorial so that it is better to view the triad above as a symptom complex which may be induced by one or more of the following factors.

1. Trauma: including road accidents, sports injuries and fights. In extreme cases there may be an acute traumatic arthritis which is extremely painful.

2. Prolonged and/or excessive mandibular opening: for example long dental appointments, choir singing or wind instrument playing.

3. Abnormalities in the dental occlusion: this is still controversial. There is no neurophysiological evidence to support a primary aetiological role for the occlusion and many people have quite gross malocclusions without developing TMJ dysfunction.

4. Dental causes: dysfunction secondary to pain, for example from caries, or erupting teeth (e.g. wisdom teeth).

5. Psychological stress: 50–70% of patients experience a stressful life event in the 6 months before onset, this being twice as common as the rate reported by control patients. These problems, concerning work, money, health, loss and interpersonal relationships, probably have a causative role. Psychological stress is thought to induce anxiety which produces increased jaw muscle activity. Experimental studies indicate that jaw muscle hyperactivity can be a cause of TMJ dysfunction pain. This is unlikely to be prompted by occlusal factors since the effect of mechanical stimulation of teeth is to reduce or inhibit jaw-closing muscle activity and there is no significant difference in the incidence of occlusal abnormalities between dysfunction patients and control subjects.

The most likely causes of jaw muscle hyperactivity are psychological or physical stress, for example life events experience or abnormal mandibular posture. Muscle hyperactivity has been demonstrated in TMJ patients during activities such as school examinations and watching horror films.

6. Arthritic changes and remodelling: these are partially but not exclusively associated with ageing and with extensive tooth loss.

7. Parafunctions, such as day-time jaw clenching or night-time tooth grinding (bruxism), are related to psychological stress (see point 5. above) and may be associated.

Joint mechanics

Studies have shown that the two heads of the lateral pterygoid muscle have separate actions. The lower head contracts during mouth opening; the superior head contracts during closing, to steady the meniscus as it moves back with the condyle into the glenoid fossa. During closing the lower head is electromyographically silent.

In TMJ dysfunction patients, the lower head of the lateral pterygoid muscle contracts during the closing phase (when it should be relaxed). It has been suggested

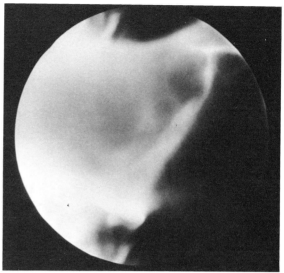

a

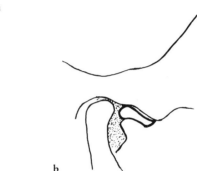

b

Fig. 9.1 (a) Tomo-arthrogram of right TMJ. Radio-opaque dye anterior to condyle in mouth-closed position suggests anterior dislocation of meniscus. (b) Tracing shows meniscus (stippled area) buckled between condyle posteriorly and upper joint space anteriorly.

that anterior displacement of the meniscus, perhaps from a tear of the posterior capsule, prevents the superior head from acting effectively. The lower head perhaps attempts to help stabilize the meniscus. This would explain why this muscle is tender on palpation in TMJ dysfunction patients.

Anterior displacement of the meniscus has been demonstrated by TMJ arthrography (Fig. 9.1) and found at operation in TMJ patients. Patients may be classified as having: no meniscus displacement (Fig. 9.2a); anterior displacement with reduction (excessive forward movement during opening which relocates on closing) (Fig. 9.2b); and anterior displacement without reduction (Fig. 9.2c), when the meniscus remains anterior to the condyle

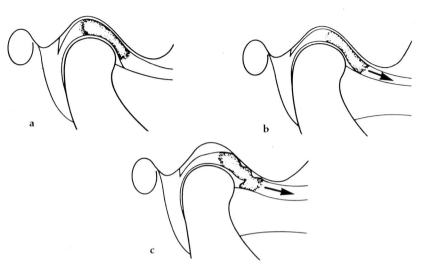

Fig. 9.2 *Possible positions of meniscus as revealed by TMJ arthrography. (a) Normal. (b) Anterior dislocation with reduction. (c) Anterior dislocation without reduction.*

in a buckled-up fashion, such that there is a reduced joint space and the articular surface of the condyle is close to the articular surface of the glenoid fossa. This latter situation predisposes to subsequent osteoarthritis.

Differential diagnosis (see also Chapter 27)

1. Referred pain from local causes such as pulpitis, periodontitis, pericoronitis or oral malignancy.
2. Local causes in adjacent anatomical structures such as the ear, sinus or salivary glands.
3. Cranial nerve disorders such as trigeminal neuralgia.
4. Vascular pain: (a) migraine or cluster headache, (b) temporal arteritis.
5. Psychogenic pain: atypical facial pain/intractable facial pain.
6. Other TMJ problems such as osteoarthritis, rheumatoid arthritis, 'loose body' deposition (see p. 95), tumours, fractures.

Treatment

It is accepted practice to relieve obvious occlusal interferences and to correct prosthetic discrepancies such as an incorrect vertical dimension. There is a high placebo response and reassurance is important.

The aims of treatment are to control pain, reduce psychological stress and eliminate TMJ and occlusal dysharmony. Ideally dental and psychological approaches should proceed simultaneously rather than separately or singly. The level of placebo response and the response from reassurance should not be underestimated. Overall, conservative measures succeed in 70–90% of cases, usually within 6 months. Some non-responders subsequently improve following surgery, especially those with obvious intra-articular pathology (osteoarthritis). The remainder may need treatment for prominent psychological problems by either medication or psychiatric therapy. This last subgroup accounts for 5–10% of patients.

The range of treatments used for TMJ dysfunction is large (indicating that many different treatments may work but that none is uniformly successful) and includes the following.

1. Dental:
    (a) reassurance/dental counselling,
    (b) occlusal covers, e.g. polythene vacuum-formed cover (Fig. 9.3),
    (c) occlusal adjustments,
    (d) occlusal reconstruction.
2. Physical:
    (a) immobilization/rest,
    (b) heat/ultrasound,
    (c) muscle exercises.
3. Medication:
    (a) local analgesics,

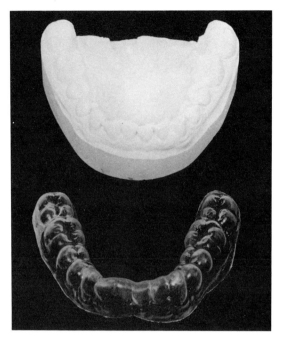

Fig. 9.3 *Polythene occlusal cover, vacuum-formed over model of lower teeth.*

(b) muscle relaxants,

(c) anxiolytics and antidepressants—benzodiazepines, tricyclic antidepressants,

(d) analgesics and non-steroidal anti-inflammatory drugs,

(e) intra-articular steroids.

4. Psychological:
   (a) psychiatric treatment,
   (b) group therapy,
   (c) behaviour modification/biofeedback,
   (d) hypnosis.
5. Surgical:
   (a) condylotomy,
   (b) high condylar shave,
   (c) capsular rearrangement,
   (d) section of auriculotemporal nerve.

OSTEOARTHRITIS (OSTEOARTHROSIS)

Osteoarthritis (OA) is a non-inflammatory condition characterized by deterioration of the articular surface of a joint and by simultaneous remodelling of the underlying bone. TMJ osteoarthritis is common in the general

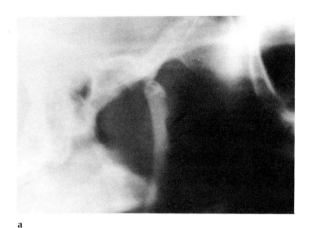

a

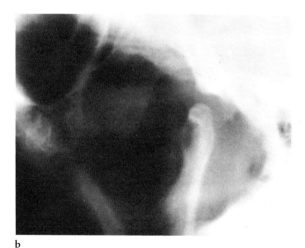

b

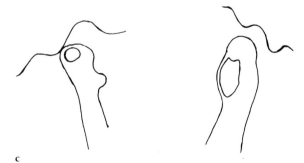

c

Fig. 9.4 *Osteoarthritis of TMJ. (a) Enlargement of right TMJ to show erosion and osteophyte formation. (b) Enlargement of left TMJ to show cystic lesion within condyle. (c) Tracing to show these features.*

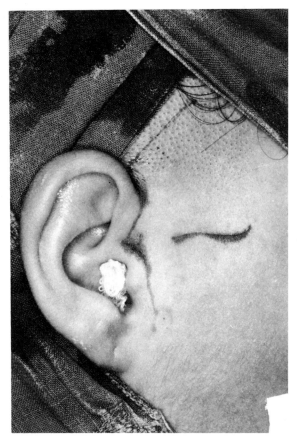

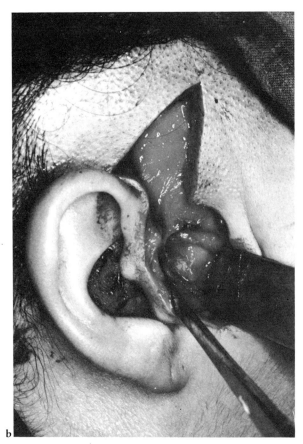

Fig. 9.5 *Preauricular approach to TMJ for high condylar shave operation. (a) Incision and glenoid fossa marked. (b) Flap raised to display lateral capsule of right TMJ. (c) Excised articular surface showing eroded surface produced by osteoarthritis.*

population, although at any specific time less than a third have experienced pain in the past 5 years. Its prevalence increases with age, as revealed by autopsy and clinical studies. The aetiological role of excessive wear and tear should not obscure the view held by many that this is an active disease process.

There is loss of glycosaminoglycan (mucopolysaccharide) from the cartilage matrix, and necrosis of chondrocytes, especially in the superficial layers. The subchondral bone becomes sclerotic and cystic lesions may appear. New bone may form in some areas (osteophytes) and bone resorbs elsewhere. The synovium may be mildly inflamed and hydroxyapatite crystals may deposit within the joint cavity.

One-third of patients with TMJ osteoarthritis are under 40 years of age and one-tenth under 25 years of age. However, as a group, OA patients are older than TMJ dysfunction patients.

The diagnostic features are:

(a) pain within the joint (rather than in the muscles),

(b) crepitus,

(c) radiological evidence of joint changes such as cystic spaces in the condyle, erosions of the articular surface and osteophytes (Fig. 9.4). It should be noted that the radiological picture of TMJ osteoarthritis is similar to that of simple condylar remodelling.

There is a relationship between longstanding TMJ dysfunction and development of subsequent OA, and the two groups of patients may not differ with respect to subjective symptoms.

Treatment is by:

(a) conservative measures (as for TMJ dysfunction),

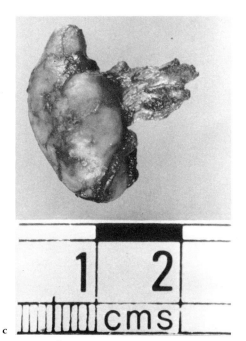

c

Fig. 9.5 (*continued*)

(b) a single intra-articular corticosteroid injection (this causes a chemical intracapsular condylectomy), or

(c) a high condylar shave operation (Fig. 9.5) to remove the articular surface.

Untreated TMJ osteoarthritis can cause chronic pain: treatments (b) and (c) are, however, quickly effective.

RHEUMATOID ARTHRITIS

Rheumatoid arthritis (RA) is a polyarthritis which can involve all synovial joints including the TMJ. It appears to be immunologically mediated: an abnormal immunoglobulin is formed in the joint tissues and an autoantibody to the abnormal globulin is produced. The autoantibody (rheumatoid factor) is usually an IgM antibody directed against IgG, and the patients with rheumatoid factor are termed seropositive. Occasionally the autoantibody is of the IgG class and fails to give a positive result on routine serological testing. Such patients are termed seronegative, though they still actually have autoantibodies. Patients with RA may also have hypergammaglobulinaemia, positive antinuclear antibodies and a raised plasma viscosity or ESR. A proliferative synovitis (pannus) which may contain lymphoid follicles, covers the articular surface and extends into subchrondral bone. There are periods of activity and periods of remission. Healing phases may be accompanied by production of scar tissue which impairs joint mobility. Increased pressure in the joint and synovium from excess fluid causes pain.

Radiographic features include soft-tissue swelling and widening of the joint space in early disease followed by osteoporosis and cyst formation in the subarticular bone.

Half to two-thirds of all RA patients have TMJ involvement, although only a small proportion complain of TMJ pain. The symptoms are then similar to TMJ dysfunction but the pain is usually located *within* the joint. Radiologically there may be little change at first, but eventually erosions are seen. Continued destruction of the condyle may lead to a 'mushroom deformity' and/or ankylosis of the TMJ. The loss of height which this causes can alter the occlusion—producing an anterior open bite (Fig. 9.6). Such changes are particularly seen in Still's disease (juvenile chronic polyarthritis).

Treatment for rheumatoid involvement of the TMJ includes the same conservative measures used for TMJ dysfunction pain.

Management includes:

(a) rest,

(b) non-steroidal anti-inflammatory agents such as aspirin,

(c) systemic steroids in severe cases.

Intra-articular steroid injections may be required and, in severe cases, release of ankylosis with reconstruction by interposition arthroplasty using, for example, silastic or titanium condylar prostheses (Fig. 9.7) is needed.

CRYSTAL DEPOSITION ('LOOSE BODIES')

Deposition of hydroxyapatite crystals within the joint space of the TMJ may occur in the following conditions.

Osteochondritis dissecans (1–3 'loose bodies').
Osteoarthritis (1–10 'loose bodies').
Chip fracture of articular surface (1–3 'loose bodies').
Synovial chondromatosis (50–500 'loose bodies') (Fig. 9.8).

Crystal deposition can cause TMJ pain. Surgical exploration of the joint may be needed if the pain does not respond to conservative treatment.

In gout, uric-acid crystals may be deposited and the radiographic appearance resembles that of osteoarthritis of the TMJ. Gout is usually treated with allopurinol.

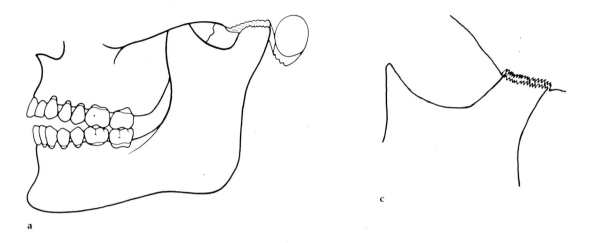

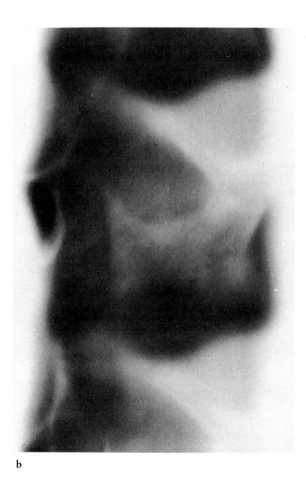

Fig. 9.6 (a) Occlusal alterations (anterior open bite) which can occur following severe rheumatoid arthritis of the TMJ. (b) Sagittal tomogram of rheumatoid ankylosis. (c) Tracing of tomographic appearance.

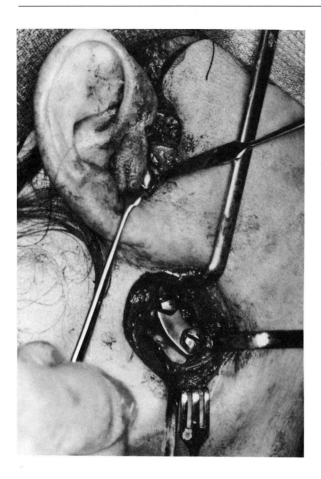

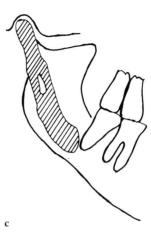

c

Fig. 9.7 (a) and (b) Use of titanium condylar prosthesis for reconstruction of the TMJ, e.g. following destruction by rheumatoid arthritis. (c) Tracing to show position of prosthesis.

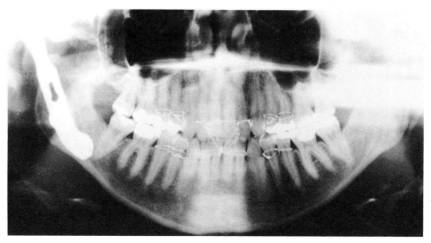

b

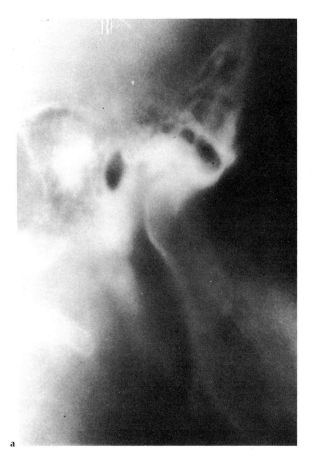

a

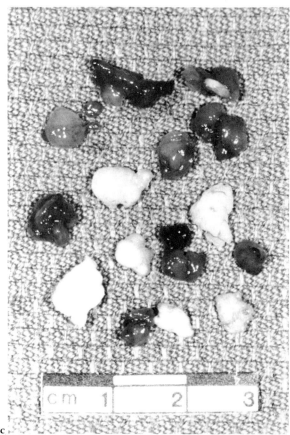

c

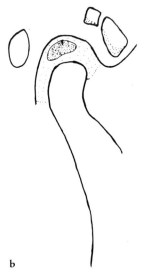

b

Fig. 9.8 *Synovial chondromatosis. (a) Sagittal tomogram of right TMJ showing calcification in joint space. (b) Tracing shows calcification in joint space and inside cavities within articular eminence. Note the auditory meatus which is shown posterior to the condyle. (c) 'Loose bodies' removed from right TMJ in various stages of calcification.*

RECURRENT DISLOCATION

The term dislocation usually refers to displacement of the condyle anterior to the articular eminence. This is usually, but not always, bilateral and the patient is unable to reposition the mandible into normal occlusion. Accompanying spasm of the mandibular muscles adds to the discomfort. If the displacement is self-reducing, the term subluxation is used. Patients frequently describe recurrent episodes which suggest a laxity of the joint. Rarely, connective tissue disorders such as the Ehlers–Danlos (see Chapter 1) or other hypermobility syndromes underly subluxation or dislocation.

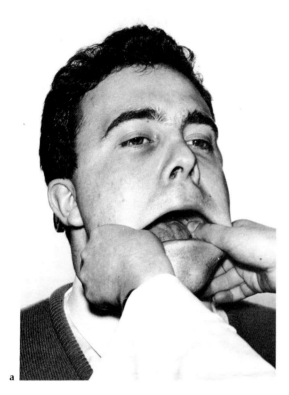

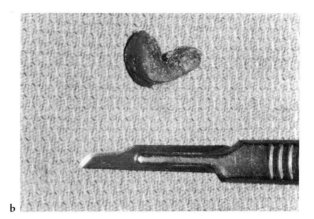

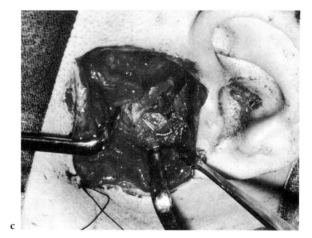

Fig. 9.9 (a) *Reduction of dislocation of the jaw.* (b) *Recurrent dislocation: iliac crest bone graft shaped for grafting to glenoid eminence;* (c) *graft wired into place anterior to left TMJ.*

Diagnosis

Clinically the jaw is locked open and protruded and the condyles can be palpated anterior to the glenoid fossae.

An orthopantomogram will confirm the abnormal condylar position(s).

Treatment

Reduction by gripping the angle of the mandible with the fingers extra-orally and the thumb on the retromolar pad intra-orally (Fig. 9.9a) is best achieved with the patient seated upright. The angle is forced down and back to take the condyle over the eminence into the glenoid fossa. Reduction is facilitated by giving a posterior superior alveolar local anaesthetic injection and also injecting local analgesic into the preauricular skin over the TMJ. Difficult cases may require sedation with intravenous benzodiazepines or general anaesthesia with muscle relaxation, before reduction is attempted.

Surgical correction of recurrent dislocation is used either to remove the eminence to facilitate reduction, or to create an obstruction to forward dislocation by placing a bone graft on the articular eminence (Fig. 9.9b,c); by tightening the capsule (plication); or by fracturing the zygomatic arch downward (Dautrey operation).

FRACTURES (see also Chapter 3)

Fractures of the mandibular condyle may be extracapsular or intracapsular. Extracapsular fractures may be undisplaced, displaced with separation or malposition at the fracture site, or dislocated with the articular head pulled out of the glenoid fossa. Intracapsular fractures cause comminution of the articular surface. Rarely, the condyle may be intruded upwards into the middle cranial fossa.

Diagnosis

Trauma to the front or side of the mandible may produce a unilateral condylar fracture such that the condyle is forced back or inwards. An oblique blow in the canine region may result in a fracture of the body of the mandible at the point of impact together with a fracture of the opposite condyle. A 'guardsman's' fracture is a midline mandibular fracture together with fractures of both condyles and results from trauma directly onto the point of the chin. On examination, the TMJ may be swollen and tender. Mouth opening is limited and uncomfortable. Sometimes there is bleeding from a skin tear anteriorly within the external auditory meatus. If blood collects on the tympanic membrane, hearing may be impaired on that side. If there is a bilateral fracture, the occlusion frequently alters and this shows as premature posterior contact with anterior open bite. Radiographs which show the neck of the condyle (orthopantomogram, reverse Townes, or transorbital views) will reveal appearances ranging from an undisplaced crack fracture of the condylar neck to a gross displacement out of the glenoid fossa (Fig. 9.10a and b).

Complications

The healing of an intracapsular fracture may be attended by unwanted ossification or fibrosis of the haematoma, which may lead to ankylosis of the TMJ (Fig. 9.10c and d). This is more likely to be seen in the child than the adult. In children, ankylosis restricts mandibular growth and, if unilateral, leads to asymmetry.

Treatment

A unilateral undisplaced or minimally displaced fracture is treated by soft diet and analgesics providing the occlusion is unaltered. Severe pain and occlusal alteration are indications for active treatment with a short period of intermaxillary fixation. Bilateral fractures are best treated similarly, to avoid a permanent occlusal discrepancy. When there is gross displacement of the condyle, open reduction and fixation with wires (Kirschner wires, Fig. 9.10d and e) or mini-bone plates may be necessary.

PROLONGED RESTRICTED MOUTH OPENING

Ankylosis

Ankylosis of the TMJ is most frequently due to trauma or infection (or both). The ankylosis may be unilateral or

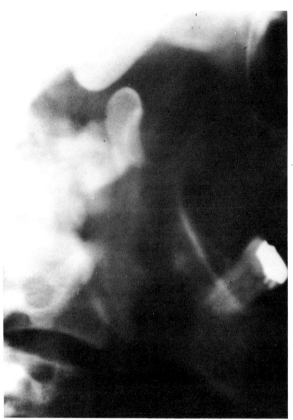

a

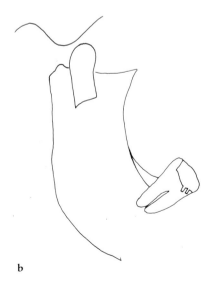

b

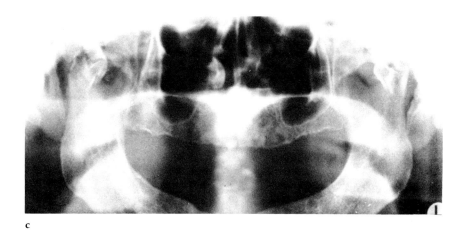

c

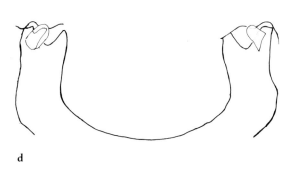

d

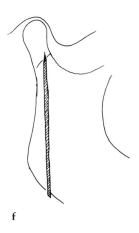

f

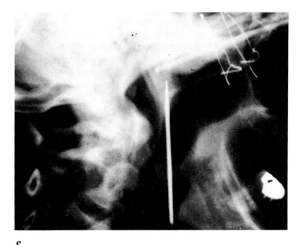

e

Fig. 9.10 (a) *Unilateral fracture dislocation of the TMJ.* (b) *Tracing to show abnormal condyle position.* (c) *Bilateral fracture dislocation of the TMJ with ankylosis.* (d) *Tracing to show abnormal positions of condyles.* (e) *Open reduction and fixation with Kirschner wire of the fracture shown in* (a). (f) *Tracing to show position of Kirschner wire.*

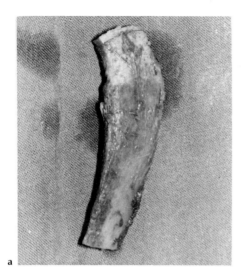

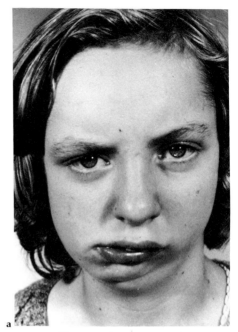

a

Fig. 9.12 See caption opposite.

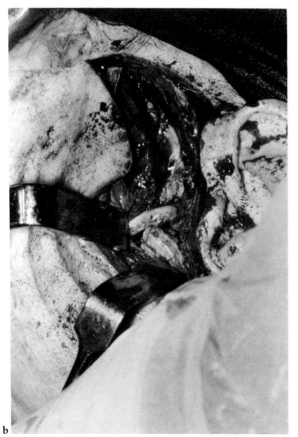

b

Fig. 9.11 Reconstruction of the TMJ with a costochondral rib graft. (a) Graft. (b) Chondral end in position against glenoid fossa, left TMJ.

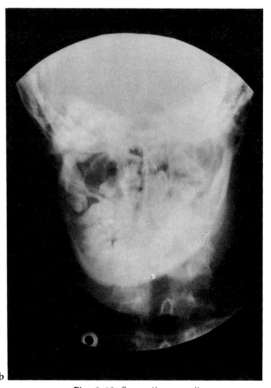

b

Fig. 9.12 See caption opposite.

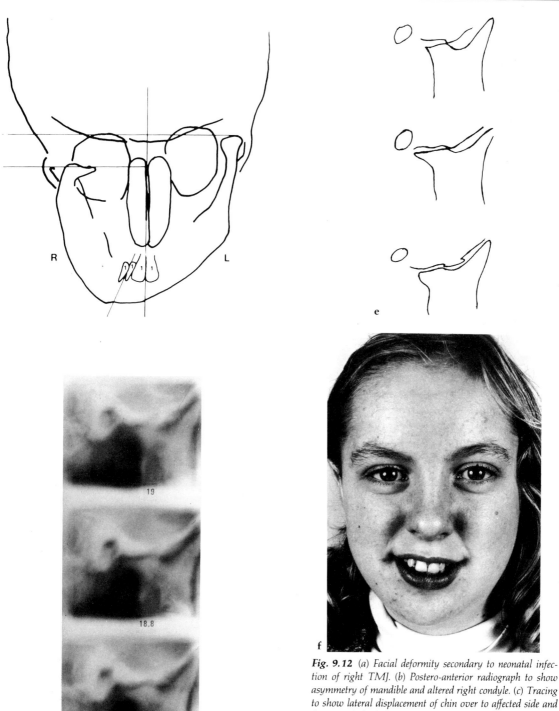

Fig. 9.12 (a) Facial deformity secondary to neonatal infection of right TMJ. (b) Postero-anterior radiograph to show asymmetry of mandible and altered right condyle. (c) Tracing to show lateral displacement of chin over to affected side and downward displacement of TMJ. (d) Sagittal tomogram of right TMJ. (e) Tracing shows deformed TMJ. (f) Improved appearance after mandibular osteotomy, bone graft and genioplasty.

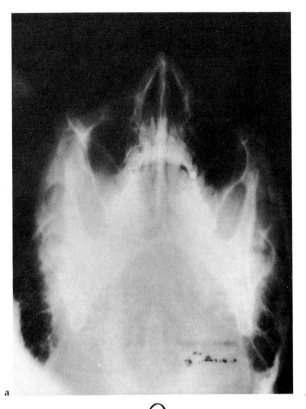

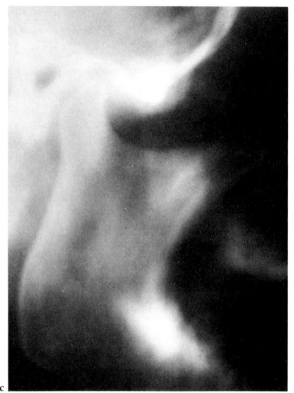

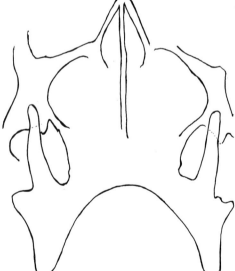

Fig. 9.13 (a) Bilateral coronoid hyperplasia seen on occipito-mental radiograph. (b) Tracing shows enlarged coronoid processes. (c) Sagittal tomogram of right coronoid process impinging on back of maxilla during attempted mouth opening. (d) Tracing of coronoid impinging on maxilla.

bilateral; intracapsular or extracapsular' (or both); and fibrous or bony (or both). In severe bony ankylosis, the ramus of the mandible may have fused to the temporal bone. Restricted mouth opening causes problems with oral hygiene and routine dental care. If unilateral, there can be asymmetry of the mandible which causes facial deformity.

Treatment involves first releasing the ankylosis and either creating a gap large enough to discourage further ankylosis or reconstructing the condyle with a costo-chondral rib graft (Fig. 9.11) or a prosthesis. Further orthognathic surgery may be required to correct the secondary deformity (Fig. 9.12).

Coronoid hyperplasia

Hyperplasia of the coronoid (Fig. 9.13) is usually but not always bilateral. There is restricted mouth opening. Radiographs such as occipitomentals and sagittal tomographs will reveal the cause. This is usually treated by intra-oral coronoidectomy. An osteochondroma of the coronoid may require both intra-oral and extra-oral access for its removal (Fig. 9.14).

Scar formation

Patients treated for oral cancer by a full course of radiotherapy involving the masticatory muscles can develop a troublesome fibrosis which gradually restricts mouth opening, and can cause considerable prosthetic problems if an obturator is to be worn. Further surgery is often hazardous because of the vascular disturbance caused by the radiotherapy which may adversely affect healing.

Other conditions

Two other conditions which progressively limit mouth opening and do not directly involve the TMJ are oral submucous fibrosis (Chapter 22) and myositis ossificans (ossification in a muscle usually after trauma).

INFECTIVE ARTHRITIS

Infective arthritis of the TMJ is uncommon. Most cases are caused by *Staphylococcus aureus* but streptococci, gonococci, *Haemophilus influenzae*, *Escherichia coli*, *Candida albicans* and actinomyces have all been reported as causes of septic TMJ arthritis. The usual route of spread is via the blood, but a penetrating injury may cause intra-articular infection. A reduced general resistance may be a predisposing factor.

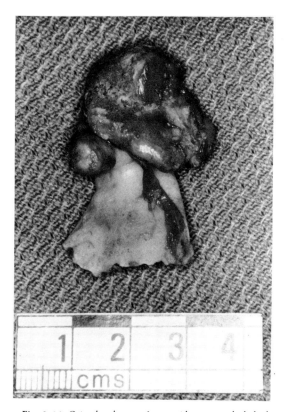

Fig. 9.14 *Osteochondroma of coronoid process which had hooked over the zygomatic arch causing total restriction of mouth opening.*

Septic arthritis in a child may lead to ankylosis and subsequent facial deformity.

CONDYLAR HYPERPLASIA

This condition is usually unilateral. There are two varieties.

1. An enlarged elongated condyle which has a relatively normal shape, with displacement of the chin towards the opposite side.

2. An enlarged distorted condyle with downward bowing of the lower border of the mandible on that side, sometimes with separation of upper and lower posterior teeth. The midline of the mandible is relatively central.

Once condylar hyperplasia has been diagnosed, follow-up over a period of time is necessary to see whether the hyperplasia has ceased to progress, especially if it is decided to avoid condylectomy and merely recorrect a distorted occlusion.

It is important to distinguish this condition from a secondary elongation of the condyle following unilateral tooth loss in childhood, which leads to adoption of a bite of accommodation that is slightly asymmetrical.

NEOPLASMS

The most common malignant involvement of the TMJ is by direct spread from a primary tumour in adjacent tissue such as the parotid gland.

TMJ primary neoplasms are uncommon. Benign lesions include osteoma and chondroma of the condylar head; giant-cell granulomas have also been reported. Malignant lesions include rhabdomyosarcoma, osteogenic sarcoma, multiple myeloma and metastatic deposits from a primary lesion elsewhere (see also Chapter 7).

TRISMUS

Limited opening of the jaw may have several causes, including the following (Fig. 9.15).

1. Extra-articular causes.
   Infection and inflammation near to, and causing spasm of, the masticatory muscles (e.g. pericoronitis).

Mandibular pain dysfunction syndrome.
Fractured condyle.
Fibrosis (caused by burns, radiotherapy, systemic sclerosis or submucous fibrosis).
Tetanus.
Tetany.
Invading neoplasms.
Myositis ossificans.
Coronoid hypertrophy.
Hysteria.
2. Intra-articular causes.
   Dislocation.
   Fracture.
   Arthritides.
   Ankylosis.

In contrast, some drugs such as metoclopramide and phenothiazines may cause facial muscle spasm inhibiting the patient from *closing* his mouth.

SURGICAL APPROACHES TO THE TMJ

The most frequently used surgical approach to the TMJ is via a preauricular incision (see Fig. 9.5a and b), the upper part of which lies within the hair line and is subsequently hidden from view when the hair regrows, the lower part lying in a fine crease just anterior to the tragal cartilage. Dissection here is in a relatively avascular plane, with the parotid gland and facial nerve anterior to this plane,

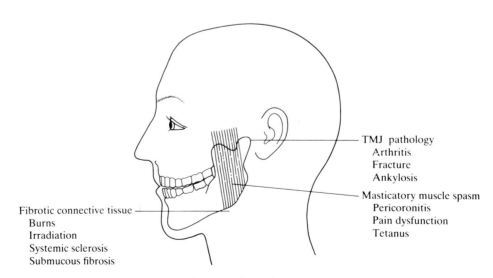

TMJ pathology
Arthritis
Fracture
Ankylosis

Masticatory muscle spasm
Pericoronitis
Pain dysfunction
Tetanus

Fibrotic connective tissue
Burns
Irradiation
Systemic sclerosis
Submucous fibrosis

Fig. 9.15 *Causes of trismus.*

providing the incision is not continued too far inferiorly. As the skin is reflected, the temporal fascia is followed as a guide down to the lateral capsule of the joint. The temporal fascia is in two layers at this level and the deeper layer is followed inferiorly. The capsule is then opened and the meniscus and upper and lower joint cavities identified as necessary.

Wider access for release of ankylosis is gained by extending the preauricular approach coronally across the scalp and also inferiorly as a submandibular approach to the ramus over the mandible. The incision crosses the facial nerve below the lobe of the ear and must therefore be kept very superficial.

Some surgeons take the lower part of the preauricular approach inside the auditory meatus (endaural approach), whilst others use a postauricular approach and turn the whole ear lobe forwards with their flap. Limited access to the condylar neck can be gained via an intra-oral wisdom tooth incision extended up the external oblique ridge of the mandible.

FURTHER READING

Clarke N. G. (1982). Occlusion and myofascial pain dysfunction: is there a relationship? *J. Am. Dent. Assoc.,* **104**: 443–446.

Helms C., Katzberg R. W., Morrish R., Dolwick M. F. (1983). Computed tomography of the temporomandibular joint meniscus. *Br. J. oral and maxillofac. Surg.,* **41**: 512–517.

Juniper R. J. (1984). Temporomandibular joint dysfunction: a theory based upon electromyographic studies of the lateral pterygoid muscle. *Br. J. oral and maxillofac. Surg.,* **22**: 1–8.

Leopard P. J. (1984). Anterior dislocation of the temporomandibular disc. *Br. J. oral and maxillofac. Surg.,* **22**: 9–17.

Norman J. E. de B. (1982). Post-traumatic disorders of the jaw joint. *Ann. Roy. Coll. Surg. (Engl.),* **64**: 29–36.

Speculand B., Goss A. N. (1985). Psychological factors in temporomandibular joint dysfunction pain: a review. *Int. J. oral surg.,* **14**: 131–137.

Speculand B., Goss A. N., Hughes A., Spence N. D., Pilowski I. (1983). Temporomandibular joint dysfunction: pain and illness behaviour. *Pain,* **17**: 139–150.

Zarb G. A., Carlsson G. E. (Eds.) (1979). *Temporomandibular joint: function and dysfunction.* Copenhagen: Munksgaard.

Diseases of the maxillary antrum

DEVELOPMENT OF THE MAXILLARY ANTRUM (SINUS)

The maxillary antrum is the first paranasal air sinus to develop, appearing at 3–4 months *in utero* as an out-pouching of the mucous membrane of the middle meatus of the nose. At birth the sinus is approximately 11 mm long, 4 mm high and 3 mm wide. By 12 years the antral floor is about level with the nasal floor. Normal adult size is reached at around 18 years of age, when the average volume is 15–30 ml and it measures approximately 3.5 cm in height by 3 cm long by 2.5 cm wide. The antral floor is then about 1 cm *below* the level of the floor of the nose.

APPLIED ANATOMY

The maxillary antrum is the largest paranasal air sinus. The antra are cavities in the body of each half of the maxilla (Fig. 10.1), each shaped like a pyramid lying on its side with the base medially forming the lateral wall of the nose and the apex laterally extending into the zygomatic part of the maxilla (and sometimes into the zygoma). The four walls of this pyramid form the floor

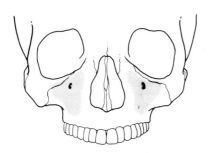

Fig. 10.1 *Size and position of maxillary antra.*

of the orbit, the alveolar process of the maxilla, the anterior surface of the maxilla, and the infratemporal surface of the maxilla.

The antral mucosa secretes a small amount of mucus which drains through a small ostium (3–4 mm diameter) formed by the uncinate process of the ethmoid and descending part of the lacrimal bone above, the palatine bone behind and the maxillary process of the inferior nasal concha below. The maxillary antrum therefore drains into the posterior middle meatus of the nose.

The posterior wall of the maxilla is pierced by several posterior superior alveolar nerves which supply the upper molar teeth. The infraorbital nerve, which supplies the cheek, runs in a ridge in the roof of the antrum.

The antral floor is close to the apices of the maxillary posterior teeth (Fig. 10.2). If the antrum is exceptionally large, all teeth posterior to the canine may be closely related, but usually the canine is unrelated to the sinus. The tooth most intimately related to the antrum is the second molar, followed by the first molar, the third molar, second premolar and first premolar. Sometimes the bony antral floor is perforated by the apices of those teeth which are therefore intimately related to the antral lining. Inflammation of the antral lining (sinusitis) can easily simulate toothache in these maxillary teeth, but the pain of sinusitis is usually persistent, worse on lying down or moving the head and associated with other features of sinusitis (p. 112).

Involvement of the antra during exodontia (see also p. 114)

As the sinus enlarges with growth, it approaches closer to the teeth and the risk of creating an oro-antral fistula when removing upper teeth, or of displacing teeth or roots into the antrum, is therefore much greater than in children. Roots of any maxillary premolar or molar tooth may be displaced into the antrum, but the complete tooth

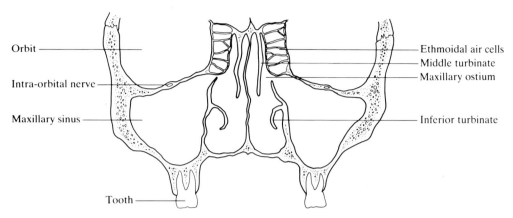

Fig. 10.2 *Coronal section of antra.*

most commonly displaced into the antrum is the unerupted upper third molar. On the other hand, small oro-antral fistulas (see p. 114) occur most frequently with extraction of the first or second molar.

A large antrum also inevitably has a thin wall and part, especially the tuberosity region, may fracture when extracting teeth. In practice this is not uncommon and the maxillary fragment may carry several teeth on it.

Maxillary sinusitis (see also p. 112)

Most sinusitis follows a viral upper respiratory tract infection, but periapical infection of a maxillary tooth may, because of the proximity of its apices to the antrum, also cause maxillary sinusitis. Once sinusitis has been established and the antrum is full of mucus and pus, drainage is difficult because, in the adult, the maxillary ostium is high on its medial wall and often above the fluid level. Attempts to assist drainage surgically by creating a fistula between the sinus and nose (intranasal antrostomy) may not be successful as the floor of the sinus is usually lower than the floor of the nose.

Malignant disease (see also p. 120)

The thin bony wall of the antrum does not easily resist the spread of a malignant neoplasm. Carcinoma of the maxillary sinus can spread in all directions: downwards into the mouth; upwards into the orbit; medially into the nose; and anteriorly into the cheek. Involvement of other structures may alert the clinician to the presence of a tumour. For instance, paraesthesia of the infra-orbital nerve may indicate that a tumour is invading the roof of

the antrum, whereas looseness of, and pain in, the maxillary teeth may point to an antral floor tumour.

INVESTIGATIONS

The most commonly used technique for imaging of the antrum is radiography, including CT scanning (Volume 1).

Conventional radiography of the antrum

Occipitomental radiography (Figs. 10.3 and 10.4)

The best radiographs for viewing the antra are occipitomental (Waters) views of the skull, which can be taken at

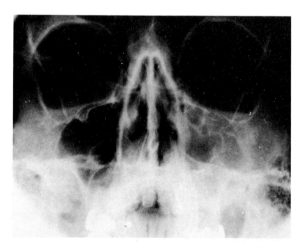

Fig. 10.3 *An opaque antrum in a patient with maxillary sinusitis.*

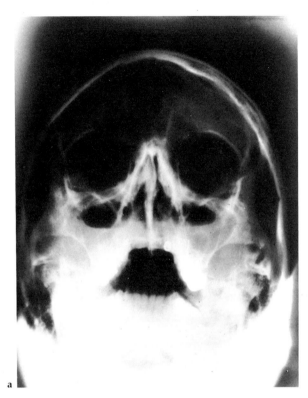

a

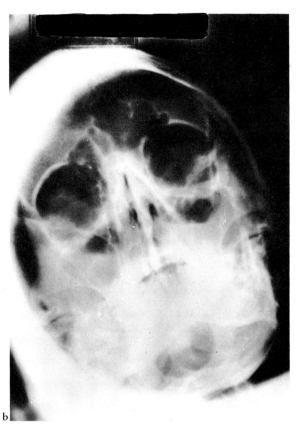

b

Fig. 10.4 (a) and (b) Bilateral maxillary sinusitis: the fluid levels are shown well by occipitomental views with the head tilted to one side. (Courtesy of Professor C. Scully.)

15° and 30°. On these radiographs an opaque antrum or a fluid level or fractures can easily be detected. Tilting the head to one side for a subsequent view may help to distinguish a fluid level—the upper surface of which remains horizontal—from a more solid lesion.

Lateral skull radiography (Fig. 10.5)

A lateral skull view is more useful than the Waters view for detecting teeth or roots lost in the antrum or beneath the antral mucosa.

Intra-oral radiography (periapical) (Fig. 10.6)

This may be helpful for showing teeth or roots in the antrum.

Panoramic radiography (Fig. 10.7)

Another useful radiograph of the antrum is the orthopantomogram although, being a tomogram, it may not always give an undistorted view. It can be most useful for detecting cysts which are well circumscribed and more radiolucent than the normal antrum. Since the contralateral antrum is also seen on this radiograph, comparison with the normal side is easy.

Upper occlusal radiography (Fig. 10.8)

An upper occlusal view is useful for detecting cysts.

Other radiographic views may fail to show cysts, and diagnosis of a cyst can be very difficult if the antrum is large with out-pouchings into the alveolar process and zygomatic bone, since these antral extensions may resemble cysts.

Tomography (Fig. 10.9)

Coronal tomography of the antrum can be useful for showing the extent of a neoplasm, particularly in the posterior and superior part of the maxilla.

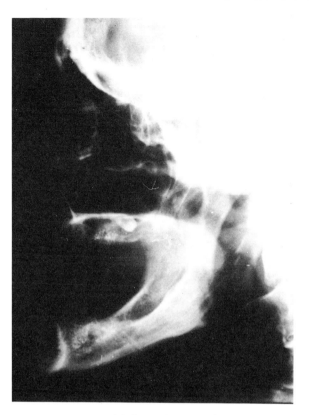

Fig. 10.5 Lateral skull view showing tooth in antrum.

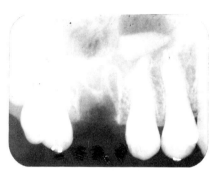

Fig. 10.6 Periapical radiograph of a root in the antrum. (Courtesy of Professor C. Scully.)

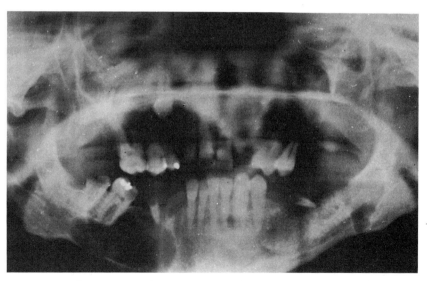

Fig. 10.7 Orthopantomogram showing cysts in each half of the maxilla and both sides of the mandible.

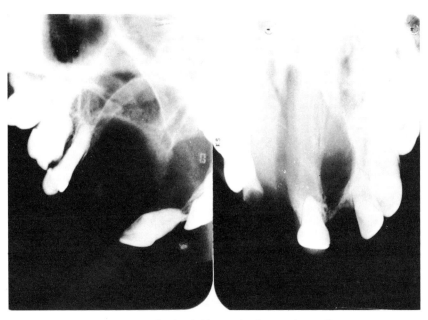

Fig. 10.8 *Upper occlusal and oblique occlusal views of a maxillary cyst.*

Computerized tomography (Fig. 10.10)

The CT scan is useful particularly in detecting the extent of spread of a malignant neoplasm of the antrum. It has the great advantage of demonstrating the posterior maxilla, the infratemporal fossa, the floor of the orbit and the nasoethmoidal sinuses—sites not readily seen with other techniques.

Other techniques

The antrum may also be examined crudely for fluid levels or tumour by transillumination. Fibre-optic endoscopy is also proving useful.

INFECTION (MAXILLARY SINUSITIS)

Acute sinusitis

Most acute sinusitis is secondary to an acute viral infection of the upper respiratory tract such as the common cold or influenza. It is caused by bacterial superinfection of the antrum. A minority of cases of sinusitis (perhaps less than 1 in 10) follow an acute periapical infection of a tooth or displacement of a tooth root into the antrum. More rarely, sinusitis may follow the introduction of foreign bodies into the antrum or result from infected water being forced retrogradely through the maxillary ostium into the sinus when diving into water.

Local factors may predispose to sinusitis, e.g. a deviated nasal septum may cause poor sinus drainage. General factors such as immune defects predispose to recurrent sinusitis.

Sinusitis is often a mixed infection with staphylococci, streptococci, and anaerobes.

Clinical features

The patient often has had an upper respiratory tract infection with an obstructed nose and a mucopurulent nasal discharge. Pain is usually experienced in the cheek and often in the upper posterior teeth. This pain is frequently aggravated by running, walking or stooping. Supra-orbital pain is sometimes also experienced if there is infection of the frontal sinus.

Diagnosis

On examination the patient may be pyrexic, the cheek may be tender to palpate, and a mucopurulent discharge may be seen beneath the middle turbinate bone on nasal

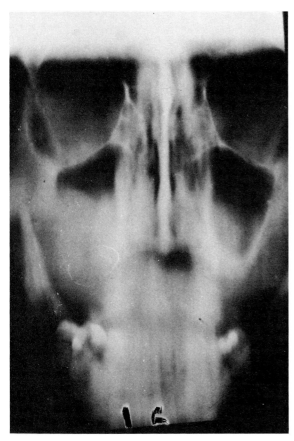

Fig. 10.9 *Coronal tomography showing a neoplasm destroying the lateral wall of the right antrum.*

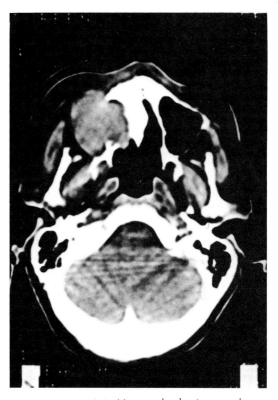

Fig. 10.10 *Computerized tomography showing a neoplasm filling the left antrum and destroying the anterior wall.*

examination. An occipitomental radiograph will often show antral opacity and sometimes a fluid level. Tilting the head laterally and taking a second film can show a fluid level since the surface of the fluid will remain horizontal but change position relative to other features (see Figs. 10.3 and 10.4).

Management

Infection should be treated by helping drainage of the antrum using nasal decongestion drops and inhalations, and with antibiotics.

Ephedrine 0.5% or 1% nasal drops or xylometazoline hydrochloride 0.1% nasal drops are the nose-drops of choice. Menthol and benzoin inhalation BP or menthol and eucalyptus inhalation BP are useful. Erythromycin or co-trimoxazole are the antibiotics of choice. Analgesics and bedrest may also be required.

Complications

Chronic sinusitis may develop. Otitis media, pneumonia and frontal sinusitis are less common complications.

Chronic sinusitis

Chronic sinusitis usually follows acute maxillary sinusitis which has failed to resolve. Factors which predispose to the development of chronic sinusitis include inadequate treatment of acute sinusitis, poor sinus drainage (for example a deviated nasal septum) and reduced host resistance.

In chronic sinusitis there is a mixed bacterial flora. The antral and nasal mucosal linings undergo hypertrophy and sometimes form polyps.

Clinical features

A patient with chronic sinusitis usually has some nasal obstruction, a post-nasal discharge (post-nasal drip) which can be seen as pus escaping behind the soft palate, a husky voice and sometimes halitosis or a bad taste, particularly if there is a foreign body in the sinus, e.g. a tooth or root.

Diagnosis

On examination there is a mucopurulent discharge in the infected side of the nose. An occipitomental radiograph may reveal one or both antra to be opaque or have thickened lining mucosa.

Management

There are three forms of treatment commonly used for chronic sinusitis.

1. *Antral washout.* The nasal mucosa is anaesthetized (with cocaine paste), a trocar and cannula are inserted into the maxillary antrum beneath the inferior turbinate, and the antrum irrigated with sterile saline. The washings are bacteriologically cultured and, if indicated, an appropriate antibiotic such as erythromycin is instilled into the antrum at a subsequent washout. If the infection does not resolve after several washouts, intranasal antrostomy is performed.

2. *Intranasal antrostomy.* A substantial opening is made into the antrum beneath the inferior turbinate, under general anaesthesia. After a few days the antrum is washed out and, if the infection does not resolve after daily washouts, the next stage is to proceed to the Caldwell–Luc operation.

3. *Caldwell–Luc operation.* Otherwise known as a radical antrostomy, the Caldwell–Luc operation consists of an approach to the antrum from the mouth (Fig. 10.11).

An incision is made in the mucoperiosteum of the canine fossa which is just behind the apex of the upper canine tooth. A window is made into the antrum using a chisel and then Hajèk's up-cutting or down-cutting forceps. Any tooth or root displaced into the antrum can usually be identified with a fibre-optic light and removed with forceps or sucker. In the case of chronic sinusitis, the antral lining and any polyps are removed. The wound is closed with interrupted sutures and an intranasal antrostomy performed if this has not already been done.

Rarely, chronic sinusitis is a consequence of an immune defect.

Other antral infections

Candidosis, mucormycosis and other fungal infections occasionally affect the antra—usually in immunosuppressed patients.

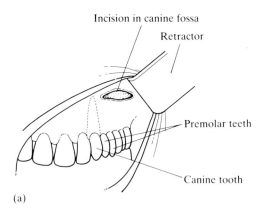

(a)

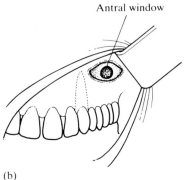

(b)

Fig. 10.11 *Caldwell–Luc operation.*

ORO-ANTRAL FISTULA

A fistula is a non-anatomical epithelial-lined tract joining two epithelial surfaces. In this instance the fistula is between the mouth (lined with squamous epithelium) and the maxillary antrum (lined with a ciliated columnar epithelium with mucous glands—respiratory epithelium).

An oro-antral fistula is most often caused by the extraction of maxillary teeth, especially the molars or premolars which are closely related to the antrum. However, facial trauma, neoplasms, osteomyelitis of the maxilla, and surgery to the maxilla may all occasionally lead to fistula formation. Major fistulae tend to occur if the maxillary tuberosity is fractured, particularly if several teeth are attached. However, such a major fistula, if sutured immediately, usually heals. Persistent oro-antral fistulae tend to occur when a molar tooth root is accidentally displaced into the maxillary sinus or when a molar tooth is extracted and a fistula created. One situation that is especially prone to fistula formation is the extraction of a single standing maxillary molar or premolar whose roots are surrounded both posteriorly and anteriorly by the maxillary antrum. The wise practitioner will, before extracting such teeth, take special note of previous fistulae that may have occurred, perhaps in a similar position on the other side.

Clinical features

Signs and symptoms from an oro-antral fistula may occur immediately after the extraction of a tooth or may take some weeks to develop.

The most common symptom is reflux of fluid from the mouth into the nose when the patient drinks; fluid then dribbles from the nose. In the early postextraction period there may be ipsilateral nose bleed (epistaxis) and, a little later, as sinusitis develops, an unpleasant ipsilateral nasal discharge, bad taste and halitosis.

Diagnosis

An obvious oro-antral fistula may be easily apparent, but often a small hole cannot be seen. A good way of testing for an established fistula is to ask the patient to squeeze his nose and then to attempt to blow it. This will force bubbles of air into his mouth through the fistula. Failing this, gentle probing with a blunt probe (e.g. a lacrimal duct dilator) will reveal the fistula. However, if it is suspected that a fistula has been newly created, it is best to assume its presence and conduct a repair without such testing. Sometimes a red 'lump' is noticed in the region of an oro-antral fistula. This 'lump' is prolapsed mucosa of the maxillary sinus (Fig. 10.12) or occasionally it may be a prolapsed antral polyp or mucosal cyst. A blunt probe will push back the prolapsed tissue and reveal an obvious fistula.

Symptoms of acute sinusitis may develop later but, in approximately one-quarter of patients who develop a fistula, there are no symptoms. This is usually because the fistula is so small that it is closed off by surrounding mucosa, particularly if it is in the buccal sulcus where the cheek may lie against it. Sometimes a fairly large fistula may be temporarily closed by a prolapse of the antral mucosa.

Management

The type of treatment indicated depends on the rapidity with which the diagnosis has been established.

1. *Treatment if the diagnosis has been made as soon as the fistula has been created.* Assuming that a tooth or tooth root has not been displaced into the antrum, the

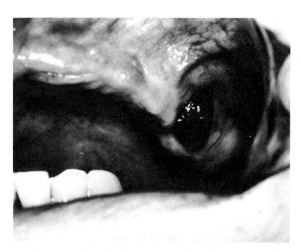

Fig. 10.12 *Antral prolapse: this is the prolapse of antral mucosa through an oro-antral fistula.*

immediate treatment is to close the tooth socket. For the experienced practitioner, the procedure is to raise and advance a buccal flap over the fistula (see below). The less experienced practitioner should simply suture the socket.

The patient should then be given prophylactic treatment against maxillary sinusitis since this would otherwise delay healing of the fistula. The patient should *not* blow his nose. Treatment includes antibiotics such as erythromycin or co-trimoxazole, nose-drops (ephedrine 0.5% or xylometazoline hydrochloride 0.1%) and inhalations (such as menthol and benzoin inhalation BP or menthol and eucalyptus inhalation BP—*see* sinusitis). Even up to 48 hours after the tooth extraction, an oro-antral fistula can be repaired by advancement of a buccal flap, but prophylactic antibiotics are indicated.

2. *Treatment if the diagnosis has been delayed more than 2 days.* If the patient is not seen until 2 or more days after fistula creation, it is unwise to attempt immediate repair because the tissues will be in a poor state. It is better to adopt conservative measures (unless the fistula is very large), since the fistula will often close spontaneously. Conservative treatment includes prophylactic antibiotics, instructing the patient not to blow his nose, and sometimes the construction of a simple acrylic plate to cover the fistula and be worn constantly for a few weeks.

If the fistula does not close spontaneously with these measures within 6 weeks, a definitive repair should be undertaken. A large fistula which is obviously never going to close spontaneously should be repaired after only 4 weeks of conservative treatment.

Surgical repair of a fistula

Maxillary sinusitis should be treated preoperatively so that postoperative healing is not impaired. A prophylactic regimen as previously mentioned should be given and, if the fistula is quite large, the patient should be given a syringe to irrigate the antrum preoperatively.

Several techniques of repair are available.

Buccal flap

Single-layer closure

Figure 10.13 illustrates this simple technique which consists of advancing a buccal flap under local or general

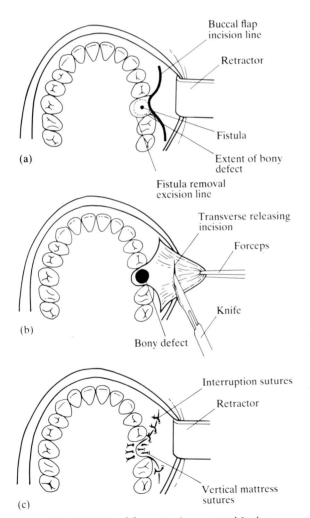

(a)

Buccal flap incision line

Retractor

Fistula

Extent of bony defect

Fistula removal excision line

Transverse releasing incision

Forceps

(b)

Knife

Bony defect

Interruption sutures

Retractor

(c)

Vertical mattress sutures

Fig. 10.13 *Buccal flap repair of an oro-antral fistula.*

anaesthesia. If, when the flap is raised, it does not easily stretch across the defect, the dense periosteum on the underside of the mucoperiosteal flap must be incised transversely to allow it to advance. The fistulous tract is excised since otherwise the wound could not be sutured over bone and would inevitably break down. The bony defect is inevitably larger than the fistula appears before operation. The buccal flap must be broad-based to ensure an adequate blood supply, and should be closed with vertical mattress sutures where possible. Sutures should be removed only after 10 days. The disadvantages of this technique are that:

(a) single-layer closure is more prone to break down than two-layer closure;

(b) where the fistula occurs between neighbouring teeth there may be insufficient bone around the fistula adjacent to the remaining teeth; this means that the repair may break down unless one or more of the neighbouring teeth are extracted, which may be necessary if surgery has failed previously;

(c) the depth of the buccal sulcus is reduced.

Two-layer closure (Fig. 10.14)

An incision is made around the fistulous tract but the mucosa is elevated, turned towards the centre and sutured together over the fistula with catgut sutures rather than excised. In practice this is not a very tidy procedure but it does close the fistula. A buccal flap is then advanced right over this primary closure and sutured with vertical mattress sutures. This technique gives a closure less likely to break down than the single-layer method, but still reduces the depth of the buccal sulcus.

Palatal flap

This technique, which does not interfere with the depth of the buccal sulcus, is rarely required. It should be carried out (as shown in Fig. 10.15) under a general anaesthetic. The exposed bone in the palate will slowly granulate and heal.

TOOTH OR ROOT DISPLACED INTO THE ANTRUM

The displacement of a tooth or tooth root into the antrum is fairly common and, of course, is usually associated with an oro-antral fistula. Sometimes the object is simply pushed beneath the antral lining. Whole

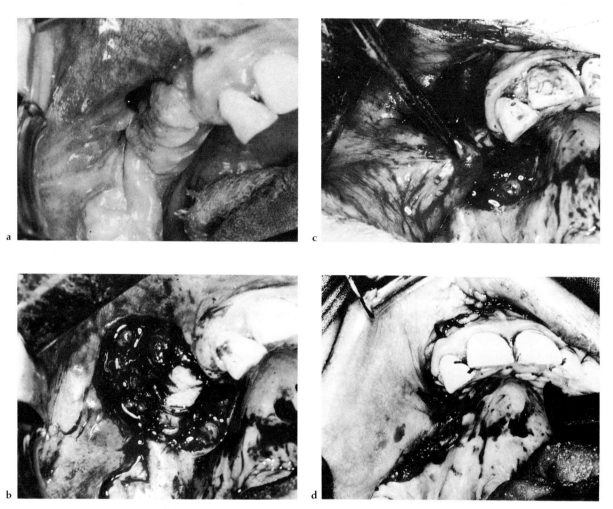

Fig. 10.14 (a) Oro-antral fistula before repair. (b) Mucosa around fistula elevated, turned towards centre and sutured. This is the first layer of closure. (c) A buccal flap is raised and advanced over the first layer. (d) The buccal flap is sutured. This is the second layer of closure.

teeth are rarely displaced into the antrum—rather, it is usually a tooth root. The diagnosis is usually straightforward, since the dentist should have seen the root disappear into the antrum when an extraction was being attempted. If the tooth fragment is small and the operator is uncertain whether the fragment has gone into the sinus or has been sucked up the sucker, radiographs must be taken in at least two planes. A tooth root displaced under the antral lining may *appear* to be in the antrum, and only a variety of views will remove any doubt as to its location. A periapical view of the socket, an upper occlusal, a lateral occlusal and a lateral skull view may locate a tooth or root in the antrum (Figs. 10.6 and 10.16).

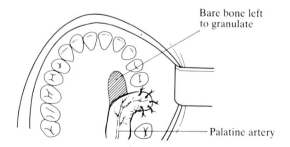

Fig. 10.15 Palatal flap repair of an oro-antral fissure.

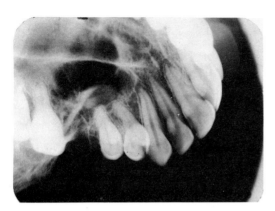

Fig. 10.16 *Root displaced into antrum. (Courtesy of Professor C. Scully.)*

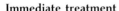

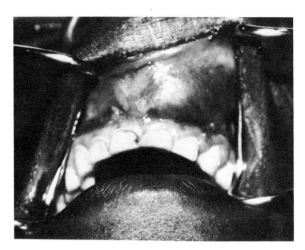

Fig. 10.17 *A maxillary cyst showing buccal expansion.*

Immediate treatment

Not infrequently, a small piece of root is pushed between an intact sinus lining and the bone. Using great care, it may be possible to find the root and extract it with forceps or a sucker. It is then wise to take post-operative radiographs to establish that the tooth root has gone and then suture the socket. If the root is definitely in the sinus itself, it may be worth attempting to suck it out blindly or even to flush it out with saline from a syringe, followed by repair of the fistula.

Later treatment

If the above procedures are unsuccessful, the patient should be referred to a specialist for closure of the fistula and removal of the root or tooth, which is carried out by a Caldwell–Luc approach (p. 114).

ANTRAL CYSTS AND BENIGN NEOPLASMS

The majority of antral cysts start not in the antrum itself but in relation to a tooth, and later encroach upon the antrum. These cysts do not usually penetrate the antral lining.

A cyst that does arise in the antrum itself is the benign mucosal cyst.

Odontogenic cysts

An odontogenic cyst may encroach upon the maxillary antrum (Chapter 5); fissural cysts rarely do so.

Periapical (radicular or dental) cysts are the most common cysts that encroach upon the antrum. Most arise from the upper lateral incisor and a large cyst may remain undetected for some time. The lateral incisor produces such cysts because the tooth is not uncommonly traumatized or carious, and the root of the lateral incisor is palatally placed so that the cysts tend to expand backwards into the antrum and remain undetected.

Cysts related to most other teeth reveal themselves as buccal expansions (Fig. 10.17).

Clinical features

Maxillary cysts present as body swellings, usually in the buccal sulcus. As the cyst expands and erodes the bone, it may be possible to indent it slightly on pressure (eggshell crackling) and, when bone is completely perforated, a fluctuant bluish swelling may appear. If the cyst is periapical, the associated tooth is usually non-vital. In the case of a dentigerous cyst or a keratocyst, there may be a tooth missing from the mouth which will be seen on radiograph to be buried.

Diagnosis

Maxillary cysts can be difficult to detect radiographically because they tend to overlie the antrum and are radiolucent. It is usually best to take several radiographs in at least two planes to determine the presence and size of a cyst overlying the antrum. Upper occlusal films, an orthopantomogram and periapical films are most useful. An occipitomental or lateral view may also be helpful.

Often a cyst is a round or curved area of radiolucency with a well-circumscribed radiopaque margin. The clarity of a cyst on a radiograph may, however, be reduced if there is bone destruction or infection.

The following points should be considered when trying to distinguish a maxillary cyst from the antrum.

1. An occlusal film is particularly helpful for diagnosing the relatively common periapical cyst on a lateral incisor tooth. A radiolucent area will be detected on one side of the palate related to the lateral incisor, with loss of the lamina dura around this tooth.

2. A cyst is a uniformly dark area whereas the normal antrum has bony markings caused by cancellous bone and neurovascular channels overlying the radiolucent area.

3. An orthopantomograph often clearly shows a well-circumscribed cyst related to the posterior teeth.

4. The margins of the antrum are thin and well defined but irregular, while the margins of a cyst are curved and regular on periapical films.

5. A benign mucosal cyst is a well-defined, dome-shaped, uniformly opaque lesion.

When there still remains doubt as to the presence of a cyst it is sometimes worth undertaking needle aspiration biopsy. Under local analgesic, a large needle is inserted into the lesion and, if liquid is aspirated, a cyst is likely (Chapter 5).

Management

Maxillary cysts should be treated, even if asymptomatic,

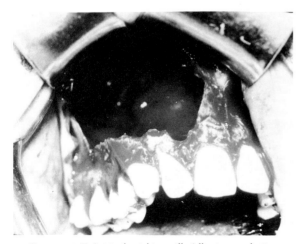

Fig. 10.18 *Defect in the right maxilla following enucleation of a dental cyst related to the lateral incisor.*

since otherwise they enlarge, may become infected and may lead to loosening of teeth. The treatment of choice is surgery under general anaesthesia, either enucleation of the cyst or marsupialization (Chapter 5).

Enucleation is the treatment of choice for most cysts (Fig. 10.18). If the lining of the antrum is punctured, as is likely when the cyst encroaches well into the antrum and particularly after infection, then the mucoperiosteum should be closed carefully to prevent the establishment of an oro-antral fistula. Prophylactic treatment against sinusitis should also be given.

Marsupialization (see Chapter 5) is particularly useful for a very large cyst which may not easily be removed surgically. In these days of safer general anaesthesia, only exceedingly unfit patients are unsuitable for such an anaesthetic and then marsupialization can be carried out as a relatively minor procedure under local analgesia.

Benign mucosal cyst

The aetiology of the benign mucosal cyst is not known, but it is generally considered that previous antral infection plays a role. The cyst is lined by ciliated columnar epithelium continuous with the antral lining. Occasionally cholesterol clefts occur in the wall. The prevalence of mucosal cysts is unclear, but perhaps they are present in up to 2% of patients who have sinus radiographs taken (Fig. 10.19).

Clinical features

The lesion is usually asymptomatic and is discovered on routine radiography as a dome-shaped shadow in an otherwise clear maxillary antrum. Occasionally, there may be vague symptoms such as 'heaviness' in the orbital or frontal region. The cysts may protrude into the nose or even the nasopharynx (antrochoanal polyp) and cause a post-nasal discharge, a blocked nose and frontal headache. It is not unknown for this cyst to prolapse through an oro-antral fistula.

Management

Treatment is rarely necessary, unless there are symptoms, when it is best to remove the cyst via a Caldwell–Luc approach.

BENIGN ANTRAL LESIONS

Benign tumours of the antrum are relatively rare.

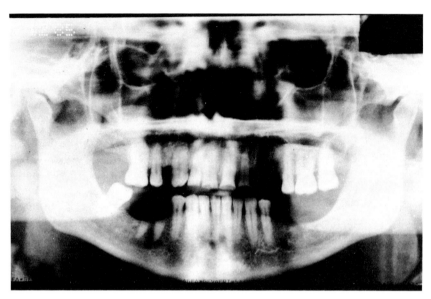

Fig. 10.19 *Mucosal cyst in right antrum.*

Osteomas

Osteomas are rare in the maxillary antrum. They are usually symptomless and detected on routine radiography. Osteomas may grow slowly and obstruct the maxillary ostium causing acute or chronic sinusitis. If large they may cause facial deformity. Surgical removal of the osteoma is required only if there are these complications.

Antrolith

This is not a tumour in the strict sense but results from calcific deposits on a foreign body in the antrum. The foreign body may be blood, pus, mucus, a root, tooth, bone fragment or items such as paper, matches, cotton wool etc. An antrolith may cause chronic sinusitis although often no symptoms are caused. Antroliths should be removed surgically.

Fibrous dysplasia (Fig. 10.20) (see also Chapter 8)

Fibrous dysplasia may encroach upon the maxillary sinus. Radiographs show a dense mass over the maxillary antrum, often with the typical 'ground glass' appearance (Chapter 8). Fibrous dysplasia is usually asymptomatic but may cause deformity.

Treatment is aimed at correcting the facial deformity surgically.

Odontogenic tumours (Fig. 10.21) (see also Chapter 6)

Any odontogenic tumour may encroach upon the maxillary antrum and should be treated in the same way as similar lesions elsewhere in the jaws.

MALIGNANT ANTRAL NEOPLASMS

A number of malignant tumours can involve the maxillary antrum but all are rare. They include the following.

1. Squamous cell carcinoma of the antrum—the most common malignant lesion. Approximately 80% of maxillary cancers are squamous cell carcinomas.
2. Other carcinomas, e.g. adenocarcinoma.
3. Lymphomas, including Burkitt's tumour.
4. Sarcomas, e.g. osteosarcoma and fibrosarcoma.
5. Salivary gland and other neoplasms arising in the palate. The maxillary antrum may, of course, be invaded by squamous carcinoma from the mouth.
6. Metastatic deposits from other carcinomas, e.g. breast or lung.

Squamous carcinoma of the antrum

The overall incidence of antral carcinoma is about 1 in 300 of all cancers. The aetiology is unclear but it is a common lesion in the Bantu tribe of South Africa where

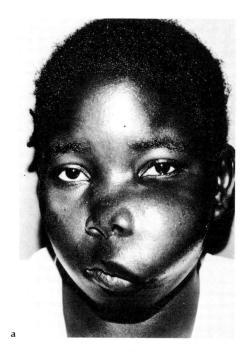

a

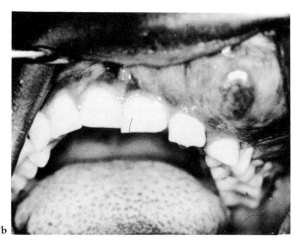

b

Fig. 10.20 (a) and (b) Fibrous dysplasia in the left maxilla.

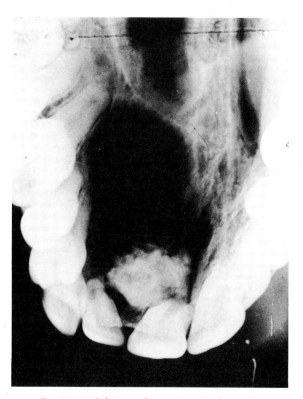

Fig. 10.21 Calcifying odontogenic cyst in the maxilla.

it may be related to the use of snuff (which contains known carcinogens). In the UK, one possible aetiological factor is exposure to wood dust, for example in woodworkers in the furniture industry.

Clinical features

Maxillary carcinoma may remain asymptomatic until it has reached quite a large size, invaded nerves and caused pain, invaded other tissues, or blocked the antral ostium. Often the first manifestations are pain in the cheek and a bloodstained discharge from the nose. Symptoms tend to vary according to the area invaded (Fig. 10.22). If the tumour invades the roof of the antrum, which of course is the floor of the orbit, involvement of the infra-orbital nerve may cause paraesthesia or anaesthesia of the cheek. Further upward growth may displace the eye forward causing proptosis, reduced eye movement and diplopia. Later on, direct invasion of the eye and the extra-ocular muscles may cause blindness and ophthalmoplegia.

Tumour invasion of the alveolus, teeth and periodontium may cause pain, root resorption and loosening of the teeth. Occasionally the blood supply to the teeth is damaged, resulting in a periapical abscess. If teeth from an invaded area are extracted, the tumour may proliferate through the tooth socket. An antral carcinoma may produce a swelling in the maxillary buccal sulcus or palate, and in the edentulous patient it may expand the alveolus. Such a patient may complain that the upper denture no longer fits properly. Examination may reveal

Carcinoma of maxillary antrum

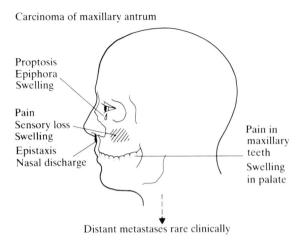

Fig. 10.22 Features of carcinoma of the antrum. (Courtesy of Professor C. Scully.)

expansion or ulceration of the palate, alveolus or buccal sulcus (Fig. 10.23).

If an antral carcinoma extends anteriorly or laterally, a swelling may appear on the cheek. The overlying skin is reddened before the tumour eventually breaks through onto the skin. Paraesthesia or anaesthesia of the infra-orbital nerve may occur.

Medial extension of the tumour to the nose may cause nasal obstruction, though mucopus or blood may escape from the nostril on the side affected. Examination of this nostril may reveal tumous proliferating inside the nose. The nasolacrimal duct may be obstructed, causing tears to run onto the face (epiphora).

Posterior extension of the tumour is uncommon but may involve the sphenopalatine ganglion and nerves in the infratemporal fossa, producing anaesthesia or paraesthesia of cheek or palate. The most common feature of posterior invasion, however, is trismus due to direct spread of the tumour into the pterygoid muscles (Chapter 9).

Diagnosis

Apart from the history, and examination of the antrum, mouth and cranial nerves, it is essential to palpate the neck for any enlarged lymph nodes suggesting metastases. Lymphatic spread from the maxillary antrum is to the retropharyngeal, submandibular and upper deep cervical lymph nodes. The latter two groups are easily palpated but the retropharyngeal nodes cannot, of course, be palpated.

Occipitomental radiographs, orthopantomograms and coronal tomograms of the antrum are all helpful and may show the bony destruction caused by a neoplasm (Figs. 10.9, 10.24 and 10.25). However, perhaps the most useful

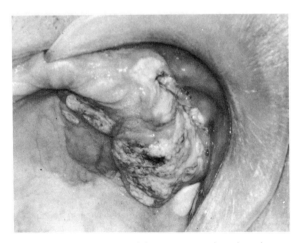

Fig. 10.23 Carcinoma of the antrum invading the palate and alveolus. (Courtesy of Professor C. Scully.)

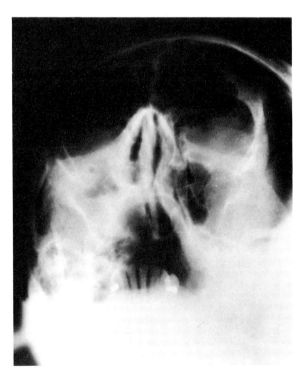

Fig. 10.24 Opacity of the right antrum that proved to be a carcinoma. (Courtesy of Professor C. Scully.)

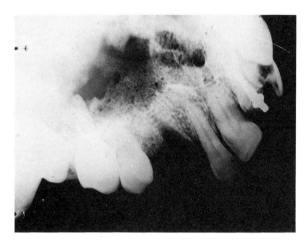

Fig. 10.25 *Squamous carcinoma arising from the antrum.*
(Courtesy of Professor C. Scully.)

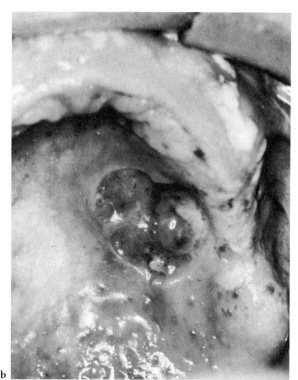

b

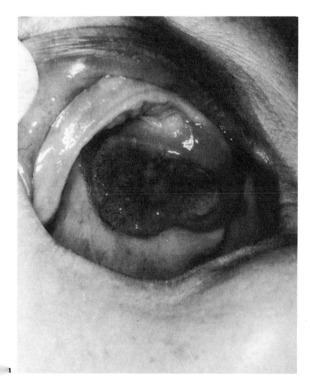

a

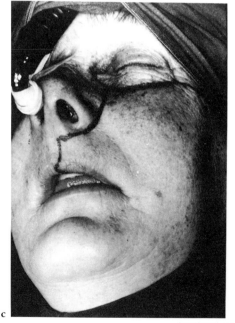

c

Fig. 10.26 *(a) Squamous cell carcinoma involving the left*
antrum. (b) The tumour following external beam radiotherapy
(teletherapy). (c) Weber–Fergusson incision line for left maxil-
lectomy. (d) Left maxillectomy. (e) A split skin graft is applied
to the maxillectomy cavity on a gutta percha bung or an
acrylic plate. (f) Skin sutured.

(continued overleaf)

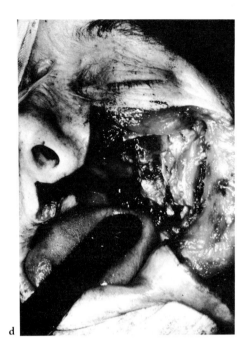

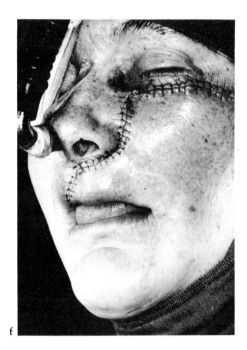

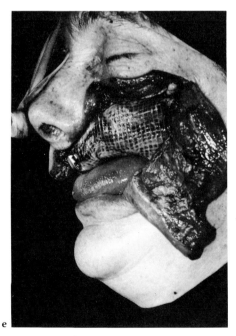

Fig. 10.26 (continued).

image is the CT scan which shows the extent of the lesion more clearly, particularly posteriorly and superiorly where conventional radiographs may not be so helpful (Fig. 10.10).

The only definitive evidence of carcinoma is, of course, a biopsy which can be performed readily if the tumour has infiltrated into the mouth. If, however, the tumour is confined to the antrum, it may be necessary to undertake a Caldwell–Luc approach to obtain a good specimen.

Staging

Attempts have been made to stage antral carcinoma so that treatment can be tailored to the degree of advancement of the tumour. It also helps the surgeon give a prognosis for the disease. The TNM classification has been used but is much more difficult to apply to antral than to oral carcinoma. The International Union against Cancer (UICC) has yet to produce a satisfactory classification of antral carcinoma.

Management (Fig. 10.26)

The best treatment for antral carcinomas is a combination of radiotherapy and surgery. A typical treatment plan is as follows.

1. Under a general anaesthetic, biopsy the lesion. Examine the patient's nose, nasopharynx, orbit and neck. Tattoo with Indian ink the periphery of the tumour, allowing a good margin of healthy tissue, e.g. 1–2 cm. Take multiple biopsies along this tattoo line to establish that the tattoo is well clear of tumour.

2. Administer a course of external beam radiotherapy, up to 60–65 Gray, which will shrink the tumour and make surgery easier.

3. Within 4–6 weeks, carry out a maxillectomy under a general anaesthetic. The limit of the surgical excision should follow the tattoo line. Line the maxillary cavity with split skin and obturate the hole in the palate (see Volume 3).

Prognosis

The prognosis varies according to the stage of the disease but is poor. The five-year survival rate for patients free of disease is of the order of 20%.

FURTHER READING

Ahmad K., Cordba R. B., Fayos J. V. (1981). Squamous cell carcinoma of the maxillary sinus. *Arch. Otolaryngol.,* **197**: 48–51.

Killey H. C., Kay L. W. (1975). *The maxillary sinus and its dental implications.* Bristol: Wright.

Powell J., Robin P. E. (1983). Cancer of the head and neck: the present state. In *Head and neck cancer* (Evans P. H. R. *et al.* eds.), pp. 3–16. New York: Alan R. Liss.

Section II
Diseases of the Oral Mucosa and Soft Tissues

Chapter
11
Development, structure and functions of oral mucosa

Oral development begins extremely early in life (on the 14th day of intra-uterine life) with the appearance of the prechordal plate in the bilaminar germ disc. The prechordal plate designates the cranial pole of the oval embryo germ disc, later to develop into the oropharyngeal membrane. The oropharyngeal membrane acts as the junction between the ectoderm that forms the epithelium of the mouth and the endoderm that forms the epithelium of the pharynx.

The connective tissue of the oral mucosa originates from the mesoderm.

ORAL MUCOSA COMPARED WITH SKIN

The oral mucosa and the skin share many similar structural features. Each consists of stratified squamous epithelium overlying a connective tissue lamina propria (Table 11.1). The oral mucosa acts as the primary organ of mastication by virtue of the reception and conveyance of all the sensory modalities, and the presence of teeth, salivary glands and taste buds. Lymphoid aggregates, which in places are organized to form the oral tonsils, may have a defensive function. By contrast, the skin also acts to regulate body temperature (eccrine sweat glands) and is a tissue of storage and insulation (fat, sebaceous glands), as well as having sensory (hairs, apocrine glands) and protective (nails, ceruminous glands) functions. Some diseases (such as pemphigus) affect all types of stratified squamous epithelium; some affect the skin alone (e.g. eczema); others affect the mouth alone (e.g. aphthae).

FUNCTIONS OF THE ORAL MUCOSA

The functions of the oral mucosa are several.

Protective

The oral mucosa not only resists mechanical stress, i.e. compression forces on the palate, shearing stresses against the gingiva and distension of all the mobile tissues, but also forms a protective barrier against micro-organisms, antigens and toxins. Since the oral mucosa is somewhat permeable, however, some substances can cross it, even under normal circumstances. The factors which influence the movement of substances across the oral mucosa are summarized in Table 11.2.

Sensory

The sensory receptors and nerves of the oral cavity receive and convey the modalities of pain, temperature, touch and taste.

Secretory and defence mechanisms

Saliva from the minor salivary glands (mucous type) of the oral mucosa functions as an efficient lubricant and buffer system and contributes IgA and other protective antibodies (see Chapter 13).

The oral mucosa is able to mount both humoral and cell-mediated immune responses. The presence of aggregates of lymphoid tissue in the oral mucosa and the high concentrations of IgG in the gingival exudate (see Volume 3) suggest that these play a significant role as an early local immune defence system (see Chapter 13).

STRUCTURE OF THE ORAL MUCOSA

Epithelium

Oral epithelial cells have a number of characteristics similar to those of cutaneous cells. They are protein-

Table 11.1
Comparison of the structural features of the oral mucosa with skin

Oral mucosa	Skin
Epithelium	
Oral epithelium	*Epidermis*
Cornified layer (at sites of keratinization	Cornified layer
	Stratum lucidum
Granular cell layer	Granular cell layer
Prickle cell layer	Prickle cell layer
Basal cell layer	Basal cell layer
Connective tissue	
Lamina propria	*Dermis*
Papillary layer: superficial connective tissue adjacent to epithelium; fine collagen fibres orientated perpendicular to epithelium	Papillary layer
Reticular layer: deeper connective tissue; thick collagen fibres with a criss-cross orientation	Reticular layer
Muscularis mucosa (soft palate only)	
Submucosa	*Hypodermis*
Contains larger arteries, veins, lymphatics, nerves and mucous glands	Large quantities of fat
Appendages and glands	
Teeth	Hairs and hair follicles
Sebaceous glands (Fordyce spots)	Sebaceous glands
Salivary glands	Apocrine glands: axilla, breast, pubis, eyelids
Taste buds	
Lymphoid tissue: lingual and palatine tonsils; lympho-epithelial tissue of soft palate, floor of mouth and ventral surface of tongue	Eccrine sweat glands
	Ceruminous glands of the external auditory meatus
	Nails

Table 11.2
Factors influencing oral mucosal permeability

Solute
  Water solubility
  Concentration gradient
  Degree of ionization
  Binding of solute to mucosal proteins

Mucosa
  Morphological barriers
    basal lamina
    keratin layer
    regional variation in mucosal thickness
  Surface-active agents, e.g. constituents of toothpaste
  Topical enzymes and mucolytic agents

Systemic factors
  Age
  Drugs, e.g. chemotherapeutic agents
  Nutritional deficiencies
  Serum-derived antibodies

site of cell division (Fig. 11.2a); the maturation compartment (spinous and granular cells) where the cells migrate superficially and become more terminally differentiated (Fig. 11.2b); and the superficial cornified compartment (Figs. 11.2c and d). The last-mentioned is composed of flattened, envelope-like structures (squames) and areas of keratinization.

The keratinized sites are either formed by

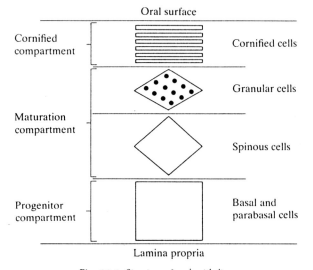

Fig. 11.1 Structure of oral epithelium.

secreting cells which retain the protein (keratin). Cell surface specializations maintain intercellular (desmosomes) and cell-to-substrate (hemi-desmosomes) cohesion. Intermediate filaments inside the cell (tonofilaments: diameter 10 nm) maintain cell shape.

The epithelial cells have been termed basal, spinous, granular or cornified, as a result either of their position in the epithelium or of their appearance (Fig. 11.1). It is now more usual, however, to speak of the epithelium as consisting of 'functional' compartments—the progenitor cell compartment (basal and parabasal cells) which is the

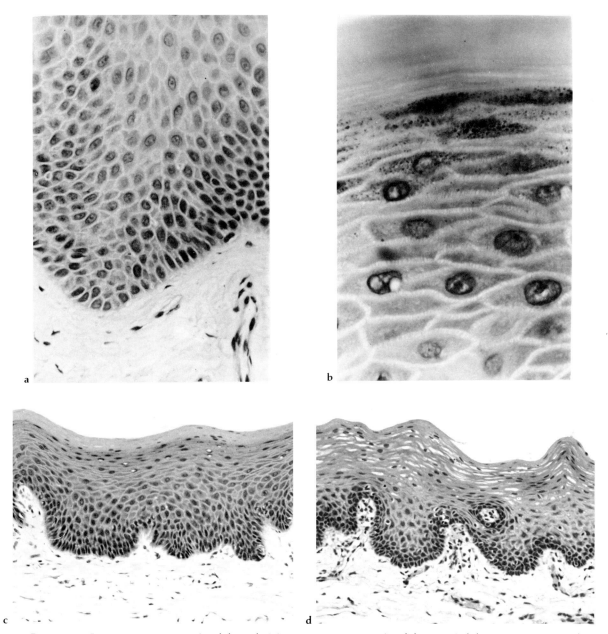

Fig. 11.2 (a) *Progenitor compartment of epithelium.* (b) *Maturation compartment of epithelium.* (c) *Orthokeratinization of cornified compartment of epithelium.* (d) *Parakeratinization of cornified compartment of epithelium.*

orthokeratosis—where all the cellular organelles (particularly the nuclei) have been lost from the cornified compartment (Fig. 11.2c)—or by parakeratosis—where remnants of nuclei and other organelles remain (Fig. 11.2d). In the non-keratinized regions of the oral mucosa, such as the buccal and floor of mouth mucosae, overt keratinization together with the typical features of the granular cells in the maturation compartment are absent. At these sites, the surface cells are flattened and contain elongated nuclei.

Table 11.3

Morphological and biochemical changes associated with keratinocyte maturation

Morphological	Biochemical
Progressive flattening of cells	Rapid decrease in DNA syn-
Increase in cell size	thesis
Progressive loss of intracel-	Gradual decrease in RNA and
lular organelles	protein synthesis
Reorientation of tonofila-	Increase in intracellular glyco-
ments (bundles—keratinized	gen (non-keratinized epithe-
epithelium; dispersed—non-	lium only)
keratinized epithelium)	Changes in intracellular water
Keratohyaline granules	content
Membrane-coated granules	Development of a fibrillar–
Cell surface changes (marked	protein matrix
folding; desmosomes; forma-	Increased expression of pem-
tion of cornified envelope)	phigus antigen
	Decreased expression of pem-
	phigoid antigen
	Increase of epidermal trans-
	glutaminase
	Increase in (γ-glutamyl)
	lysine cross-links

During epithelial maturation, the cells of both keratinized and non-keratinized epithelia change from a cuboidal (basal cell) to a flattened (corneocyte) morphology before being lost at the epithelial surface (desquamation). The morphological and biochemical changes associated with this transition are shown in Table 11.3, but, in general terms, there is an increase in cell size; a progressive decrease in the intracellular organelles, which most probably accounts for the decreases in DNA, RNA and protein synthesis; but an increase in cell surface specializations such as desmosomes. Intracellular membrane-coated granules (Odland bodies) become evident in the spinous and granular layers of both keratinized and non-keratinized epithelia, but it is unclear whether they are lysosomes, part of the Golgi complex, or infoldings of the cell membrane. Keratohyaline granules are also present in keratinized and non-keratinized epithelia and are thought to represent keratin precursors in the stratum corneum and to influence the formation of a thickened plasma membrane during terminal differentiation. Keratinized epithelium is characterized by the aggregation and organization of tonofilament bundles and the development of a thickened cell membrane. The flexibility of non-keratinized epithelium has been attributed to an increase in intracellular water content, marked folding of the cell membrane, a dispersed orientation of tonofilaments and a mucinous nature of the intercellular substance.

Characteristics and functions of other cells, the non-keratinocytes, found in the oral epithelium are summarized in Table 11.4. Melanocytes produce melanin; dendritic cells process antigens; Merkel cells are sensitive to tactile stimuli. Inflammatory cells in the oral epithelium may act in a direct immune capacity or non-specifically.

Basement membrane

The junction between the epithelium and the underlying connective tissue is marked by the basement membrane.

Table 11.4

Intraepithelial non-keratinocytes

Cell	Origin	Characteristics	Function
Melanocyte	Neural crest	Dendritic cell; no tonofilaments or desmosomes or keratinization; basal distribution	Production of the pigment melanin and transfer to keratinocytes
Langerhans' cell	Bone marrow	Dendritic cell; no tonofilaments or desmosomes or keratinization; Birbeck granule (function unknown); suprabasal distribution	Antigen-presenting cell
Merkel cell	Neural	Non-dendritic; tonofilaments; desmosomes; characteristic electron dense vesicle (function unknown); basal distribution	Epithelial sensory receptor
Inflammatory cells	Bone marrow	Various leukocytes	Defensive

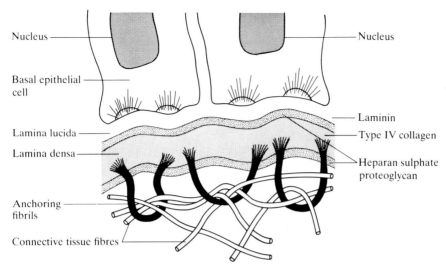

Fig. 11.3 *Ultrastructure of the basal lamina complex.*

Under the light microscope this is an apparently relatively structureless zone (1–2 μm wide), staining strongly with periodic acid-Schiff and silver stains but when viewed with an electron microscope, the basement membrane is clearly a complex of fibrils and matrices (Fig. 11.3) and is therefore often termed the basal lamina or basal lamina complex.

The basal lamina is organized morphologically into two major zones: the lamina lucida which is an electron-lucent region, 20–40 nm wide, located just below the epithelial cells; and the lamina densa, a zone 20–100 nm wide, electron dense and containing a meshwork of fine filaments. Associated with the lamina densa are anchoring fibrils which form loops through which run the collagen fibrils of the connective tissue.

The basement membrane acts mechanically to attach

Table 11.5
Components of basement membranes

Component	Distribution	Purported function
Type IV collagen (non-fibrillar, felt-like mesh)	Lamina densa	Tensile strength and elasticity of the matrix
Proteoglycan—heparan sulphate	Bounds lamina densa	Anionic and restricts the passage of proteins
Glycoproteins		
Laminin	Lamina lucida	Mediates the attachment of epithelial cells to type IV collagen
Fibronectin	Transient deposition in lamina densa	May serve to attach fibroblasts, collagen and proteoglycans to basement membrane
Bullous pemphigoid antigen	Closely associated with cell surfaces of basal epithelial cells	? Involved in cell-matrix interactions and adhesion
Entactin		Basal cell attachment
Epidermolysis bullosa antigen		?

the epithelium to the connective tissue; as a barrier to filter metabolites at a molecular level; and has an important role during tissue regeneration after injury.

Basement membranes are made up of several distinct glycoproteins which fulfil specific functions (Table 11.5).

Lamina propria

Cells

The predominant cell type in the lamina propria is the fibroblast—an elongated, spindle-shaped cell with an oval nucleus and parallel bundles of cytoplasmic filaments (actin, myosin) aligned in the long axis of each cell. Features evident in fibroblasts that are common to all protein-secreting cells include rough endoplasmic reticulum, a well-defined Golgi system and numerous mitochondria. Fibroblasts produce and degrade collagen, elastin and proteoglycans of the extracellular matrix.

Other cells in the connective tissue are defensive. Macrophages are not only phagocytic but are also antigen-presenting cells. Granulocytes are also phagocytic. Lymphocytes function in humoral (B-lymphocytes) and cell-mediated (T-lymphocytes) immunity. Plasma cells differentiate from B-lymphocytes and synthesize and secrete immunoglobulins. Mast cells function both as the primary effector of immediate-type hypersensitivity and also play a role in cell-mediated immunity (Chapter 13).

Finally, in common with other mesenchymal tissues, the connective tissue of the oral mucosa contains fat, nerves (neurones, Schwann cells) and vascular and lymphatic channels (endothelial cells, pericytes).

Extracellular matrix

The extracellular matrix contains three major fibre-forming proteins—collagen, elastin and fibronectin—which are interwoven in a hydrated gel-like ground substance formed by a network of glycosoaminoglycan chains.

The fibre-forming proteins

The collagens are a family of highly characteristic fibrous proteins (see also Chapter 1). Collagens are composed of three polypeptide α-chains which are wound around each

Table 11.6
Mammalian collagens

Type	Distribution
I	Skin, bone, dentine
Trimer	Skin, dentine, eye, chondrocytes
II	Cartilage, vitreous humour
III	Reticulin fibres, aorta
IV	Basal lamina
V	Muscle, lung, placenta

other in a regular helix to generate a rope-like collagen molecule. Several genetically distinct collagen α-chains have been defined and various combinations of these give rise to the main collagens—types I, II, III, IV and V (Table 11.6). A schematic summary of the various steps involved in collagen synthesis is given in Fig. 11.4. After being secreted into the extracellular space, types I, II and III collagen molecules assemble into ordered polymers—collagen fibrils—which are clearly visible with the electron microscope. Such fibrils are often grouped into larger bundles which can be seen under the light microscope as collagen fibres. Collagen fibres provide tensile strength and help to organize the extracellular matrix. Type IV collagen (the main collagen in basal laminae) and type V molecules (small amounts in basal laminae) do not form fibrils and their arrangement in tissues is uncertain.

The property of recoil after transient stretch of the oral mucosa is attributable to a network of elastic fibres in the connective tissue. The main component of elastic fibres is elastin which, like collagen, is unusually rich in proline and glycine but, unlike collagen, contains little hydroxyproline and no hydroxylysine. Elastin molecules are secreted by fibroblasts and smooth muscle cells and exist as random-coiled structures with extensive cross-linking—features which allow them to stretch and recoil like an elastic band.

The other non-collagen glycoproteins of the extracellular matrix have been relatively neglected until recently. Much is now known about fibronectin, a fibre-forming glycoprotein which may play a significant role in cell adhesion and cell migration. It exists in the form of large aggregates in the extracellular space, and small quantities are bound to the surfaces of fibroblasts. Fibronectin appears to provide a bridge between the intracellular actin filaments of fibroblasts and the macromolecules of collagen and hyaluronic acid in the extracellular matrix.

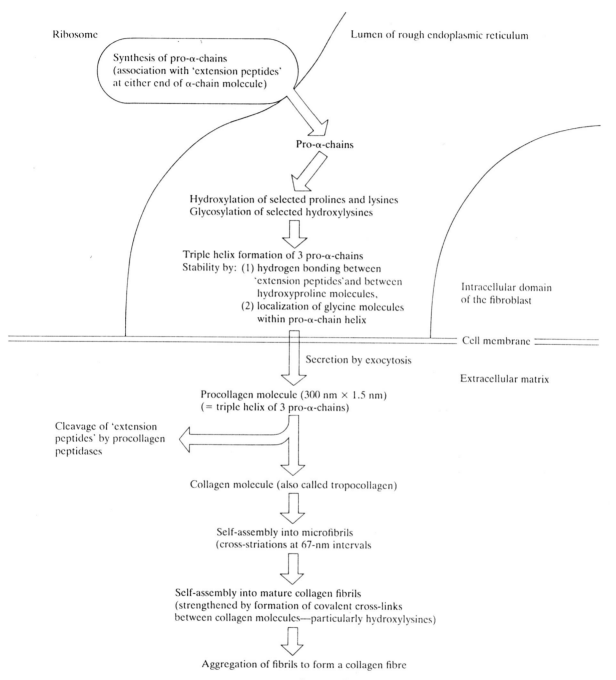

Ribosome

Lumen of rough endoplasmic reticulum

Synthesis of pro-α-chains
(association with 'extension peptides'
at either end of α-chain molecule)

Pro-α-chains

Hydroxylation of selected prolines and lysines
Glycosylation of selected hydroxylysines

Triple helix formation of 3 pro-α-chains
Stability by: (1) hydrogen bonding between
'extension peptides' and between
hydroxyproline molecules,
(2) localization of glycine molecules
within pro-α-chain helix

Intracellular domain
of the fibroblast

Cell membrane

Secretion by exocytosis

Extracellular matrix

Procollagen molecule (300 nm × 1.5 nm)
(= triple helix of 3 pro-α-chains)

Cleavage of 'extension
peptides' by procollagen
peptidases

Collagen molecule (also called tropocollagen)

Self-assembly into microfibrils
(cross-striations at 67-nm intervals

Self-assembly into mature collagen fibrils
(strengthened by formation of covalent cross-links
between collagen molecules—particularly hydroxylysines)

Aggregation of fibrils to form a collagen fibre

Fig. 11.4 *Collagen synthesis.*

Ground substance

Glycosoaminoglycans (GAGs), formerly known as muco-polysaccharides, are long, unbranched polysaccharide chains of repeating disaccharide units. One of the two sugar residues in the repeating disaccharide is always an amino sugar, i.e. N-acetylglucosamine or N-acetylgalactosamine. The GAGs are highly negatively charged due to the presence of sulphate or carboxyl groups, or both, on many of the sugar residues. Various groups of GAGs have been distinguished by their sugar residues, the type of linkage between these residues and the number and location of sulphate groups. These are hyaluronic acid (in which no sugars are sulphated), chondroitin-4-sulphate, chondroitin-6-sulphate, dermatan sulphate, heparan sulphate and keratan sulphate.

Hyaluronic acid exists as a single, very long carbohydrate chain of several thousand sugar residues in a regular repeating sequence of disaccharide units. All the other GAGs, however, are covalently linked to protein to form proteoglycans (formerly called mucoproteins). In contrast to typical glycoproteins, proteoglycans are much larger and contain more carbohydrate in the form of many long, unbranched GAG chains, usually without terminal sialic acid. In principle, proteoglycans have the potential for almost limitless heterogeneity because they can differ markedly in protein content, molecular size, number and type of GAG chains per molecule and the spatial arrangements of their side groups. Proteoglycans, however, do share the common properties of occupying a huge volume for their mass and of being hydrophilic. In forming hydrated gels, proteoglycans create a swelling pressure (turgor) in the extracellular matrix that resists compressive forces (in contrast to collagen fibrils that resist stretching forces). Furthermore, it is now recognized that proteoglycans and GAGs can function as molecular or cellular sieves.

REGIONAL DIFFERENCES IN THE ORAL MUCOSA

There are considerable variations in the structure of the oral mucosa at different sites, a feature which is thought to reflect regional differences of function.

Conventionally, the mucosa is divided into masticatory, lining and specialized types (Table 11.7). The masticatory mucosa (hard palate, gingiva) shows adaptations to the forces of pressure and friction, as reflected by its keratinized epithelium, numerous tall rete ridges and connective tissue papillae and the little, if any, submucosa. By contrast, the lining type of oral mucosa (buccal, labial and alveolar mucosa, floor of mouth, ventral surface of tongue, soft palate, lips) is subject to stretching and is characterized by non-keratinized epithelium, broad rete ridges and connective tissue papillae, and abundant elastic fibres in the lamina propria. Specialized mucosa covers the dorsum of the tongue and is adapted for the sense of taste, the interaction between tongue and palate during mastication (compression), and also the forces of distension. There is a keratinized epithelium, numerous rete ridges and connective tissue papillae, abundant elastic and collagen fibres in the lamina propria and an absence of submucosa, with the surface firmly attached to the underlying muscle.

THE DYNAMICS OF ORAL EPITHELIUM

Descriptions of the oral mucosa traditionally have been of an anatomical nature. This section attempts to illustrate the dynamic nature of the oral mucosa by examining some of the recent advances in cell renewal, differentiation, epithelial–mesenchymal interactions and immune functions.

Cell renewal

Cell division takes place in the progenitor compartment, and conventionally the cell life cycle has been divided into the following four phases.

	Approximate duration	Variation
M—mitosis	1 hour	Constant
G1—post-mitotic phase	Hours–weeks	Variable
S—DNA synthesis	8 hours	Constant
G2—post-DNA synthesis phase	3–4 hours	Constant

A so-called G0 phase has been postulated between M and G1 and is thought to be that period of indeterminate length in which each daughter cell determines its prospective fate of either further cell division or terminal differentiation.

A more recent concept of cell renewal in epithelial tissues, which is gaining increasing acceptance, proposes the existence of epithelial proliferative units. In the epidermis, these proliferative units appear to lie under the large hexagonal surface squames of keratin, but the oral epithelium does not seem to have a similarly regular pattern, except perhaps in relation to the proliferative compartment of the filiform papillae of the tongue. The proliferative unit in the oral epithelium appears to be the epithelial ridge bounded by the connective tissue papillae on either side. According to the hypothesis, each epithelial proliferative unit shelters the basal cells, among which are a stem cell—a cell with extensive self-renewal capacity, which extends throughout the whole (or most) of the life span of the organism and which is ultimately responsible for all the cell replacement that occurs under steady state conditions. The stem cell divides to give both a further stem cell and a daughter cell. The latter passes into a transit compartment where it undergoes a limited number of amplification divisions (perhaps three to four) before remaining for a period of time in the basal layer in a post-mitotic state. If the functional stem cell is killed, the column maintains its

integrity by raising one of the daughter cells to stem cell status, i.e. a number of *potential* stem cells exist. The older the cell the less the probability of its being able to become a functional stem cell. Eventually, the age of the cell is such that it is irreversibly committed to differentiation, after which a few divisions may still occur before terminal maturation.

The mechanisms that control the balance between epithelial cell proliferation and maturation are unclear, but the following have been implicated: epithelial chalones acting by way of a negative feedback mechanism; cyclic nucleotides (cAMP and cGMP) forming second messengers in the epithelial cell's response to pharmacological agents such as adrenaline, prostaglandins and corticosteroids; and epidermal growth factor which promotes

Table 11.7

Functional adaptations of the oral mucosa

Lining mucosa	Masticatory mucosa	Specialized mucosa
Site		
Soft palate, ventral surface of tongue, floor of mouth, labial and buccal mucosa, aveolar mucosa, lips	Gingiva, hard palate	Dorsal surface of tongue
Functional demands		
Mobility and distension	Compression and friction	Taste, tongue–palate interaction, mobility and distension
Epithelium		
Thin, non-keratinized stratified squamous epithelium	Thick, keratinized stratified squamous epithelium	Thick, keratinized stratified squamous epithelium
Infrequent, broad, short rete ridges	Numerous, tall, narrow rete ridges	Numerous broad rete ridges
Lamina propria		
Short papillae	Long papillae	Long papillae
Abundant elastic fibres	Thick dense collagen bands which merge with periosteum of bone—'mucoperiosteum'	Elastic and collagen fibres associated with connective tissue fibres of muscle bundles
Infrequent collagen fibres	Elastic fibres absent	
Ventrum of tongue: minor salivary glands		Dorsum of tongue: minor salivary glands (von Ebner), lymphoid tissue, taste buds
Submucosa		
Diffuse connective tissue	Surface firmly attached to cementum (gingiva) or periosteum (hard palate)	Surface firmly attached to underlying muscle
Irregular distribution of minor salivary glands, sebaceous glands and fat	1. Gingiva—no distinct layer	Dorsum of tongue—no distinct layer
	2. Hard palate anterior—fat; posterior—minor salivary glands	

proliferation and differentiation of epithelial cells. More recently, it has been suggested that the stem cell character is maintained by its contact with the basal lamina complex and that the changes leading to terminal differentiation begin by loss of cell contact with the lamina.

Differentiation

Epithelial differentiation is the process whereby a living epithelial cell (keratinocyte) in the progenitor cell compartment matures and eventually changes into a flattened dead cell in the stratum corneum. The process is attributable to two separate but related phenomena, namely keratinization and the formation of an intracellular cornified envelope.

Keratinization

The keratins are a family of water-insoluble proteins (40–70 kilodaltons, kd) that form the intermediate filaments (tonofilaments) in epithelial cells. The cells of the stratum corneum contain large quantities of keratin filaments which become organized in an intracellular matrix termed filaggrin, a histidine-rich protein derived from the keratohyaline granules found in close association with the tonofilament bundles (keratinized epithelium only) and responsible for organizing the keratin filaments into the supramolecular bundles so characteristic of the stratum corneum.

Keratin polypeptides are now known to be present in all epithelial cells, not simply in the superficial layers. The keratin filaments vary in composition in simple, stratified or keratinized epithelia (Table 11.8). The epidermis contains 67-kd and 56-kd polypeptides which are markers of keratinizing tissue, as well as 50-kd and 58-kd polypeptides characteristic of stratified epithelium. Certain keratin polypeptides are synthesized in different layers of the epithelium—the 56-kd and 67-kd polypeptides in suprabasal cells and the 50-kd and 58-kd proteins in the basal layer. A similar pattern of keratinization may be present in oral epithelia (Figs. 11.5 and 11.6).

Cornified envelope formation

In addition to cell keratinization, the plasma membrane of the superficial cells becomes thickened and strengthened on its intracellular surface. The enzyme transglutaminase, located in the epithelial granular layer, catalyses the formation of epsilon (γ-glutamyl) lysine and disulphide bonds which covalently cross-link a soluble cytoplasmic precursor termed involucrin (keratolinin). It has been suggested that the precursor proteins linked by disulphide bonds may be derived from keratohyaline granules found in close association with ribosomes (keratinized and non-keratinized epithelia). The resultant polymer forms the cornified envelope that lines the inner aspect of the plasma membrane of the keratinocytes in the stratum corneum.

There may also be molecular changes at the cell surface itself during differentiation. Carbohydrates in the epithelial cell membrane not only show a regional variation in their expression, but their nature and composition change during epithelial maturation. It has been proposed that these cell surface carbohydrates may function in intercellular adhesion and may possibly be involved in cell responses to hormones, vitamins and other types of chemical signal.

Table 11.8

Molecular weights (kd) of keratin polypeptides identified in simple, non-keratinized and keratinized epithelia

Epithelium				
Simple	Non-keratinized	Keratinized	Location	Marker
40	40			Epithelium
46	46			
	50	50	Basal	Stratification
	52			
		56	Suprabasal	Keratinization
	58		Basal	Stratification
		65–67	Suprabasal	Keratinization

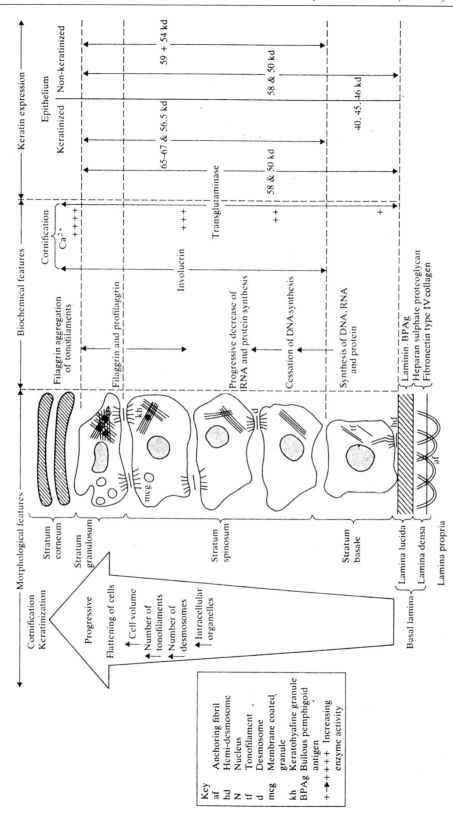

Fig. 11.5 *Keratinocyte differentiation. (Courtesy of Dr J. Luker.)*

Keratin types and pairs

I   II

Stratified (oral)

    10 ------ 1   Cornified epithelium

    12 ------ 3   (Cornea only)

    13 ------ 4   (Non-cornified epithelium

    16 ------ 6   Fast turnover epithelium
                (cornified and some non-cornified sites)

    14 ------ 5   All stratified epithelium
                (may also be present suprabasally)

    17

Simple (lining, secretory, early embryonic)

      7

    18 ------ 8   Merkel cell population only
                (gingivae, hard palate)

    19   Mainly simple epithelium
                (some basal cells in non-cornified
                oral epithelia, e.g. buccal)

Suprabasal cells

Basal cells

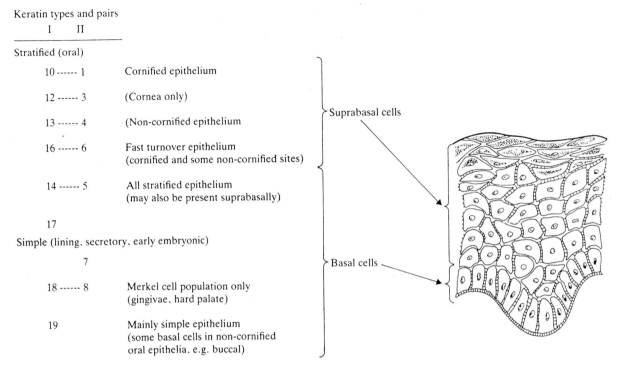

Fig. 11.6 *Expression of keratins in oral epithelium.*

Epithelial–mesenchymal interactions

In most tissue interactions, possibly including the oral mucosa, the mesenchyme (connective tissue) controls the expression of epithelial morphogenesis and cytodifferentiation. Whether this is a specific direct effect by the connective tissue or a permissive effect whereby the mesenchyme 'allows' the full expression of a predetermined epithelial phenotype is unclear. Further, the mechanism by which such information may be transferred from connective tissue to epithelium is unclear, but possible inductive signals include direct cell–cell contact, the diffusion of chemical substances, and cell–matrix interactions.

Clearly, the dominant role attributed to the connective tissue is likely to be an oversimplification. The spectrum of responses between epithelium and mesenchyme may well reflect: (i) the strength of the inductive stimulus, (ii) the nature of the responding tissue, and (iii) the source of the interactants. It seems possible, therefore, that the developmental response of interacting tissues may be specified by either the inducing or the responding tissues.

Immune functions (see also Chapter 13)

The skin is an integral and active element of the immune system and it is likely that the oral mucosa also functions in this capacity.

The cellular and molecular components of the skin's response to an antigenic challenge are summarized in Figure 11.7. Foreign antigens penetrate the superficial layers of the epithelium and bind to dendritic antigen-presenting cells in the epithelium. Two types of epithelial dendritic cells have been identified, Langerhans' cells and Granstein cells. Langerhans' cells present antigen to specific 'helper' T-lymphocytes, whereas Granstein cells interact similarly with 'suppressor' T-lymphocytes. The helper and suppressor responses are in approximate balance, but normally the overall result is a helper-positive signal. The mechanism of antigen presentation by dendritic cells is unknown, but T-cells recognize antigen on the dendritic cell only when it is in association with gene products of the major histocompatibility complex (MHC): this is known as MHC-restricted specificity. In other words, it is essential that dendritic cells are

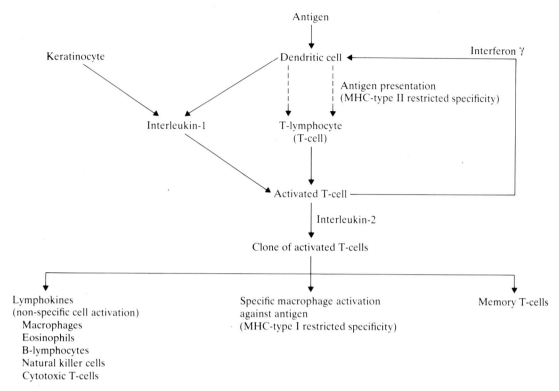

Fig. 11.7 *Immune system in mucosa.*

genetically identical to the responding T-cells; simple diffusion of unprocessed antigen to lymph nodes and T-cells is not immunogenic.

In addition to being presented with an antigen, the responding T-cells also receive a complementary signal in the form of a cytokine, termed interleukin-1, secreted both by keratinocytes and dendritic cells. This prompts the activated T-cells to secrete a lymphokine—interleukin-2—which binds to additional antigen-responsive T-cells and causes them to proliferate, dramatically increasing the number of T-cells capable of responding to the antigenic challenge. A further lymphokine which potentiates this system is γ-interferon, which is released by activated T-cells and stimulates dendritic cells and possibly keratinocytes to enhance antigen presentation.

Activated T-cells evoke either a specific immunological response to the antigenic challenge via macrophages, a phenomenon again restricted by MHC specificity, or, alternatively, they activate a number of different defence cells by releasing lymphokines.

SPECIALIZED AREAS OF THE ORAL MUCOSA

The tongue

The mucosa of the dorsum of the tongue is a modified type of masticatory mucosa which subserves both mechanical (mastication) and sensory (taste) functions. The tongue is divided by a V-shaped groove, the sulcus terminalis, into an anterior two-thirds and a posterior third (Fig. 11.8). Various papillae are found on the dorsum of the tongue.

Filiform papillae

These papillae, distributed over the entire anterior surface, are cone-shaped structures covered by keratinized epithelium. During mastication, they form an abrasive surface against which the food bolus is compressed against the hard palate (Fig. 11.9).

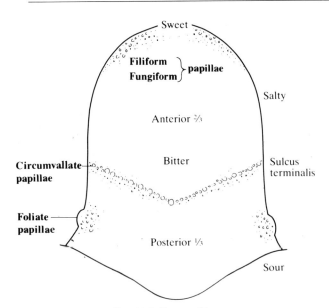

Fig. 11.8 *Dorsum of tongue.*

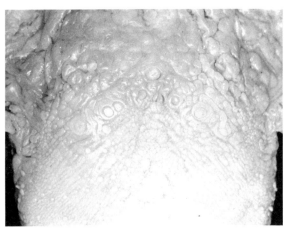

Fig. 11.10 *Circumvallate papillae, post-mortem specimen. (Courtesy of Professor C. Scully.)*

Fungiform papillae

Fungiform papillae are isolated, mushroom-shaped, red structures, which are covered by non-keratinized epithelium and scattered between the numerous filiform papillae (Fig. 11.9). Taste buds are present on their surface.

Circumvallate papillae

Adjacent and anterior to the sulcus terminalis are 8–12 large papillae (Fig. 11.10), each surrounded by a deep groove into which open the ducts of the glands of von Ebner (serous minor salivary glands). The superior surface of these circumvallate papillae is covered by keratinized epithelium, whereas the epithelium covering the lateral walls is non-keratinized and contains taste buds. (Taste is discussed in Chapter 29.)

Foliate papillae

These papillae consist of 4–11 parallel ridges, alternating with deep grooves in the mucosa, on the lateral margins on the posterior part of the tongue (Fig. 11.11).

Taste buds are present in the epithelium of the lateral walls of the ridges.

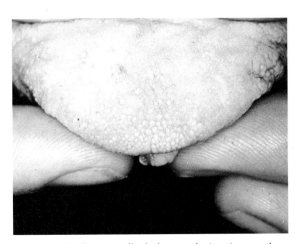

Fig. 11.9 *Filiform papillae lie between the fungiform papillae. (Courtesy of Professor C. Scully.)*

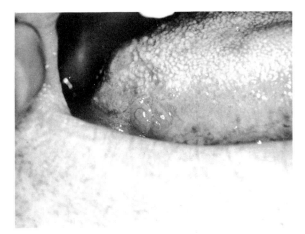

Fig. 11.11 *Foliate papillae. (Courtesy of Professor C. Scully.)*

Lingual tonsil

The lingual tonsils, consisting of round or oval prominences with intervening lingual crypts lined by non-keratinized epithelium, are part of Waldeyer's ring of lymphoid tissue and contain aggregates of lymphoid tissue which function in a primary immune capacity.

The junction of the oral mucosa and teeth

The dentogingival junction represents a unique anatomical feature concerned with the attachment of the oral mucosa to the tooth (Volume 3). A schematic diagram of the anatomical features of this junction in health is shown in Fig. 11.12. The junction is composed of keratinized gingival epithelium on the external oral surface, non-keratinized crevicular/sulcular epithelium forming a cuff-like gingival crevice (0.5–3.0 mm depth) surrounding the tooth, and non-keratinized junctional epithelium which is adherent to the enamel and extends apically to the amelocemental junction at the time of tooth eruption. The junctional epithelium consists of layers of flattened squamous cells lying parallel to the tooth surface and is unique in that it is bounded both on its tooth and lamina propria aspects by basement membranes. The cells of the junctional epithelium have a high turnover rate, an abundance of intracellular organelles and wide intercellular spaces with few desmosomes. Many of these features have been attributed to an inflammatory infiltrate in the underlying lamina propria, and indeed neutrophils migrate through the junctional epithelium in response to chemotactic stimuli, and into the gingival crevice.

The nature of the biological mechanism which unites the cells of the junctional epithelium to the tooth surface is unknown. The morphological components of the epithelial attachment are hemi-desmosomes, which are formed at the cell surface of the junctional epithelium, and a basement membrane complex identical to that described above. In addition, at the end of amelogenesis, the enamel surface is covered by the reduced enamel epithelium which not only contributes to the formation of the junctional epithelium, but secretes a structureless organic layer termed the primary enamel cuticle. However, the relationship between the primary enamel cuticle and components of the lamina densa, such as fibronectin, collagen type IV and the proteoglycan heparan sulphate, has not been elucidated. Furthermore, it is not clear whether the lamina lucida of the junctional epithelium differs from that of basement membrane complexes at other sites. Such information is likely to be of great importance because it underlies the initial events involved in periodontal disease.

NEUROVASCULAR SUPPLY OF THE ORAL MUCOSA

Blood supply

The blood supply of the oral mucosa is extremely rich and is derived from arteries in the submucosa and reticular layer of the lamina propria. The vessels subdivide to form arterioles and an extensive capillary network subjacent to the epithelium. Capillary loops pass upwards into the connective tissue papillae. The vascularity undoubtedly contributes to the more rapid healing of the oral mucosa when compared with the skin. However, unlike skin, the oral mucosa lacks arteriovenous shunts and is thought not to play a role in temperature regulation in humans.

Nerve supply

The sensory functions of the oral mucosa, like those of the skin, include the reception and conveyance of pain, cold, heat, touch and pressure. Unique to the oral cavity is the sense of taste. With the exceptions of taste and possibly touch, stimuli are received by specialized nerve endings (Meissner's corpuscles, Krause's end-bulbs, Ruffini corpuscles, etc.) or free nerve endings either within the epithelium or in the superficial lamina

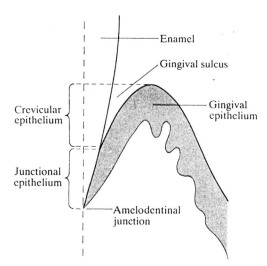

Fig. 11.12 *Diagrammatic representation of the junction of mucosa and tooth.*

propria. Specific receptors are not exclusively associated with a particular modality, but are more numerous in anterior than posterior regions of the oral mucosa, and sensitivity parallels this distribution. Sensory nerve plexuses are located immediately beneath the basement membrane and at the junction of the papillary and reticular layers of the lamina propria. Stimuli are transmitted via non-myelinated nerves and are conveyed to the central nervous system essentially by the trigeminal nerve (V cranial nerve) and afferent fibres of the IX and X cranial nerves.

Stimuli from receptors evoke a number of reflex actions which include withdrawal, swallowing, gagging, retching and minor salivary gland control. Responses involving higher centres in the CNS may include the activation of the thirst mechanism.

FURTHER READING

Alberts B., Bray D., Lewis J., Raff, M., Roberts K., Watson, J. D. (1983). *Molecular biology of the cell.* New York: Garland Publishing.

Heathcote J. G., Grant M. E. (1981). The molecular organisation of basement membranes. In *International review of connective tissue research,* Vol. 9, pp. 191–264. New York: Academic Press.

Hume W. J., Potten C. S. (1979). Advances in epithelial kinetics—An oral view. *J. oral Pathol.,* **8**: 3–22.

Meyer J., Squier C. A., Gerson S. J. (1984). *The structure and function of oral mucosa.* Oxford: Pergamon Press.

Morgan P. R., Shirlaw P. J., Johnson N. W., Leigh I. M., Lane E. B. (1987). Potential applications of anti-keratin antibodies in oral diagnosis. *J. oral Pathol.,* **16**: 212–222.

Ten Cate A. R. (1985). *Oral histology,* 2nd edn. St Louis, Missouri: C. V. Mosby.

Chapter 12 · Developmental disorders

Though a large number of developmental disorders of oral soft tissues have been described, most are very rare. There may, however, be a genetic basis to some more common disorders such as recurrent aphthae (Chapter 14). Only the more common developmental disorders and those that do not appear elsewhere in this volume are described here.

FORDYCE SPOTS

Fordyce spots are yellowish soft granules which are sebaceous glands beneath the oral mucosa. They are extremely common. They are usually seen in the buccal mucosa, particularly inside the commissures (Fig. 12.1), but also in the retromolar regions and lips—especially the upper. They seem to be more obvious in males, in patients with greasy skin and in the elderly.

Fordyce spots are totally benign, though the occasional patient becomes concerned about them or they are mistaken for thrush or lichen planus (Chapter 19).

LEUCOEDEMA

This is not a mucosal disease but simply the description of very faint whitish lines in some normal buccal mucosae, seen very often in Blacks. The whitish lines disappear if the mucosa is stretched—a diagnostic test.

WHITE SPONGE NAEVUS

Also known as pachydermia oralis and white folded gingivostomatosis, white sponge naevus is a rare benign familial disorder of mucosae. Usually inherited as an autosomal dominant trait, it is totally symptomless.

Table 12.1

Some rare genetically determined mucosal lesions

	Inheritance	Manifestations	
		Oral	Other
Pachyonychia congenita	AD	Keratosis	Hyperkeratotic palms and soles, thickened nails
Dyskeratosis congenita	X linked or AR	White lesions, risk of carcinoma	Skin pigmentation, nail dystrophy, aplastic anaemia
Focal oral and cutaneous hyper-keratosis (tylosis)	AD	Leukoplakia, oesophageal carcinoma	Hyperkeratotic palms and soles
Dyskeratosis follicularis (Darier–White's disease)	AD	Papules	Skin papules

AD = autosomal dominant; AR = autosomal recessive.

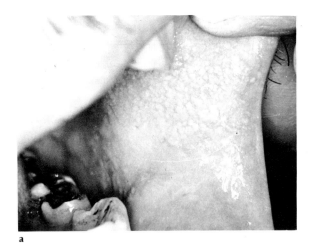

a

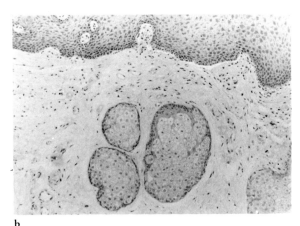

b

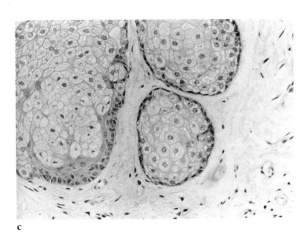

c

Fig. 12.1 Fordyce spots: (a) shown in the buccal mucosa—
the typical site; (b) sebaceous glands; (c) high power to show
the sebaceous glands.

Clinical features

The oral mucosa is almost invariably involved in white
sponge naevus. Shaggy or folded white lesions typically
affect the buccal mucosa bilaterally but may also involve
other areas (Fig. 12.2a).

Similar lesions may also affect the upper respiratory
tract, genitalia and anus.

Diagnosis

The family history and examination are usually adequate
to make the diagnosis but there may be confusion with
other white lesions (Table 12.1, Chapter 19), in which
case a biopsy is indicated. Histologically, the lesion
typically consists of hyperplastic epithelium in which
gross oedema causes a basket-weave appearance (Fig.
12.2b).

Management

Reassurance is all that is required.

EPIDERMOLYSIS BULLOSA

Epidermolysis bullosa is a rare genetically determined
disorder related to a defect in the epidermolysis bullosa
antigen found in epithelial basal lamina (Chapter 11).

Clinical features

There are several subgroups of epidermolysis bullosa
with different prognoses, but the essential feature is
vesiculation in response to even minor trauma. In the
more severe types, oral bullae appear in the infant as
soon as suckling begins. The skin also blisters.

The other essential feature is scarring and this may
cause severe disability such as limb deformities, micro-
stomia and trismus (Fig. 12.3). Enamel hypoplasia may be
seen.

Management

Oral hygiene requires careful attention. Trauma should
be minimized and drugs such as phenytoin may help
reduce the blistering. Specialist care is required.

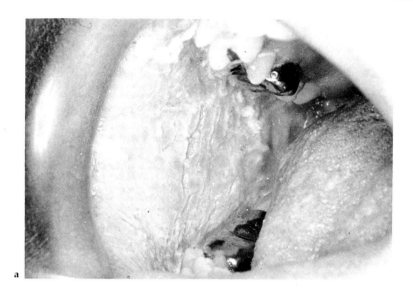

a

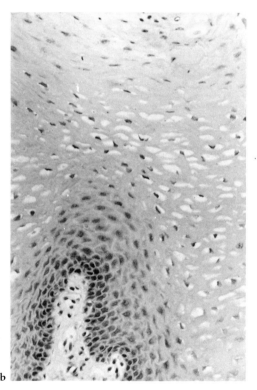

b

Fig. 12.2 White sponge naevus: (a) showing the corrugated white appearance in the buccal mucosa; (b) photomicrograph showing the basket-weave appearance caused by intra-epithelial oedema.

ECTODERMAL DYSPLASIA

Inability to sweat (hypohidrosis); thin, often blond scalp hair, eyelashes and eyebrows (hypotrichosis); and conical or missing teeth (hypodontia) characterize hypohidrotic ectodermal dysplasia. There is also soft, thin skin, frontal bossing and a depressed nasal bridge (Volume 3). Affected children may require dentures.

ACRODERMATITIS ENTEROPATHICA

This is a rare genetically determined disorder of zinc metabolism causing mouth ulceration and candidosis, rashes around body orifices, and alopecia.

PORPHYRIA

Porphyrias constitute a group of rare disorders of porphyrin metabolism. Erythropoietic porphyria may cause reddish discoloration of both the deciduous and permanent dentitions, hirsutism, and skin blisters. Hepatic porphyria predisposes to mouth blisters (and is a contraindication to the use of intravenous barbiturates: Volume 1).

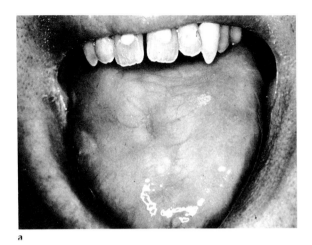

a

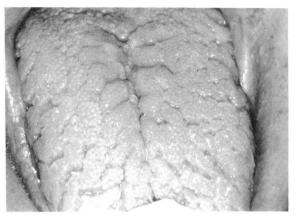

Fig. 12.4 *Fissured tongue.*

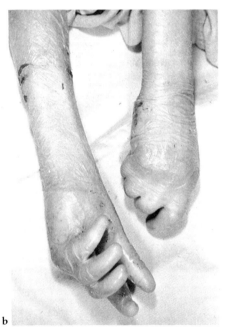

b

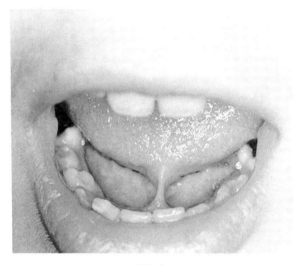

Fig. 12.5 *Ankyloglossia (tongue-tie).*

Fig. 12.3 *(a) Scarring and depapillation and (b) scarring and limb deformities in epidermolysis bullosa.*

GENETICALLY DETERMINED DISORDERS AFFECTING THE TONGUE

Fissured tongue

The cause of a fissured tongue (plicated or scrotal tongue) is unclear, but it is an extremely common condition. It is occasionally associated with, for example, erythema migrans, but the condition is otherwise of no consequence (Fig. 12.4).

Patients with Down's syndrome often have a fissured tongue.

Ankyloglossia

Ankyloglossia, or tongue-tie, is an uncommon isolated anomaly in which the lingual fraenum is tight and the tongue cannot be fully protruded (Fig. 12.5). Speech is *not* usually affected but the ability to cleanse the buccal sulcus with the tongue is. If necessary, surgery to the fraenum can readily relieve ankyloglossia.

Erythema migrans (see Chapter 17)

Median rhomboid glossitis (see Chapter 18)

GENETICALLY DETERMINED DISORDERS AFFECTING THE PALATE

Few mucosal disorders specifically affect the palate.

Cleft palate is discussed fully in Volume 4; bifid uvula (Fig. 12.6) is probably an extremely minor manifestation which may be associated with a submucous cleft.

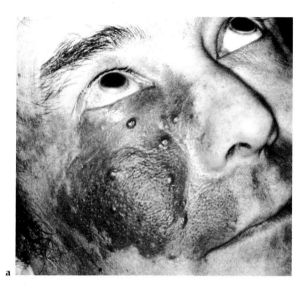

a

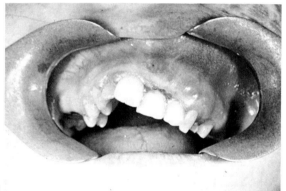

b

Fig. 12.7 Sturge–Weber syndrome.

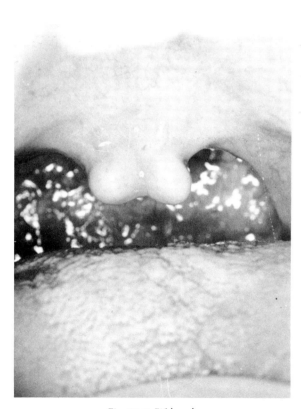

Fig. 12.6 Bifid uvula.

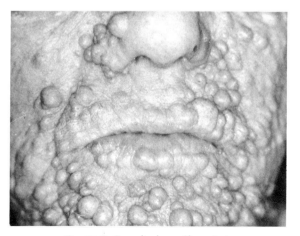

Fig. 12.8 Generalized neurofibromatosis.

GENETICALLY DETERMINED DISORDERS OF THE GINGIVA

Hereditary gingival fibromatosis is discussed in Chapter 21. Gingival swelling may also be seen in mucopolysaccharidoses.

OTHER RARE GENETICALLY DETERMINED DISORDERS
(see also Table 12.1)

Chronic mucocutaneous candidosis (see Chapter 19)

Ehlers–Danlos syndrome (see Chapter 1)

Peutz–Jeghers syndrome (see Chapter 20)

Phakomatoses

This is the term given to a range of disorders affecting ectoderm, with neurological manifestations and sometimes with mental handicap. They include the following.

1. *Sturge–Weber syndrome.* The Sturge–Weber syndrome consists of haemangioma in the trigeminal region and extending into the leptomeninges with subsequent intracranial calcification, epilepsy and hemiplegia (Fig. 12.7). The haemangioma may involve the mouth and may bleed during surgery.

2. *Von Recklinghausen's neurofibromatosis.* Generalized neurofibromatosis may, if there are intracerebral neurofibromas, cause epilepsy. There may be brownish café-au-lait patches of pigmentation on the skin. Neurofibromas may be found on the face and intra-orally (Fig. 12.8).

3. *Tuberous sclerosis (epiloia).* Various hamartomas affecting especially the brain, kidneys and heart are seen in tuberous sclerosis but the most obvious features are fibromas at the base of the nails (subungual fibromas) and skin nodules in the nasolabial fold (adenoma sebaceum).

There is often a minor degree of enamel hypoplasia.

FURTHER READING

Baden E., Jones J. R., Khedekar R., Burns W. A. (1984). Neurofibromatosis of the tongue: a light and electron-microscopic study with review of the literature from 1849–1981. *J. oral Med.,* **39**: 157–164.

Jorgenson R. J., Levin L. S. (1981). White sponge naevus. *Arch. Dermatol.,* **117**: 73–76.

13   *Aspects of mucosal immunology*

This chapter is a *brief* synopsis of immunology. The main function of the immune response is to provide defence against infection, and patients with defective immune responses often suffer from repeated and severe infections.

NATURAL IMMUNITY

When a micro-organism attempts to invade the body, it must overcome two main lines of defence before having any damaging effect upon the tissues. The first *and most important* line of defence—natural immunity—consists of various anatomical and physiological factors that react in the same way with every foreign substance (antigen). Because natural immunity cannot distinguish between antigens it is said to have no *specificity*. The integrity of skin and mucosa, and secretions such as saliva, constitute the main host defences against infection.

ACQUIRED IMMUNITY

The body's second line of defence—acquired immunity—consists of several systems that *can* distinguish between antigens in a highly *specific* manner. In addition, by possessing a *memory*, their destructive efficiency, both in speed of onset and size of immune response, increases with each subsequent exposure to the same antigen. *Specificity and memory are thus the main features of a response that is immunological in nature.*

The immune system is composed of three interrelated elements, namely the humoral, cell-mediated and phagocytic systems. The humoral system generates antibodies which are proteins (immunoglobulins) that result in destruction of antigens. The cell-mediated system generates lymphokines, which are substances that influence the activities of other cells—especially leucocytes. Both the humoral and cell-mediated systems aid the destruction of antigens by phagocytic cells such as polymorphonuclear leucocytes and macrophages (Fig. 13.1).

Humoral system

Once an antigen has overcome the body's initial defence measures it is engulfed by antigen-presenting cells (APCs). The APCs (mainly macrophages and Langerhans' cells) process the antigen, place it on their cell surface and release a short-acting hormone (a cytokine), interleukin-1 (IL-1). The processed antigen, along with various receptors (class II HLA antigens) of the APC, is presented to T-helper cells which are activated by this and IL-1, and the T-cells induce B-lymphocytes to proliferate and differentiate into either memory B-cells or plasma cells. The memory B-cells ensure that, on subsequent exposure to the same antigen, the response by the humoral system is both more rapid and more effective. Plasma cells generate antibody that is highly specific for the antigen which was initially engulfed by the APC.

Antibodies are glycoproteins known as immunoglobulins (Ig). The various immunoglobulins and their functions are outlined in Table 13.1, but their main actions are to destroy antigens by neutralizing them, having activated complement (see below) to lyse them, or by inducing phagocytosis (see below). IgM is predominantly intravascular; IgG appears in all tissue fluids; and IgA is found mainly in external secretions (e.g. saliva).

Cell-mediated system

While most bacteria induce a humoral immune response, viruses, fungi and mycobacteria activate the cell-mediated immune system. Following antigen processing, the APCs stimulate T-lymphocytes to proliferate, release interleukin-2 (IL-2), and divide into three cell types:

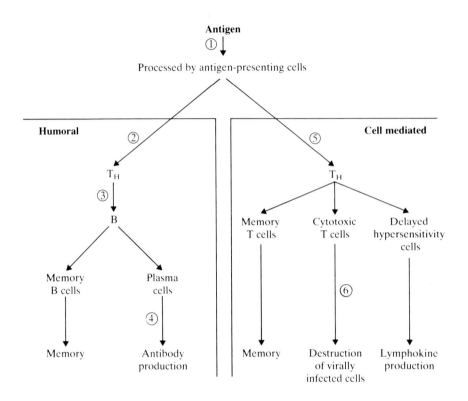

① After by-passing the natural immune system, the antigen undergoes processing by antigen-presenting cells such as macrophages and dendrite cells.

Humoral immunity

② T helper cells are stimulated to multiply.
③ The enlarged pool of T helper cells stimulates B lymphocytes to multiply and differentiate into B memory cells and plasma cells.
④ The plasma cells synthesize and secrete antibody specific for the antigen that initiated this series of reactions.

Cell-mediated immunity

⑤ The modified antigen stimulates T helper cells (T_4 cells) to multiply and differentiate into memory T cells, cytotoxic T cells and delayed hypersensitivity cells.
⑥ The cytotoxic T cells destroy any virally infected host cells. Delayed hypersensitivity cells produce lymphokines.

These reactions occur at the site of antigen accumulation and/or in local lymph nodes. The reactions of T helper cells may be dampened down by T suppressor (T_8 cells) cells.

Fig. 13.1 *Humoral and cell-mediated immune systems.*

Table 13.1
Immunoglobulin classification

	Class (isotype)				
	IgG	IgA	IgM	IgD	IgE
Heavy-chain name	γ (At least four gamma subclasses are known)*	α (At least two alpha subclasses are known)†	μ	δ	ε
Light-chain name	κ or λ in all classes	Several subclasses are known			
Extra chains		J chain and secretory component			
Functions	Activates complement, crosses placenta; main immunoglobulin formed in secondary response	Secretions, immune response to pathogens that enter by respiratory or gastrointestinal tracts	Early antibody, activate complement, powerful agglutinin and haemolysin	? Membrane receptor on lymphocytes	Allergic responses, sensitize mast cells in anaphylaxis
Normal serum concentration (mg%)	700–1500	150–400	60–170	3.0	0.01–0.03

* IgG1, IgG2, IgG3 and IgG4.
† IgA1 and IgA2.
  IgA in serum tends to polymerize to form dimers and larger molecular weight polymers.

delayed hypersensitivity cells (Tdh; these produce lymphokines, short-acting hormones that alter the action of other cells); cytotoxic T-cells (Tc; important in the destruction of graft tissue and virally infected host cells); and memory T-lymphocytes. Macrophages and natural killer (NK) cells are also involved in cell-mediated immunity. IL-2 induces proliferation both of T-cells and NK-cells. Other lymphokines ensure that the concentration of monocytes at the site of the invading microorganism increases and also stimulate increased phagocytosis. In addition they prevent further spread of viral infections; alter fibroblast, macrophage and osteoclast activity; and activate cytotoxic T-cells. NK cells have spontaneous cytotoxicity to virally infected cells.

A further type of cytotoxic lymphocyte (killer or K-cells) is a mediator of cytotoxicity but is also dependent on antibody for killing (antibody dependent cellular cytotoxicity, ADCC).

Phagocytic system
The principal cell types of the phagocytic system are polymorphonuclear leucocytes (PMNLs) and macrophages. Phagocytes adhere to vascular endothelium in inflammatory sites, pass to the site of inflammation by chemotaxis, and engulf (phagocytose) an invading antigen which they destroy with powerful digestive enzymes and oxidizing agents.

Chemotaxis can be influenced both by complement activation (IgG and IgM antibodies activate the classical complement pathway when they react with antigens) and by lymphokines such as macrophage migration inhibition factor (MIF). Phagocytosis is increased by opsonization (coating) of the antigen by antibodies and/or certain complement components (C3b), or by increasing the phagocytic activity of the cells, for example by the action of the lymphokine MAF (macrophage-arming factor; Fig. 13.2).

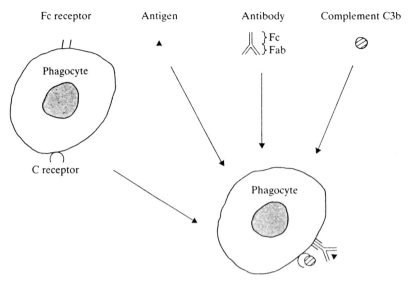

Fig. 13.2 *Phagocytosis. (Courtesy of Professor C. Scully.)*

Complement

This group of plasma glycoproteins serves as a means of amplifying the responses of the immune system. When activated, complement components cause vasodilatation and increased vascular permeability (i.e. inflammation) and can enhance chemotaxis and phagocytosis by PMNLs and macrophages. Complement can be activated via either a classical or alternative pathway. The classical pathway is activated by antigen binding to either IgG or IgM antibodies. The alternative pathway is activated by antigens of high molecular weight (e.g. bacterial and fungal cell walls and lipopolysaccharide or endotoxin), in the absence of antibody (Fig. 13.3), and therefore acts as a defence system even where antibodies are not present, e.g. in neonates who have yet to develop immunity.

When activated by either pathway, complement can enhance leukocyte chemotaxis by increasing blood vessel wall permeability (C3a and C5a) and by producing chemotactic agents (C5a). Phagocytosis by PMNLs and macrophages is increased by the binding of C3b-coated (opsonized) micro-organisms to their cell surface. The activated final product of both complement pathways causes lysis of micro-organisms (Fig. 13.3).

Complement activation, therefore, produces inflammation and, where there is inflammation present, complement has usually been activated.

IMMUNOLOGY OF THE ORAL CAVITY

In the mouth, aspects of both the natural and acquired immune systems protect the teeth, gingiva, mucosa and other tissues.

Natural immunity of the oral cavity

The mucosa prevents penetration of most antigens but the epithelium is permeable to some low molecular weight substances (Chapter 11). Movement of the cheeks, lips and tongue during speech and swallowing ensures that most foreign material is passed backwards to the pharynx and swallowed. This muscular activity is a highly efficient cleaning mechanism and in patients with facial paralysis there is a rapid build-up of oral debris.

Gingival crevicular fluid has a slight washing action, clearing bacteria and debris from the gingival sulcus, and also contains lysozyme and various proteolytic enzymes which may serve a protective function.

Saliva physically deters the attachment of bacteria to oral surfaces, causes their aggregation, has a washing action and, through various non-specific components, has a protective role (Chapter 23). For example, lysozyme breaks down the mucopolysaccharide of bacterial cell walls; thiocyanate and peroxidases convert bacterially derived peroxide into an effective antibacterial agent; and various mucins may be antimicrobial.

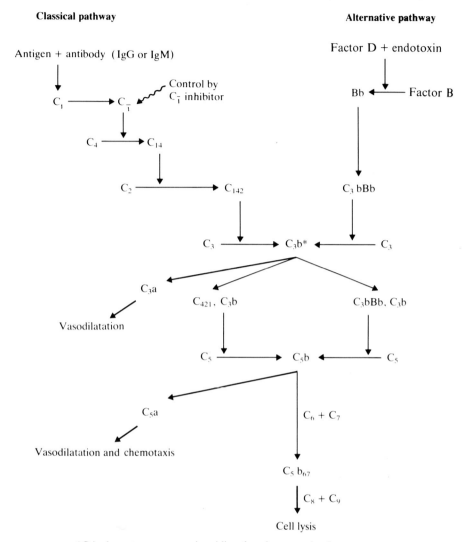

Classical pathway

Antigen + antibody (IgG or IgM)

$C_1 \longrightarrow C_{\bar{1}}$ — Control by $C_{\bar{1}}$ inhibitor

$C_4 \longrightarrow C_{14}$

$C_2 \longrightarrow C_{142}$

$C_3 \longrightarrow C_3b^*$

C_3a

Vasodilatation

C_{421}, C_3b

$C_5 \longrightarrow C_5b$

C_5a

Vasodilatation and chemotaxis

$C_6 + C_7$

$C_5 b_{67}$

$C_8 + C_9$

Cell lysis

Alternative pathway

Factor D + endotoxin

Bb ← Factor B

$C_3 bBb$

C_3

C_3bBb, C_3b

C_5

*C_3b also acts as an opsonin, aiding the phagocytosis of antigens by phagocytes.

Fig. 13.3 *Pathways of complement activation.*

The sensation of taste is a useful protective mechanism, since it ensures harmful agents such as strong acids and alkalis do not reach the gastrointestinal tract. The importance of saliva to oral health is shown by the tendency of patients with dry mouth (xerostomia) to develop caries, candidosis and sialadenitis (Chapter 23).

Acquired immunity of the oral cavity

All immune defences contribute to mucosal defence, and patients with immune defects are liable to develop oral ulcers, infections and periodontal damage (Fig. 13.4). This section discusses features unique to the oral cavity; mucosal immunity is further discussed in Chapter 11.

Saliva (see also Chapter 23)

Saliva contains large amounts of IgA antibodies synthesized by plasma cells in both the major and minor

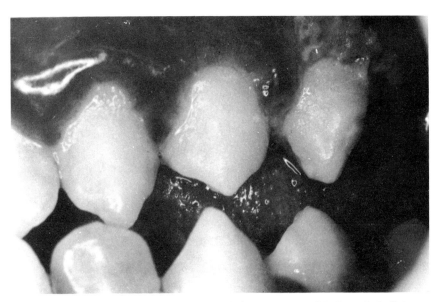

Fig. 13.4 *Gingivitis and ulcers in neutrophil defect. (Courtesy of Professor C. Scully.)*

salivary glands. The acinar cells produce a secretory component (transport piece) which is needed to ensure transport of IgA into the saliva and ensures antibodies are not broken down by salivary or gastric proteolytic enzymes. The main immunoglobulin in saliva is therefore secretory IgA (sIgA) and differs from serum IgA in that it contains secretory component.

IgA antibodies have an agglutinating action and also prevent attachment of bacteria to mucosal surfaces and teeth. Although the exact contribution to oral defence made by salivary IgA antibodies is difficult to estimate, some patients who have IgA deficiency do suffer from oral infections and, conversely, it is possible in animals to induce salivary IgA antibodies to organisms such as *Streptococcus mutans* and protect those animals against experimental caries. This is the basis of some experimental caries vaccines (Volume 3).

Salivary tissue derives its B-cells from the gastro-intestinal-associated lymphoid tissue (GALT) system. This part of the humoral immune system is solely concerned with the production of IgA-type antibodies of mucosal and glandular tissues. The primary response of the GALT system occurs in the lymphoid tissue of the intestine (Peyer's patches). This generates B-lymphocytes which pass to the mesenteric lymph nodes, and eventually to the peripheral circulation. The B-cells then preferentially migrate to the mucosal/glandular tissue and, following differentiation into plasma cells, synthe-

size antibodies specific to the tissue's needs. A major problem with the GALT system is its poor immunological memory, such that secondary immune responses are usually weak and ineffective. This is one of the factors that has hampered the development of a suitable caries vaccine.

Gingival crevice

All aspects of the acquired immune system may be of importance in the protection of the gingival tissues since bacterial colonization of the gingival crevice induces an accumulation within the gingival tissues of polymorphonuclear leucocytes, followed by lymphocytes (particularly B-cells) and plasma cells.

In normal healthy gingival and mucosal tissue there are always a few lymphocytes present (mainly T-cells). In addition, PMNLs constantly migrate from local blood vessels into the gingival crevice and, to a small extent, across mucosa. This normal physiological movement greatly increases when there is bacterial accumulation, since the bacteria and antigen–antibody reactions generate various chemotactically active agents.

Gingival PMNLs may have a protective role. Within a few days of bacterial plaque accumulation they form a layer between the surface of the junctional epithelium and the advancing bacterial front. The gingival PMNLs phagocytose bacteria in the crevice, migrate into the oral cavity and pass to the pharynx. That phagocytes are essential for mucosal health is shown by the fact that patients with low numbers of phagocytes (for example those with neutropenia or agranulocytopenia), and those with poorly functional PMNLs (for example with leukaemia or chronic granulomatous disease) are predisposed to severe gingivitis and rapid periodontal breakdown, as well as oral ulceration (Fig. 13.4).

As well as protecting the gingival tissues, PMNLs may, paradoxically, cause tissue damage since they release small amounts of lysosomal enzymes and oxidizing agents during phagocytosis which may cause some local tissue destruction. Overall, however, gingival PMNLs appear to be protective rather than destructive.

While both T- and B-lymphocytes are present in chronic periodontal lesions, their exact role in periodontal immunology is unknown. Certainly humoral immunity is important, since IgG-type antibodies are always present in gingival fluid. These antibodies are derived both from passive transudation from blood plasma and from local synthesis by plasma cells. When periodontal destruction occurs, levels of antibodies specific for periodontally pathogenic bacteria rise both in serum and gingival fluid. For example, *Actinobacillus actinomycetemcomitans* (Aa) specific antibodies are greatly increased in patients with localized juvenile periodontitis (see Volume 3).

The mechanism of action of IgG antibodies is unclear. *In vitro*, they slow the passage of bacterial toxins across epithelial surfaces and can inactivate many of the tissue-damaging agents produced by bacteria (for example the leucotoxin of Aa). However, they may also accentuate periodontal destruction since, in localized juvenile periodontitis, it has been observed that periodontal lesions in patients with both Aa and specific antibody are more likely to undergo further breakdown than sites where either antibody or antigen alone is present.

Little is known about the role of cell-mediated immunity in periodontal disease. Antigens of periodontal bacteria can induce lymphokine release *in vitro*, but it is not known if this is true *in vivo*. It is conceivable that lymphokines such as osteoclast-activating factor (OAF) as well as other factors such as prostaglandins may indirectly accentuate breakdown of the periodontium.

IMMUNE REACTIONS

Broadly speaking, there are four main types of immune reaction (types I to IV). All are manifestations of a humoral response except type IV which is a cell-mediated reaction (Table 13.2).

Table 13.2
Hypersensitivity reactions

	Type I (anaphylactic)	Type II (cytotoxic)	Type III (toxic complex)	Type IV (cell-mediated)
Mechanism	Antigen causes release of pharmacologic mediators of anaphylaxis from mast cells	Antibody combining with cellular antigens causes activation of complement which causes cytolysis	Antibody and soluble antigen form insoluble complexes that deposit at various sites, and cause activation of complement causing inflammation etc.	Immune lymphoid cell reaction with antigenic cells or proteins causes: (a) direct killing of antigenic cells, (b) production of mediators causing accumulation of monocytes etc., the liberation of lysosomal enzymes and inflammation
Examples	Penicillin allergy, anaphylaxis	Systemic lupus erythematosus, rheumatic fever, pemphigus	Serum sickness (antigen excess) Arthur phenomenon (antibody excess)	Allograft rejection

Type I is an anaphylactic (immediate hypersensitivity) type of response, mediated by IgE antibodies, and is responsible for asthma, angioedema and anaphylaxis. The antigen reacts with IgE antibodies on the surface of mast cells, causing them to release various products, such as histamine and leukotrienes, that cause vasodilatation and bronchoconstriction.

Type II is a cytotoxic type of response, often mediated by complement activation subsequent to binding of IgG or IgM antibodies to antigens on a cell surface. This type of response occurs in autoimmune diseases such as pemphigus.

Type III is an immune complex reaction in which serum complexes (often of antigen and antibody) deposit in tissues. Immune complexes are implicated in many connective tissue diseases where they may, by complement activation, cause lesions.

Type IV (delayed hypersensitivity) is a T-cell-mediated reaction; a classic example is formation of a granuloma such as in tuberculosis, where T-cells accumulate and their lymphokines cause macrophages to accumulate. Some of the macrophages fuse and produce giant cells.

Although four types of immune reaction are distinguished, mixed reactions are implicated in many diseases

FURTHER READING

Dolby A. E. (1986). The host defence system of the mouth. In *Immunological aspects of oral diseases* (L. Ivanyi, Ed.) pp. 1–12. Lancaster: MTP Press.

Chapter 14

The sore mouth: 1. Traumatic and recurrent aphthous ulcers

Most patients make a fairly clear distinction between localized sore areas in the mouth (usually ulcers) and more generalized soreness (usually widespead ulceration, atrophy or inflammation). More problematical are those complaining of soreness of the mouth—usually of the tongue particularly—without any sort of visible lesion; some of these patients have organic disease but in many

Table 14.1
Causes of mouth ulcers

Local causes (e.g. trauma)
Recurrent aphthae (and Behçet's syndrome)
Malignant neoplasms (Chapter 15)
Ulcers associated with systemic disease (Chapter 16)

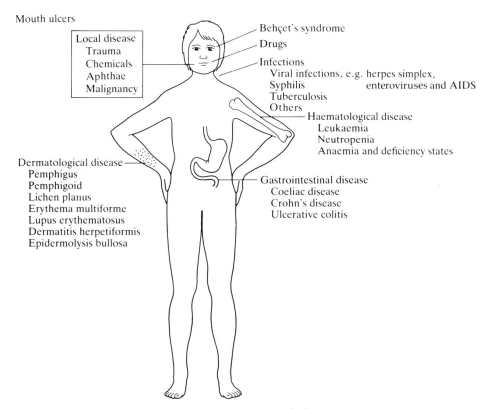

Mouth ulcers

Local disease
Trauma
Chemicals
Aphthae
Malignancy

Behçet's syndrome
Drugs
Infections
  Viral infections, e.g. herpes simplex,
  Syphilis   enteroviruses and AIDS
  Tuberculosis
  Others
      Haematological disease
        Leukaemia
        Neutropenia
        Anaemia and deficiency states

Dermatological disease
  Pemphigus
  Pemphigoid
  Lichen planus
  Erythema multiforme
  Lupus erythematosus
  Dermatitis herpetiformis
  Epidermolysis bullosa

Gastrointestinal disease
  Coeliac disease
  Crohn's disease
  Ulcerative colitis

Fig. 14.1 *Causes of mouth ulcers.*

159

there is a psychogenic basis (Chapter 27). Paradoxically, the common condition of 'denture sore mouth' is rarely sore.

Oral ulcers are the most common cause of a sore mouth. Usually traumatic in origin or of unknown aetiology (aphthous ulcers, aphthae, recurrent aphthous stomatitis) and of little systemic significance, ulcers may also be the result of more serious disease such as malignant neoplasms, infections, disorders of the skin, blood or gastrointestinal tract, or drugs (Table 14.1, Fig. 14.1). Occasionally, ulcers are self-induced by biting or deliberate trauma.

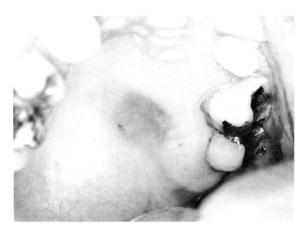

Fig. 14.3 Burn in the palate.

ORAL ULCERATION OF LOCAL AETIOLOGY

Trauma and a range of micro-organisms are ever present in the oral cavity and it is perhaps surprising that oral ulceration due to these factors is not more frequent. Accidental cheek-biting or facial trauma may cause ulceration in any individual; the history is usually quite clear and a single ulcer of short duration (5–10 days) is present. Ulceration due to biting, often of an anaesthetized lower lip or tongue following a dental regional local analgesic, is a common problem in young children (Fig. 14.2 and Volume 1).

Orthodontic appliances or, more commonly, dentures (especially if new) are responsible for many oral ulcers. These ulcers are usually clearly related to the appliance

and will readily heal in a few days if the appliance is removed.

Other local causes of ulceration include burns (Fig. 14.3), especially of the tongue and palate (e.g. pizza burn of the palate), and the holding of medicaments or drugs (e.g. aspirin) against the mucosa.

The possibility of other causes of trauma should always be borne in mind. Child abuse may cause ulcers, especially over the labial fraenae (Volume 1). Self-mutilation may be seen in some psychologically disturbed patients (Fig. 14.4), in some psychiatric diseases, in some mentally handicapped patients, and in some rare syndromes (see Fig. 32.12, and Chapter 33).

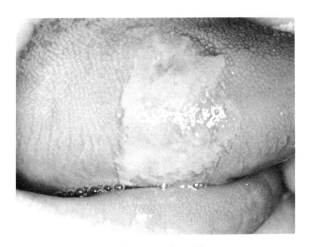

Fig. 14.2 Traumatic ulcer of the tongue.

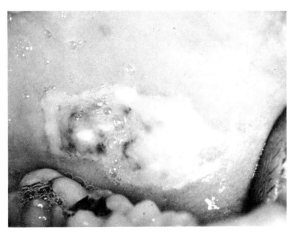

Fig. 14.4 Deliberate cheek-biting in an attention-seeking hysterical patient.

Management

Most ulcers of local cause heal spontaneously within 7 to 10 days if the cause is removed. Maintenance of good oral hygiene and the use of hot saline mouthbaths and a 0.2% chlorhexidine gluconate mouthwash aid healing. A benzydamine mouthwash may give some relief.

Patients should be reviewed within 3 weeks to ensure healing has occurred. *Any ulcer lasting for more than 2–3 weeks should be regarded with suspicion and biopsied if it does not heal after removal of obvious irritants—it may be a neoplasm or other serious disorder.*

RECURRENT APHTHOUS STOMATITIS

Recurrent aphthous stomatitis (RAS) is characterized by episodes of ulcers from childhood or adolescence, each lasting from 1 to about 4 weeks before healing. Aphthae typically are small, round or ovoid ulcers with a circumscribed margin, erythematous halo, and a yellow or grey floor (Fig. 14.5). RAS in most patients resolves spontaneously with age.

This is a common disease which probably afflicts some 20–30% of the population. There is a high prevalence in higher socio-economic classes.

There are three main types of RAS; the most common are minor aphthous ulcers which account for 80% of all RAS. Some 10% of patients with RAS have major aphthous ulcers, and a further 10% suffer from a herpetiform type of ulceration (Table 14.2).

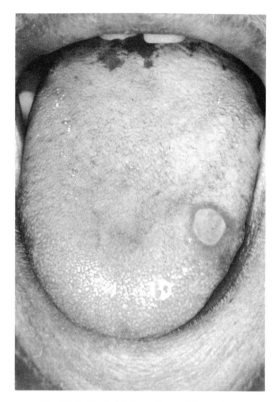

Fig. 14.5 *Typical features of an aphthous ulcer.*

Table 14.2
Main features of recurrent aphthous stomatitis

	Minor aphthae	Major aphthae	Herpetiform ulcers
Age of onset	Childhood or adolescence	Childhood or adolescence	Young adult
Ulcer size	2–4 mm	May be 10 mm	Initially tiny but ulcers coalesce
Number of ulcers	Up to about 6	Up to about 6	10–100
Sites affected	Mainly vestibule, labial, buccal mucosa and floor of mouth; rarely, dorsum of tongue, gingiva or palate	Any site	Any site but often on ventrum of tongue
Duration of each ulcer	Up to 10 days	Up to 1 month	Up to 1 month
Other comments	The most common type of aphthae	May heal with scarring	Affect females predominantly

Clinical features

Minor aphthous ulcers (Mikulicz ulcers)

Minor aphthous ulcers (MiAU or MiRAS) occur mainly in the 10–40-year age group, and often cause minimal symptoms. MiAU are small round or ovoid ulcers, 2–4 mm in diameter, which are found mainly on the non-keratinized mobile mucosa of the lips, cheeks, floor of the mouth, sulci or ventrum of the tongue. They are only uncommonly seen on the keratinized mucosa of the palate or dorsum of the tongue. Only a few ulcers (one to six) appear at a time; they heal in 7–10 days and recur at intervals of 1–4 months. MiAU are round or ovoid in most situations, but are often more linear when in the buccal sulcus—a common site. The ulcer floor is initially yellowish but assumes a greyish hue as healing and epithelialization proceed. The ulcers are surrounded by an erythematous halo and some oedema, but when MiAU heal they leave little or no evidence of scarring (Fig. 14.6).

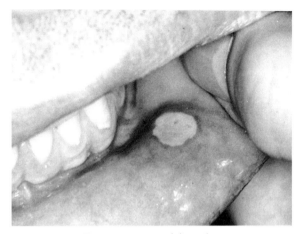

Fig. 14.6 *Minor aphthous ulcer.*

Major aphthous ulcers (Sutton's ulcers)

Previously known as periadenitis mucosa necrotica recurrens (PMNR), major aphthous ulcers (MjAU or MajRAS) tend to be more of a problem to the patient. They are larger, of longer duration, of more frequent recurrence, and often more painful than minor ulcers. They reach a large size, usually about 1 cm in diameter or even larger. MjAU are found on any area of the oral mucosa, including the keratinized dorsum of the tongue or palate. Usually only a few ulcers (one to six) occur at one time; they heal slowly over 10–40 days, and recur extremely frequently. The MjAU are round or ovoid-like minor ulcers, but they are larger and associated with surrounding oedema (Fig. 14.7). The ulcers may heal with scarring (Fig. 14.8). Occasionally a raised erythrocyte sedimentation rate or plasma viscosity is found.

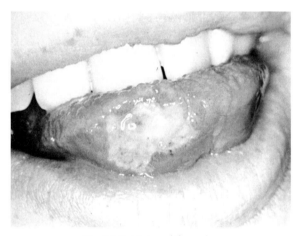

Fig. 14.7 *Major aphthous ulcer.*

Herpetiform ulceration

Herpetiform ulceration (HU) is found in a slightly older age group than the other RAS, and there is a marked female predominance. These ulcers are often extremely painful and recur so frequently that ulceration may be virtually continuous. HU begins with vesiculation which passes rapidly into multiple minute, pinhead sized discrete ulcers (Fig. 14.9). The ulcers, which involve any oral site including the keratinized mucosa, increase in size and coalesce to leave large, round, ragged ulcers which heal in 10 days or longer.

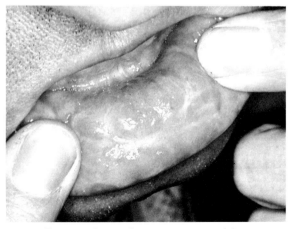

Fig. 14.8 *Scarring from previous major aphthae.*

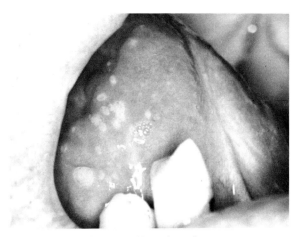

Fig. 14.9 *Herpetiform ulcers.*

Aetiology

The aetiology of RAS is not entirely clear, but many causes have been suggested. A positive family history is found in about one-third of cases and recent reports of an increased frequency of HLA-A2, A11, B12 and DR2 may support a genetic basis for susceptibility to ulceration in some patients.

There are associated factors in some patients (Table 14.3). An important finding is that a minority (about 10%) of patients with RAS have underlying haematological abnormalities, usually a low serum iron or ferritin, or deficiency of folate or of vitamin B12. While in some cases deficiencies may result from poor intake because of the oral ulceration, a number are true deficiencies due to blood loss or a malabsorption state (e.g. some 3% of RAS patients have coeliac disease). Such patients often have a relevant medical history such as gastrointestinal symptoms or a relevant drug history, and their RAS often are of recent onset, possibly at a late age. The patients may have other oral lesions due to the deficiency (e.g. glossitis). The RAS in such patients may respond to correction of the deficiency state, but the cause of the deficiency should always first be established and treated if possible.

There is no evidence that RAS is an autoimmune disease: there is no known association with systemic autoimmune disorders; none of the common autoantibodies is found; and RAS tends to resolve spontaneously with increasing age. In most instances the serum immunoglobulin levels are normal. However, IgA and IgG may be increased and immune complexes may be found in some patients.

Cell-mediated immune mechanisms appear to be involved in the pathogenesis of RAS (Fig. 14.10). Mononuclear cells, T-cells and NK-cells may be involved. In the lesions, T-helper cells predominate early on, with some NK-cells. Cytotoxic cells then appear in the lesions and there is evidence for an antibody-dependent cellular cytotoxicity reaction. It now seems likely that

Table 14.3

Systemic and other factors that may occasionally underly or be associated with recurrent aphthous stomatitis

Factor	Comments
Behçet's syndrome	Association of RAS with uveitis and genital ulcers; a multisystem disease predominantly affecting males; prognosis may be poor
Haematinic deficiency	In some studies, 10–20% of patients with RAS have deficiencies of iron, folic acid or vitamin B12; the cause of the deficiency must be established; replacement therapy *may* help RAS
Gastrointestinal disease	Disorders causing malabsorption of haematinics (pernicious anaemia, coeliac disease and Crohn's disease) may precipitate RAS in a small minority
Endocrine factors	In some women RAS are clearly related to a fall in progestogens in the late (luteal) phase of the menstrual cycle; hormone therapy may be beneficial.
Immunodeficiency	A few patients with RAS have an immune defect such as AIDS
Other factors	Trauma, certain foods, stress and cessation of smoking may play a part

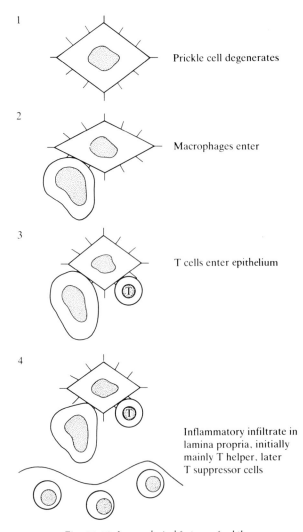

1   Prickle cell degenerates

2   Macrophages enter

3   T cells enter epithelium

4   Inflammatory infiltrate in lamina propria, initially mainly T helper, later T suppressor cells

Fig. 14.10 *Immunological features of aphthae.*

there is a minor degree of immunological dysregulation underlying aphthae.

Attempts to implicate a variety of viruses or bacteria in the aetiology of RAS have largely been unsuccessful, but cross-reacting antigens between the oral mucosa and micro-organisms such as *Streptococcus sanguis* or its L form (lacking a cell wall) may be involved (Table 14.4).

Other aetiological factors in RAS include those related to emotion and trauma, both of which may influence the pattern of ulceration. Cessation of smoking appears to precipitate ulceration in some patients, but the mechanism is unclear. Other patients have ulceration in associ-

ation with the menstrual cycle, while the occasional patient has a food allergy.

Ulcers similar to aphthae may be a manifestation of AIDS or AIDS-related complexes.

Diagnosis

Recurrent aphthous stomatitis is diagnosed on the basis of the history and clinical features. Biopsy is indicated only where some other cause of ulceration is suspected. There are no specific diagnostic tests.

Management

It is important to exclude any systemic involvement such as Behçet's syndrome (see below), or a systemic predisposing factor. Therefore, the history and examination should be directed towards excluding disorders of the skin, eyes, joints, genitalia and gastrointestinal tract. A blood sample should be sent for a full blood picture, haemoglobin, white cell count and differential, red cell indices, iron studies and, possibly, red cell folate and serum vitamin B12, since RAS may be the first or only clinical manifestation of, for example, coeliac disease.

Therapy, while highly effective in some patients, still leaves much to be desired. Underlying predisposing factors should be corrected where possible. Oral hygiene should be maintained at a high standard and is assisted by the use of 0.2% chlorhexidine gluconate aqueous mouthwash. Some patients find one of the numerous available proprietary preparations useful, but for most it is an expensive and frustrating search for relief. A topical tetracycline mouthwash such as a Mysteclin capsule emptied into 5 ml of water (tetracycline 250 mg + nystatin 250 000 units) may be useful in those with HU but, in most cases of RAS, topical corticosteroids are more useful (Table 14.5). Hydrocortisone hemisuccinate (Corlan) pellets 2.5 mg four times daily, and triamcinolone acetonide in carboxymethyl cellulose (Adcortyl in Orabase) four times daily are useful preparations which appear not to cause adrenocortical suppression. Rarely are stronger topical or systemic corticosteroids required.

Fortunately, the natural history of RAS is one of eventual remission in most cases. The occasional patient who relates ulcers to the menstrual cycle or to an oral contraceptive may benefit from supression of ovulation with a progestogen, or a change of oral contraceptive. If there is an obvious relationship to certain foods, these should be excluded from the diet.

Newer therapies for RAS such as carbenoxolone,

Table 14.4
Recurrent aphthous stomatitis: hypotheses on aetiology

Hypothesis	Evidence For	Against
Autoantibodies cytotoxic to oral epithelium	Antibodies to fetal oral mucosa	Not a constant finding; antibodies may be the result, not cause, of ulcers
Antibodies cross-reactive against *Strep. sanguis* or viruses, and mucosa	Cross-reactivity with certain strains only	Reduced cellular response to *Strep. sanguis*
Mononuclear cells cytotoxic to oral epithelium	Cells cytotoxic to epithelium have been isolated	—
Disturbed cellular immunity	Reduced lymphocyte transformation; association of RAS with herpes labialis; association of RAS with immunodeficiencies	—

Table 14.5
Topical corticosteroids for oral use

Examples of topical corticosteroid preparations*	Proprietary name	Dose	Comments
Hydrocortisone hemisuccinate pellets 2.5 mg	Corlan	1 pellet dissolved in mouth q.d.s.	No significant systemic absorption; often effective
Triamcinolone acetonide in Orabase	Adcortyl in Orabase	Apply to ulcer q.d.s.	Adheres best to dried mucosa; also provides mechanical protection; of little value for ulcers on tongue or palate

* More potent steroids may be needed but should only be used in hospital practice because of systemic absorption and possible adrenal suppression.

benzydamine, dapsone, colchicine and thalidomide remain to be fully evaluated and, it is hoped, will be more successful than the recently tried dicromoglycate and levamisole which have not been well accepted by most clinicians.

BEHÇET'S SYNDROME

Not all cases of RAS occur in isolation. An important rare group of patients suffer from Behçet's syndrome—the association of RAS with genital ulceration, eye disease (especially iridocyclitis) and a number of other systemic manifestations (Table 14.6; Fig. 14.11). Most patients are males, usually in their third or fourth decade. There is a high prevalence of Behçet's syndrome in people from around the Mediterranean, the Middle East and Japan.

Recurrent aphthous stomatitis is found in 98% of patients with Behçet's syndrome and is the usual initial manifestation, but only a very small percentage of patients with RAS progress to Behçet's syndrome. At present, it cannot be determined which patients are at risk or when the transition may occur (Fig. 14.12), but recent

Table 14.6
Features of Behçet's syndrome

Oral	Aphthae
Genital	Ulcers
Neuro-ocular	Iridocyclitis Retinal vasculitis Optic atrophy Syndromes resembling disseminated sclerosis, pseudobulbar palsy or neurosyphilis Others
Dermatological	Pustules Erythema nodosum Pathergy
Others	Proteinuria and haematuria Thrombosis of venae cavae Aneurysms Arthralgia

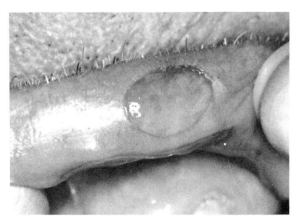

Fig. 14.12 *Aphthous ulcer in Behçet's syndrome.*

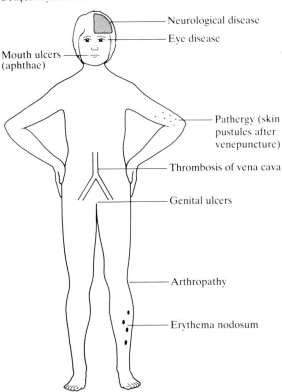

Fig. 14.11 *Main features of Behçet's syndrome.*

Behçet's syndrome

Neurological disease
Eye disease
Mouth ulcers (aphthae)
Pathergy (skin pustules after venepuncture)
Thrombosis of vena cava
Genital ulcers
Arthropathy
Erythema nodosum

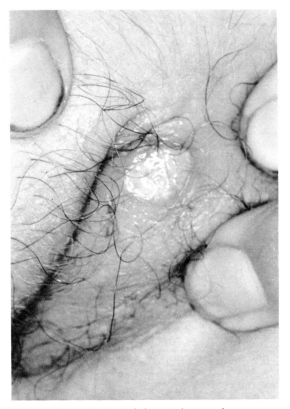

Fig. 14.13 *Genital ulcer in Behçet's syndrome.*

Table 14.7
*Oculomucocutaneous syndromes**

| Disease | Main lesions | | |
	Oral and genital	Ocular	Skin
Behçet's syndrome	Aphthae	Uveitis	Erythema nodosum
Erythema multiforme	Erosions	Erosions	Target lesions
Mucous membrane pemphigoid	Bullae Erosions	Erosions Scarring	Occasional bullae
Reiter's syndrome	Ulcers Urethritis	Conjunctivitis	Keratoderma blenorrhagica

* Ulcerative colitis may also cause oral, cutaneous and eye lesions.

HLA findings, such as the association with HLA B5, BW51 and DR7, and immunological findings may eventually help in this respect.

Genital ulcers are especially common in females with Behçet's syndrome, and resemble RAS (Fig. 14.13). The most common ocular manifestation is relapsing iridocyclitis, but uveitis, retinal vascular changes, and optic atrophy may occur. Both eyes are eventually involved and blindness may result.

Skin lesions (pustules, erythema nodosum), arthropathies, thromboses, neurological lesions, and gastrointestinal involvement may also occur. Venepuncture is, in some patients, followed by pustulation, but this phenomenon (pathergy), said to be characteristic of Behçet's syndrome, is not seen often in UK patients.

Aetiology

As in the focal forms of RAS, the aetiology of Behçet's syndrome is uncertain. There are immunological changes similar to those seen in patients with MiAU and MjAU, with various T-lymphocyte abnormalities (especially T-suppressor cell dysfunction), changes in serum complement, and increased polymorphonuclear leucocyte motility. There is also evidence that mononuclear cells may initiate antibody-dependent cellular cytotoxicity to oral epithelial cells, and evidence of disturbance of NK-cell activity. A viral aetiology (? herpes simplex) has been proposed but remains to be proven. As in RAS, there are weak associations with HLA types.

Many of the features of Behçet's syndrome (erythema nodosum, arthralgia, uveitis) are common to established immune complex diseases and, indeed, immune complexes (usually antigen–antibody complexes) are found in the sera. However, the antigen responsible has not been identified.

Diagnosis

Behçet's syndrome is diagnosed on clinical grounds alone. Activity of the disease may be assessed by serum levels of acute phase proteins or antibodies to intermediate filaments (Chapter 11): both are raised in active Behçet's disease.

Management

In the face of such serious complications, patients with suspected Behçet's syndrome should be referred early on for specialist advice. Other causes of oculomucocutaneous syndromes (Table 14.7) should be excluded. The available therapy includes mainly colchicine, systemic corticosteroids and azathioprine. However, the multiplicity of therapies, now including levamisole, thalidomide, dapsone and cyclosporin, confirms their overall low level of success.

FURTHER READING

Barnes C. G. (1984). Behçet's syndrome. *J. Roy. Soc. Med.*, **77**: 816–819.

Grattan C. E. H., Scully C. (1986). Oral ulceration: a diagnostic problem. *Br. med. J.*, **292**: 1093–1094.

Rennie J. R., Reade P. C., Hay K. D., Scully C. (1985). Recurrent aphthous stomatitis. *Br. dent. J.,* **159**: 361–367.

Rogers R. S. (1981). Recurrent aphthous stomatitis and Behçet's syndrome. In *Immunodermatology* (R. Safai and R. A. Good, Eds.) p. 345. New York: Plenum Press.

Scully C. (1980). Recent advances in oral medicine. *Br. J. Hosp. Med.,* **10**: 490.

Scully C. (1983). An update on mouth ulcers. *Dent. Update,* **10**: 141–152.

Scully C., Cawson R. A. (1987). *Medical problems in dentistry.* Bristol: Wright.

Scully C., Cawson R. A. (1988). *Colour aids to oral medicine.* Edinburgh and London: Churchill-Livingstone.

Scully C., Flint S. (1988). *An atlas of stomatology.* London: Martin Dunitz (in press).

Chapter
15

The sore mouth: 2. Malignant ulcers

Malignant neoplasms may present as mouth ulcers and, even if ulcerated, are often but not always painful. About 90% of oral malignant tumours are squamous carcinomas. Most carcinomas appear to arise in apparently normal mucosa, but a few cases are preceded by clinically obvious premalignant lesions, especially erythroplasia (red patch), leukoplakia (white patch), or a speckled leukoplakia (red and white), and many others are associated with such lesions. Erythroplasia in particular, but also leukoplakia, betel-nut chewing, erosive lichen planus, syphilitic glossitis, submucous fibrosis, iron deficiency or previous oral malignancy may predispose to carcinoma (Chapters 18 and 19).

The most common sites involved by carcinoma are the lower lip, the lateral margin of the tongue and the floor of the mouth. The clinical appearance of carcinomas is highly variable and not all appear as ulcers; they may be in the form of a red or white area, a lump, fissuring or ulceration often with rolled edges (Figs. 15.1–15.9). Lymph node examination is of paramount importance to detect metastases (see Chapter 31). Salivary gland tumours, malignant melanomas, leukaemias, lymphomas, Kaposi's sarcoma and other malignant neoplasms occasionally involve the oral cavity. Usually presenting as a rapidly growing mass which ulcerates. Any chronic lesion should be regarded with suspicion, especially if there are appearances as above, induration, fixation to underlying tissues, any recent changes in appearance, associated lymphadenopathy, or no obvious explanation for the lesion (Fig. 15.10).

A specialist opinion should be sought at an early stage. Pain is a *late* feature in malignancy and any suspicious lesion, including any ulcer not healing within 2–3 weeks, *must* be biopsied.

ORAL SQUAMOUS CARCINOMA

Incidence

Though in Western countries oral cancer accounts for less than 3% of all malignant tumours, it is a significant world health problem. In parts of South East Asia, particularly India, some 40% of malignancy is oral cancer.

Geographic factors

In Asia, the incidence of oral cancer varies widely in

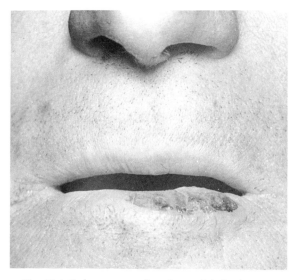

Fig. 15.1 *Early squamous cell carcinoma of the lip showing resemblance to herpes labialis.*

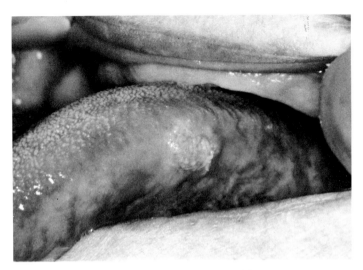

Fig. 15.2 *Early squamous carcinoma of the tongue.*

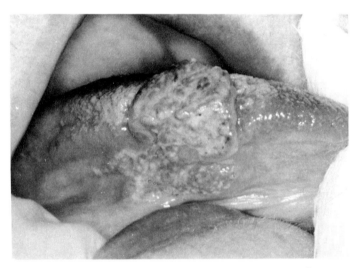

Fig. 15.3 *More advanced squamous carcinoma of the tongue showing multinodular surface. This is the most usual site and appearance of intra-oral carcinoma.*

different areas and in different races within one geographical area.

The incidence of oral cancer in the Western world also varies between countries and between different regions of the same country. Newfoundland, for example, has the highest incidence in the West, with about ten times the incidence of oral carcinoma in the UK. Oral cancer in the UK is more than twice as common in Scotland than in England and Wales and, for example, even within Scotland there are regional differences. In most parts of the UK and elsewhere in the West the incidence of oral cancer has been falling but may now be rising.

The reason(s)—genetic or environmental—for these geographical differences are not yet completely understood. Some possible factors are discussed below.

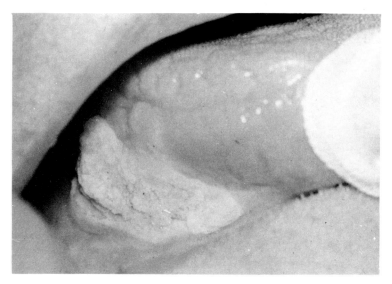

Fig. 15.4 *Carcinoma presenting as a non-ulcerated white lesion. As can be seen, it is difficult to determine whether the origin is on the tongue or floor of mouth.*

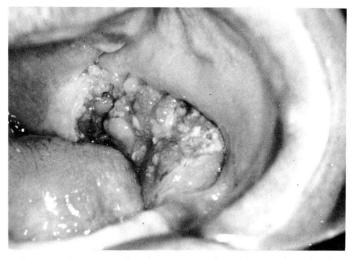

Fig. 15.5 *Carcinoma of buccal mucosa: an indurated lump with a red and white nodular surface.*

Site of tumour

Nearly 30% of all oral cancers affect the lip: some 25% affect the tongue—the common intra-oral site. In some ways labial carcinoma can be regarded as a somewhat different disease to intra-oral carcinoma; lip cancer cer-

tainly has a more defined aetiology and far better prognosis than intra-oral cancers.

The majority of intra-oral cancers involve the lateral border of the tongue and/or the floor of the mouth, but the very invasive nature of these tumours makes difficult the precise definition of the site of origin (Fig. 15.4)

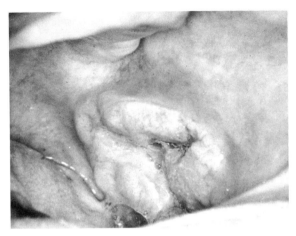

Fig. 15.6 *Carcinoma of buccal mucosa: this carcinoma has a smoother surface than that in Fig. 15.5 with a deep fissure.*

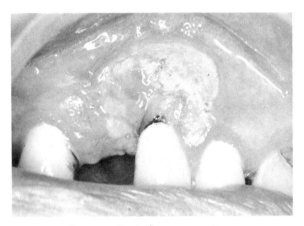

Fig. 15.8 *Gingival squamous carcinoma.*

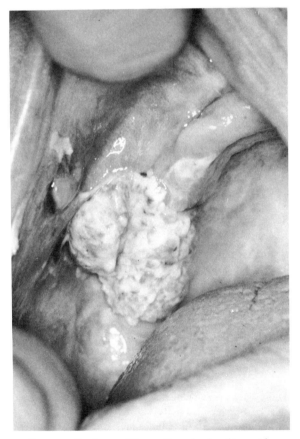

Fig. 15.7 *Carcinoma of the maxillary alveolus: this must be distinguished from an antral carcinoma invading the alveolus (see Chapter 10).*

Nevertheless, most arise from the lower part of the mouth (the 'graveyard area'—see Fig. 15.4), raising questions as to why this site appears predisposed to tumour development (see below).

Aetiology (Fig. 15.11)

The aetiology of oral cancer has not been clearly defined, but often a combination of tobacco, alcohol and liver cirrhosis has been implicated. These and other factors are discussed below.

Premalignancy

In a *minority* of patients who develop oral cancer, the tumour arises from clinically definable premalignant lesions such as erythroplasia, some types of leukoplakia or erosive lichen planus (see Chapters 18 and 19). Many tumours, however, arise from clinically normal mucosa. Premalignant systemic conditions, especially Plummer–Vinson (Patterson–Kelly) syndrome, underly a minority of cases of oral cancer. This syndrome involves the association of iron deficiency with achlorhydria; spoon-shaped nails (koilonychia); and dysphagia due to a post-cricoid web. It predisposes to oral and oesophageal cancer.

Racial factors

Racial factors appear to influence the development of oral cancer, though this may be as much through different habits and environmental factors (e.g. dietary) as through

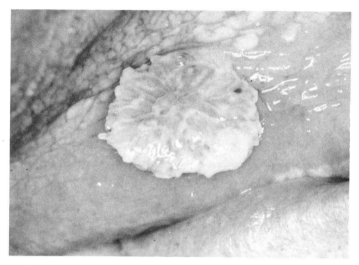

Fig. 15.9 *Exophytic verrucous type of carcinoma showing resemblance to a papilloma.*

Oral carcinoma

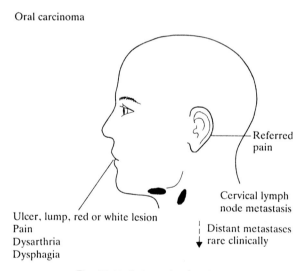

Referred pain

Cervical lymph node metastasis

Ulcer, lump, red or white lesion
Pain
Dysarthria
Dysphagia

Distant metastases rare clinically

Fig. 15.10 *Features of oral carcinoma.*

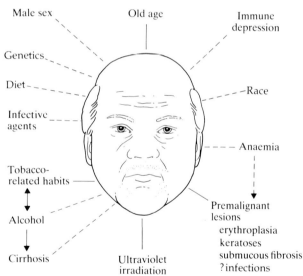

Male sex

Old age

Immune depression

Genetics

Diet

Infective agents

Tobacco-related habits

Alcohol

Cirrhosis

Race

Anaemia

Premalignant lesions
  erythroplasia
  keratoses
  submucous fibrosis
  ?infections

Ultraviolet irradiation

Fig. 15.11 *Factors predisposing to oral squamous carcinoma.*

genetic factors. The traditional way to examine these factors has been to compare tumour incidence rates in racial groups in their homeland and in countries into which they have immigrated. In Singapore, for example, the incidence of oral cancer among Indians is about threefold that of Chinese but about as frequent as in Indians in India. However, a change in place or country of abode does not necessarily lead to changes in local environmental factors (e.g. diet or habits) and, in any event, good controlled studies have yet to be carried out.

In the case of lip cancer in Hong Kong, the incidence is at least fives times higher in Westerners than in the Chinese. However, lip cancer is far less frequent in Westerners living in the West—suggesting that the difference is environmental, probably actinic radiation from the ultraviolet of sunlight (see below).

In the British Isles the highest prevalence of oral cancer seems to be amongst the Celtic descendants, but environmental factors (for example smoking and alcohol consumption) might be responsible.

There appear to be no large-scale studies into the genetic basis (if any) of oral cancer.

Age

Oral cancer in the West predominantly affects those between the ages of 55 and 75 years. Whether this age factor is a function of a long latent period following exposure to some cancer-producing (oncogenic) agent or to chronic exposure to an agent, or whether it is related to some decrease in host resistance, such as the decreasing immune responses in old age, is unclear. Oral cancer is occasionally seen in younger persons and it is interesting that it may be a *rare* complication of the acquired immune deficiency syndrome (AIDS, Volume 1).

Sex of patient

Over the past 50 years or so there has been a gradual decline in overall incidence of oral cancer in the West (see above), almost entirely due to a decline in the number of males affected. Earlier in the century, oral cancer affected males ten times more frequently than females but this ratio has dropped to the extent that the incidence in males is now less than double that in females in many countries. For most sites affected the ratio is changing towards equal incidences in males and females.

Questions again arise as to the reason(s) for the change in sex distribution (see below).

General health and defensive responses

Chronic renal failure appears to predispose to oral leukoplakia and there are associations between liver dysfunction and oral cancer. Animal studies have shown that liver damage (by various factors, including alcohol) can enhance chemically induced oral cancer.

Iron deficiency in humans, as in the Patterson–Kelly (Plummer–Vinson syndrome) of sideropenia, achlorhydria and glossitis, appears to predispose to oral, pharyngeal and oesophageal carcinoma. In animals, iron deficiency appears to accelerate chemically induced oral carcinogenesis. Other dietary factors such as vitamin A may be protective.

Patients with acquired immune deficiency syndrome may rarely develop oral cancer (Volume 1). There is no good evidence of a relationship between oral cancer and other immune deficiency states, although there is a predisposition to lip carcinoma in patients with drug-induced immunosuppression. Patients with oral cancer have a range of immune defects but some might be secondary to the disease and do not necessarily predispose to the tumour.

Host responses of *some* kind must, to a degree, be influential on cancer development since there are differences in predisposition to malignancy between humans existing in identical environmental conditions and differences in susceptibility of different animals to carcinogens.

Environmental factors

Traditionally, oral cancer has been said to be caused by smoking, spirits and spices, as well as syphilis and sepsis. The evidence is reviewed here.

Habits

1. *Pipe smoking.* In the UK, pipe smoking may be associated with nicotinic stomatitis (Chapter 19), a benign non-premalignant condition. There is some evidence from other countries that pipe smoking may be associated with a predisposition to lip carcinoma.

2. *Cigarette smoking.* Smokers of more than 40 cigarettes per day appear to be about five times more likely to develop oral cancer than are non-smokers. The precise role of cigarette smoking in oral cancer is surprisingly difficult to define, not least because many heavy smokers also drink alcohol and can have other complicating factors. However, studies of those who abstain from such habits (e.g. Mormons, Seventh Day Adventists) have shown a lower incidence of oral cancer in those groups. Smoking and alcohol appear to have a synergistic effect in the aetiology of oral cancer. Nevertheless, it has to be remembered that the increasing incidence of smoking since the Second World War has been associated with a falling rate of oral cancer in males.

Reverse smoking—where the lighted end is held in the mouth, as in parts of India—is linked with a high incidence of oral cancer, particularly of the hard palate, an otherwise unusual site.

3. *Cigar smoking.* Cigar smoking may predispose to oral cancer and some studies have shown an association with floor of mouth leukoplakia in woman cigar smokers (Chapter 19).

4. *Bidi smoking.* Bidi is a type of cigarette made of tobacco rolled in a dried temburni leaf. It is smoked in India and emits larger amounts of potential carcinogens than most Western cigarettes. Bidi smoking is associated with a high incidence of leukoplakia, particularly at the commissures, and oral cancer.

5. *Tobacco chewing.* Tobacco chewing predisposes to oral cancer in Western countries. In parts of Asia, tobacco is chewed or held in the mouth for long periods, along with a variety of ingredients in a 'betel quid'. This often contains betel vine leaf, betel nut, catachu, and slaked lime together with tobacco. This habit appears to predispose to oral cancer, particularly when it is started early in life and is used frequently and for prolonged periods. In Pakistan, for example, betel chewing together with smoking increases the risk of oral cancer by about 25 times.

6. *Snuff dipping.* Women in the south-east of the USA who place snuff in the buccal sulcus have been shown to be predisposed to developing gingival and alveolar carcinoma close to where the snuff is placed. Currently there is concern that the use of smokeless tobacco such as Skoal-Bandits may predispose to similar lesions (Fig. 15.12).

7. *Mouthwashes.* There have been suggestions, based on a very small number of patients, and which further studies have failed to confirm, that the frequent use of proprietary alcohol-containing mouthwashes over prolonged periods predisposes to oral cancer, but only in those patients who neither smoke nor drink alcohol.

8. *Alcohol.* Several, but not all, studies have shown an association between high alcohol consumption and oral cancer. Many alcoholic drinks contain cogeners and some local brews may contain carcinogens that are responsible for oral cancer. For example, in parts of France, such as Brittany, there is a close relationship between the consumption of the alcoholic drink Calvados (a pot-stilled spirit) and cancer of the oesophagus and mouth. Indeed, Brittany has the highest incidence of oral cancer in Western Europe.

Again it should be noted that many patients who may drink alcohol heavily may have liver dysfunction and may also smoke tobacco a great deal.

Oral sepsis

There is evidence that chronic mucosal irritation in animals enhances chemically-induced oral carconoma. Many patients with oral carcinoma have oral cancerous lesions closely related to a denture flange or to a sharp or carious tooth, but there is no study that unequivocally demonstrates that these dental factors are aetiological. However, oral cancer is uncommon in a well-cared-for mouth.

The relationship may be more with smoking and drinking habits of patients with oral carcinoma who also may have a low interest in oral hygiene and oral care. Nevertheless there are anecdotal case reports of oral cancer apparently related to chronic irritation.

Occupational factors

The relationship between buccal cancer and snuff dipping, a habit practised because of a ban on smoking at work, is discussed above. The relationship between lip cancer and exposure to sunlight in outdoor workers is dicussed below.

Some workers in the UK textile industry are at risk from oral cancer, apparently related to exposure to dust from carding raw cotton and wool. Woodworkers are predisposed to develop carcinoma of the paranasal sinuses, especially ethmoid cancer, but also antral carcinoma.

Infective agents

Syphilis

Tertiary syphilis may cause a diffuse glossitis or keratosis—particularly of the dorsum of the tongue (Chapter 19). However, although early studies showed positive syphilis serology in a small minority of patients with oral carcinoma, they failed to point out that this was not higher than in control patients without oral cancer. Many patients with tertiary syphilis (now rare) were also

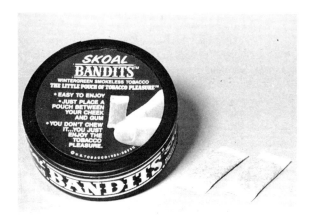

Fig. 15.12 *Smokeless tobacco.*

heavy smokers and drinkers, factors equally likely to be incriminated in the aetiology of oral cancer. Arsenicals or other agents used in the treatment of syphilis may have been implicated.

Candida albicans

Some leukoplakias, especially commissural and speckled leukoplakias (the more highly premalignant forms), may be infected with *C. albicans*. This appears not to be simply a secondary infection of a damaged, already dysplastic, epithelium, but *C. albicans* may induce the dysplasia.

Viral infections

There is very weak evidence of an association between herpes simplex virus and oral carcinoma, particularly labial carcinoma. Recurrent herpetic lesions and labial carcinoma often present at similar sites and there are anecdotal reports of development of carcinoma at sites of recurrent herpes labialis. There is some serological evidence of higher titres of herpes antibodies in oral cancer patients than in controls, but these seem related to smoking habits. The evidence at present does not necessarily implicate nor exonerate herpes simplex in the aetiology. In tissue culture, the virus can induce malignant transformation.

Papillomaviruses have been detected in some leucoplakias and some oral cancers but are also found in other non-malignant lesions, and their role, if any, in oncogenesis of oral cancer is unclear.

Other oncogenic viruses such as adenoviruses have been proven not to be associated with oral cancer.

In contrast there is evidence associating various herpesviruses with other malignant neoplasms of the head and neck. Epstein–Barr virus is strongly implicated in the development of Burkitt's lymphoma and in nasopharyngeal carcinoma. Cytomegalovirus may be implicated in Kaposi's sarcoma.

Actinic radiation

There is a higher incidence of lip cancer in outdoor workers and rural populations than in office workers or urban populations, indicating a relationship with exposure to sunlight (and ultraviolet irradiation). In Newfoundland, for example, the incidence of lip cancer is four times higher in fishermen than in males of similar age but different occupation.

Other studies have shown the predisposition of fair-skinned people to develop lip cancer (as well as skin cancer and melanoma) in sunny climates. The fact that lip cancer involves the more exposed lower lip rather than the upper lip also supports a relationship with actinic radiation.

This is not an entirely unequivocal finding, however, and recent studies have shown variations in incidence in three southern USA cities on the same latitude, and a *lower* incidence of lip cancer in the sunnier parts of Finland.

PROGNOSIS FOR ORAL CANCER

Despite the fact that oral cancer should be one of the most readily detected neoplasms because of the easy access for clinical and biopsy examination, the prognosis of intra-oral carcinoma is still little better than that for lung cancer, i.e. a five-year survival of only about 30%.

The following factors adversely influence prognosis.

1. *Site of tumour.* The prognosis is worst where the floor of mouth, alveolus, posterior tongue or maxilla is involved. Conversely, carcinoma of the lip has an excellent prognosis, with a five-year survival of over 70%.

2. *Stage.* Most oral cancer presents at a stage when there is little clinical evidence of local metastases to lymph nodes. Only very rarely are distant metastases detectable at presentation. Nevertheless, most tumours are relatively advanced (T2 or more: considering they should be detectable at a much earlier stage. The larger the size of the tumour and the presence of metastases also adversely affect prognosis.

Patients are still presenting and being referred for treatment after inordinate delays of months or years, while some practitioners try in vain to treat persistent ulcers with a variety of medications, failing to appreciate the seriousness of the situation.

Any ulcer, unusual lump, red patch or white patch or enlarged cervical node which persists for more than 3 weeks should be seen by a specialist, who will almost invariably biopsy the lesion.

3. *Histological lack of differentiation.* Poorly differentiated or anaplastic carcinomas appear to have a worse prognosis than well-differentiated tumours.

4. *Sex of patient.* The prognosis is usually worse for male patients—possibly because of the somewhat later presentation for treatment, or because of associated medical problems. Many patients with oral cancer are heavy smokers and drinkers, and some have cirrhosis and nutritional defects.

5. *Age of patient.* The poor general health of some aged patients may limit their resistance to the disease or its

treatment. Age may necessitate modification in therapy leading to less effective treatment of the neoplasm, but, apart from this, age *per se* does not appear to influence survival.

Treatment

The major impact that treatment has had on the prognosis of oral cancer to date has been in relation to improved anaesthetic and medical care. Surgical reconstruction has also been markedly improved and there are fewer side-effects from modern radiotherapy.

DIAGNOSIS OF ORAL CANCER

Any patient with an ulcer, unusual lump, red patch or white patch or enlarged cervical lymph node that persists for more than 3 weeks should be suspected of having a neoplasm until proven otherwise (see Fig. 15.10).

Inspection and examination

Features which suggest malignancy include the following.

1. The presence of erythroplasia.
2. A granular appearance or an ulcer with fissuring or raised exophytic margins.
3. The presence of abnormal blood vessels supplying a lump.
4. Induration beneath a lesion, i.e. a firm infiltration beneath the mucosa, or hardness in a lymph node.
5. Fixation of the lesion (or node) to deeper tissues or to overlying skin or mucosa.
6. Cervical lymph node enlargement (see below; Figs. 15.13–15.15).

As always, the whole mucosa should be examined as there may be widespread dysplastic mucosa ('field change') or even a second neoplasm (Fig. 15.16), and the cervical lymph nodes must be examined for enlargement, hard consistency or fixation to deeper tissue. Enlarged nodes in a patient with oral carcinoma may be caused by infection, reactive hyperplasia secondary to the tumour, or metastatic disease (see also Chapter 31).

Biopsy (Volume 1)

An incisional biopsy is invariably required. The biopsy should be sufficiently large to include enough suspect and apparently normal tissue to give the pathologist a chance

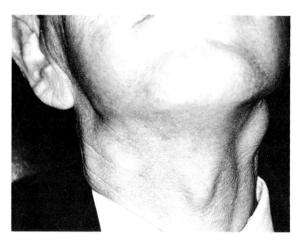

Fig. 15.13 *Cervical lymph node metastasis in a patient with oral squamous carcinoma.*

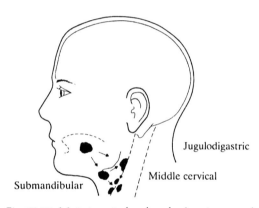

Fig. 15.14 *Mestastases to lymph nodes from tumours of lateral border of tongue/floor of mouth. (Lesions near midline may metastasize bilaterally.)*

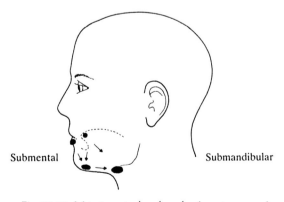

Fig. 15.15 *Metastases to lymph nodes from tumours of lower lip or tip of tongue. (Lesions near midline may metastasize bilaterally.)*

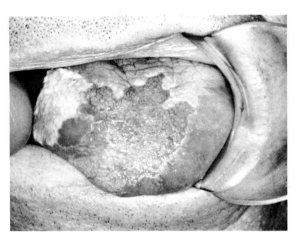

Fig. 15.16 *'Field change': this patient has already had a carcinoma of the right buccal mucosa, excised and skin grafted. He now has mixed white and red lesions over the whole tongue and in both buccal mucosae. Biopsy of the red lesion revealed a second carcinoma.*

to make a diagnosis and not to have to request a further specimen. Most patients tolerate (physically *and* psychologically) *one* biopsy session, although it is never a particularly pleasant experience. Most biopsy wounds,, whether 0.5 cm (too small) or 1.5 cm long (usually adequate), heal within 7–10 days. Therefore it is better to take at least one ample specimen. Since red rather than white areas are most likely to show dysplasia, a biopsy should be taken of the former.

If the pathology report denies malignancy, and yet clinically that is still the diagnosis, then a re-biopsy is indicated. Some clinicians always take several biopsies at the first visit in order to avoid the delay and aggravation resulting from a negative pathology report for a patient who is strongly suspected to be suffering from a malignant neoplasm.

Various attempts to highlight clinically probable dysplastic areas before biopsy, e.g. by the use of toluidine blue dye, have, unfortunately, not proved to be reliable, but may be of some help where there is widespread 'field change'.

An *excisional* biopsy should be avoided unless the lesion is minute since this is unlikely to have excised an adequately wide margin of tissue if the lesion *is* malignant, but will have destroyed for the surgeon or radiotherapist clinical evidence of the site and character of the lesion.

Exfoliative cytology of oral mucosal lesions is, by and large, valueless. It cannot be depended upon to give a reliable diagnosis in any of the serious disorders (e.g.

carcinoma, pemphigus) for which it has, in the past, been recommended, and it is time-consuming. Virtually the only value is to increase the pathologist's revenue!

Suspect lymph nodes are best biopsied by *needle* biopsy, using a fine-bore needle to aspirate cells for cytological examination. False negative results are possible, but the danger of incisional biopsy is that it may seed malignant cells into the wound. In practical terms, ipsilateral enlarged regional lymph nodes in a patient with an obvious oral carcinoma are likely to include metastases (or at least micrometastases) and will need treatment.

REFERRAL TO A SPECIALIST

One of the most difficult clinical situations in which to find oneself is with the patient in whom you suspect serious disease and who insists (rightly) on a full explanation as to why you wish to refer him for a second opinion. As you do *not* know for sure, it is unwise for you to suggest a serious diagnosis to the patient. Better that you admit ignorance about the field and say that you are trained more to be suspicious but doubt the lesion is anything to worry about, though you would be failing in your duty if you did not ask for a second opinion. That is what you would do for a member of your family—why should the patient be treated any the less? If you *are* concerned phone or write for an *urgent* opinion.

TISSUE CHANGES IN CARCINOMA

The essential feature distinguishing carcinoma from premalignant lesions is the *invasion* of malignant epithelium through the basement membrane and into deeper tissues in carcinoma. A variety of epithelial cellular abnormalities and disordered stratification (dysplasia, dyskeratosis, or atypia) are also present (Figs. 15.17–15.20). Invading carcinoma cells infiltrate the lamina propria and spread in many directions to underlying tissues such as muscle and bone. Histological sections show finger-like projections of the tumour into deeper tissues, with irregular 'islets' where projections have been sectioned at different angles. In more highly differentiated tumours, premature keratinization results in concentric rings of keratin (cell nests) (Fig. 15.20).

Cellular abnormalities include the presence of cells of varying size and shape (pleomorphism), and intense nuclear staining (hyperchromatism), often with prominent nucleoli, indicating active protein synthesis. The

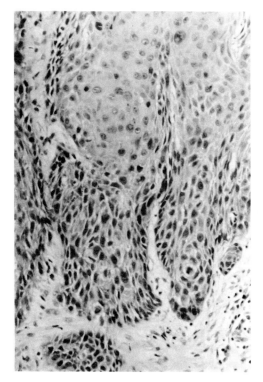

Fig. 15.17 *Epithelial dysplasia showing disordered stratification, cellular pleomorphism and increased nuclear:cytoplasmic ratio of malignant cells.*

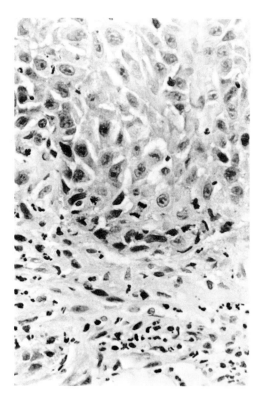

Fig. 15.18 *Epithelial atypia showing also abnormal and multiple mitoses, and enlarged nucleoli.*

nuclei enlarge at the expense of the cytoplasm (increased nuclear:cytoplasmic ratio) and there is evidence both of frequent and bizarre cell division (increased mitoses and abnormal mitoses) (Figs. 15.7–15.20).

Disordering of the epithelium in carcinoma makes it difficult for the pathologist to identify clearly separate basal and spinous layers (irregular stratification). The nuclei are in unusual positions within the cells (loss of polarity) and there is loss of intercellular adherence. These features are evidence of disordered maturation.

The lamina propria is not simply passive during the invasion by the malignant epithelium, but responds with an inflammatory reaction showing an infiltrate of mononuclear cells (lymphocytes and macrophages and a few plasma cells). Opinions vary as to whether these cells effectively function in defence against tumours or, indeed, whether they facilitate spread, but the prognosis appears better where there is a dense mononuclear cell infiltrate.

The tumour metastasizes primarily via the lymphatics (Fig. 15.21).

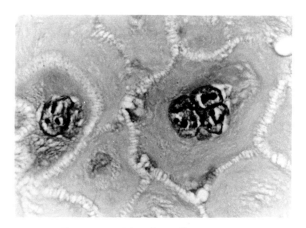

Fig. 15.19 *Multinucleate cells in carcinoma.*

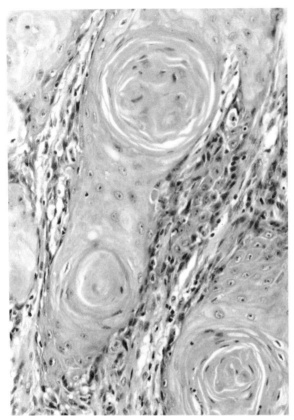

Fig. 15.20 *Cell nests in squamous carcinoma.*

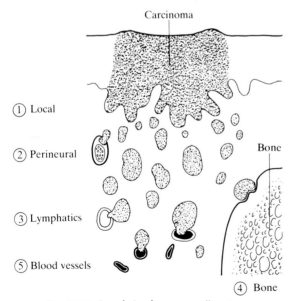

Fig. 15.21 *Spread of oral squamous cell carcinoma.*

MANAGEMENT OF ORAL CANCER

Cancer to many, if not most, patients is a term that forebodes disaster—not unreasonably, since most have had relatives or friends who have died of the disease. The prognosis, at least of intra-oral carcinoma, is not especially good, but little is gained by expressing this to the patient or relative. On the other hand, early lesions in otherwise healthy patients, especially those in sites such as the lip, have such a good prognosis that they can be said to be 'curable'. Therefore, when the diagnosis has been established, it is reasonable to discuss with patient and relatives that:

(a) tumours differ in their degree of malignancy;
(b) their tumour has been detected at an early stage (hopefully);
(c) treatment is continually improving;
(d) you have referred them to the best possible centre for treatment.

You must leave discussion of actual treatment to the surgeon/oncologist concerned, as only he or she is in a position to give accurate facts to the patient.

TREATMENT OF ORAL CANCER

The treatment of oral cancer involves one or a combination of:

(a) radiotherapy,
(b) surgery, and occasionally
(c) chemotherapy.

The many variables, such as local resources, expertise and referral patterns, as well as the variable nature of oral cancer patients in terms of, for example, site, stage of disease and medical problems, mean that there have been very few unequivocal controlled trials of treatment.

A most important factor in deciding the modality or combination to be used should always be to ensure that the cure is better than the disease, i.e. the *quality* of life should be considered rather than simply the quantity.

Patients with oral cancer who die of their disease will almost always do so either because of failure to control the primary tumour or because of metastatic tumour in the cervical lymph nodes. Death due to distant metastasis is unusual. This means that in planning treatment for a patient with oral cancer, the regional lymph nodes must be considered. Thirty per cent of patients present with palpably enlarged cervical lymph nodes with meta-

Table 15.1

Factors influencing choice of treatment modality	Choice of treatment
Site of tumour	
Lip	Radiotherapy or surgery can give up to 90% cure
Tip of tongue	Radiotherapy often used for moderate-sized lesions; surgery used for very small or very large lesions
Lateral tongue	Surgery used for very small or very deep lesions or where bone involved; radiotherapy for other lesions
Floor of mouth	Radiotherapy often preferred except for large tumours with bone involvement where surgery and radiotherapy used
Buccal mucosa	Radiotherapy often preferred
Bone involvement	Surgery preferred
Field change present	Surgery preferred
Cervical lymph node involvement	Radiotherapy plus surgery often preferred
Verrucous carcinoma	Surgery preferred

stases and, of those who do not, a further 25% will go on to develop metastases in nodes within 2 years. For many patients, therefore, their initial treatment must include treatment of the lymph nodes in the neck. For patients with clinically enlarged nodes, the treatment of choice is radical neck dissection, with postoperative radiotherapy if there is extracapsular spread or multiple node involvement. The neck dissection is continued upwards to include the primary site in continuity if the primary cancer is of the tongue, floor of mouth or lower alveolus.

In view of the high incidence of subsequent lymph node metastases, there is debate as to whether even a patient with no enlarged cervical lymph nodes should be treated prophylactically. However, although prophylactic neck dissection has been advocated, this concept has not been universally accepted since it is a procedure with considerable morbidity and there is little actual evidence of improved survival or cure rates. Moderate-dose radiotherapy (40 Gray) is sometimes used to 'sterilize' such necks.

It is only for primary cancers without obvious lymph node involvement or for inoperable tumours that radiotherapy is used as the sole modality of treatment for oral carcinoma (Table 15.1).

Chemotherapy is, at present, of very limited value in the treatment of oral cancer, and most centres use a combination of radiotherapy and surgery. A few salient points are discussed below.

Radiotherapy

The advantages of radiotherapy include:

(a) cure without the disadvantages of surgery—in *some* patients;

(b) even if radiotherapy fails, surgery can still be used.

Disadvantages include mainly:

(a) the fact that surgery is more difficult and hazardous on tissues that have been irradiated;

(b) the immediate and later side-effects of radiotherapy (see Volume 1 and p. 182)—these are somewhat reduced with modern techniques.

Radiotherapy can be given by either of the following.

1. External beam radiation (or teletherapy) by supervoltage therapy using:
    telecobalt (rays of over 1 megavolt, MV), or
    linear accelerator (x-rays of over 4 MV), or
    betatron (electron beam of over 8 MV).
2. Interstitial therapy (or plesiotherapy) by radionuclide implants of iridium-192 (or occasionally caesium-137).

In general, plesiotherapy (Fig. 15.22) is both more effective than teletherapy and causes fewer complications, but its use is limited by local anatomy. There have been attempts to improve the efficacy of teletherapy by

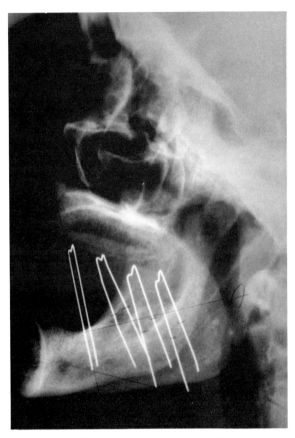

Fig. 15.22 *Radionuclide needle implants (iridium wire) in the tongue to irradiate a carcinoma of the tongue.*

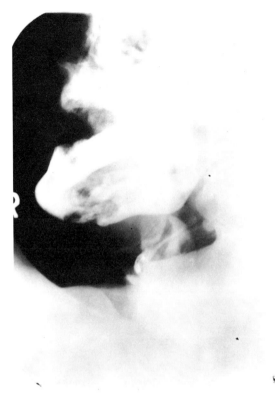

Fig. 15.23 *Osteoradionecrosis of the mandible.*

increasing the sensitivity of tumour cells to radiation by raising the oxygen concentration within the tumour (by hyperbaric oxygen or by infusions of hydrogen peroxide); by using electron-affinic chemicals (radio-sensitizers such as vitamin K analogues or misonidazole); or by using radiation that depends less on the presence of oxygen within the tumour for it to be tumoricidal (neutron therapy). Neutron therapy, however, actually offers little advantage except that bone is damaged less.

Dental management of patients receiving radiotherapy to the head and neck

The complications of dental treatment after radiotherapy (especially after teletherapy) can be such that planned treatment must be carried out before irradiation. Oral hygiene should be meticulous, preventive dental care

instituted and restorative procedures carried out at this stage.

1. *Extractions.* Necrosis of bone and the jaw, particularly the mandible, is a potentially serious complication of irradiation endarteritis. Dental extractions can lead to intractable osteomyelitis (Chapter 4 and Volume 1).

Irradiation-associated osteomyelitis (osteoradionecrosis: Fig. 15.23) may also occasionally be precipitated by mucosal ulceration caused by a denture and therefore some specialists even refuse to permit patients to wear dentures.

Osteoradionecrosis is not such a serious problem now, as megavoltage radiotherapy has less effect on bone than did orthovoltage therapy. Osteoradionecrosis appears to develop mainly in patients receiving more than 60 Gray, particularly to the floor of the mouth and mandible. Osteomyelitis may follow months or years after radiotherapy, and is heralded by pain and swelling. The area of involved bone is often small (less than 2 cm diameter) and, with antibiotics, the signs and symptoms of

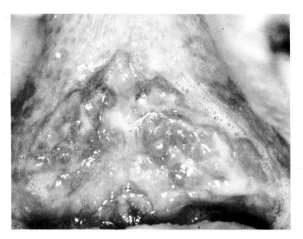

Fig. 15.24 *Radiation mucositis and xerostomia after external beam radiotherapy involving the mouth and salivary glands.*

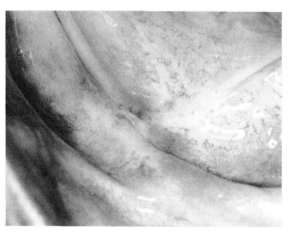

Fig. 15.25 *Post-radiation scarring and telangiectasia in the floor of the mouth.*

inflammation may clear within a few weeks. Complete resolution can, however, take 2 or more years.

Most patients with oral carcinoma are of middle age or over and many have poorly maintained dentitions. In such patients, teeth in the radiation path should be extracted or a total clearance may be preferable. It is not always necessary to extract all the teeth before radiotherapy. The patient may have such a healthy dentition and such good oral hygiene that dental complications are unlikely. Alternatively, clearance before irradiation may not be practicable, because the patient is too old or ill, or the prognosis is too poor.

The time interval permitted between extractions and radiotherapy is invariably a compromise because of the need to start radiotherapy. No bone should be left exposed in the mouth when radiotherapy begins since, once the blood supply is damaged by radiotherapy, wound healing is jeopardized. An interval of at least 2 weeks between extracting the teeth and starting radiotherapy is advised. If the patient has already completed radiotherapy, extractions should be carried out before endarteritis obliterans becomes established, i.e. within 6 months of the irradiation.

If extractions are unavoidable, trauma should be kept to a minimum, raising the periosteum as little as possible and ensuring that sharp bone edges are removed. Prophylactic antibiotics should be given in adequate doses for 4 weeks at least.

2 *Mucositis.* Mucosal erythema, followed by sloughing with pain, dysphagia and soreness, becomes maximal 2–4 weeks after radiotherapy starts, but usually subsides in a further 2–3 weeks after completion (Fig. 15.24). Scarring and dilated capillaries (telangiectasia) may later be seen (Fig. 15.25).

Mucositis may be relieved by using warm normal saline mouthwashes and lignocaine viscous 2%. A 0.2% aqueous chlorhexidine mouthwash maintains oral hygiene and a benzydamine rinse or saliva substitute such as carboxymethylcellulose may provide some symptomatic relief, particularly at meal times.

3. *Xerostomia.* Radiotherapy of tumours of the naso- and oropharynx is especially liable to damage the salivary glands, depress salivary secretion and result in saliva of higher viscosity but lower pH (see Fig. 15.24). Salivary secretion diminishes within a week of radiotherapy, but some salivary function may return after many months.

The dryness of the mouth is managed as for Sjögren's syndrome (Chapter 25), but palliation with liberal use of artificial saliva is usually the best that can be achieved.

4. *Loss of taste.* Hypogeusia (loss of taste) follows radiation damage to the taste buds. Taste may start to recover within 2–4 months. If more than 60 Gray have been given, loss of taste is usually permanent.

5. *Infections.* Xerostomia predisposes to inflammatory periodontal disease, caries, oral candidosis and ascending acute sialadenitis (see Chapters 24 and 25).

6. *Radiation caries and dental hypersensitivity.* Patients frequently take a sloppy cariogenic diet because of the dry sore mouth and loss of taste. Irradiation also directly

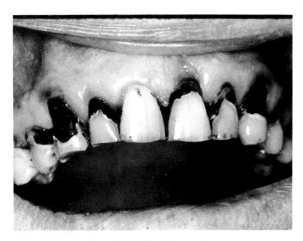

Fig. 15.26 *Radiation caries.*

damages the teeth, which may become hypersensitive. These factors combine to cause rampant dental caries, involving any site, including incisal edges and cervical margins. Caries begins at any time between about 2 and 10 months after radiotherapy, and may eventually result in the crown breaking off the root (Fig. 15.26).

Radiation caries and dental hypersensitivity can be controlled with daily topical fluoride applications (sodium fluoride mouthwash, stannous fluoride gel or acidulated fluoride phosphate gel). Occasionally, full-cover acrylic splints are used to protect the teeth. Patients must be given practical guidance about diet, with avoidance of sweets and sweet confectionery and the use of sugar substitutes (e.g. saccharin) whenever possible.

Mucosal trauma from dentures may predispose to osteomyelitis and some specialists therefore insist that dentures be abandoned. If dentures are required, they should be fitted at about 6 months after radiotherapy, when initial mucositis subsides and there is only early fibrosis.

7. *Candidosis.* Candidosis is common after radiotherapy. Antifungal drugs such as miconazole gel 250 mg/5 ml, or nystatin suspension 100 000 u/ml as a mouthwash should be given four times daily.

8. *Trismus.* Progressive endarteritis following radiotherapy leads to replacement fibrosis of the masticatory muscles, apparent 3–6 months after radiotherapy. Trismus may be reduced by instituting jaw-opening exercises with tongue spatulas or wedges used three times a day.

Surgery

Advantages of surgery include the following.

1. There is the possibility of complete excision and histological examination of the tumour with a wide margin of healthy tissue, particularly where bone is involved.

2. There is the possibility of excision and histological examination of enlarged cervical lymph nodes.

3. It can be used for radioresistant tumours.

4. Salvage surgery following failed radiotherapy is possible.

Disadvantages include the following:

1. Perioperative morbidity and mortality.

2. Aesthetic and functional defects may be produced.

Modern techniques have significantly decreased these disadvantages, but the fact remains that surgery always carries the risk of some morbidity and mortality. Another disadvantage is that salvage radiotherapy is rarely effective after failed surgery.

Surgical excision of oral cancer can only be successful where the whole tumour is excised. This requires excision of the total tumour mass plus a margin of 1.5–2.0 cm of clinically normal tissue and there must be histological verification of tumour-free margins. It is unreasonable to carry out extensive surgery unless the tumour can be completely excised. The perioperative risks associated with such sometimes extensive and mutilating procedures have been reduced particularly by advances in anaesthesia and medical and intensive care.

There must be, as far as possible, restoration of normal anatomy in order to restore normal aesthetics and function. Fortunately, many major surgical and prosthetic advances have been, and are being, made in this field.

Excised tissue is, where necessary, replaced by the following means.

1. *Pedicle flaps.* Initially, forehead or deltopectoral flaps were used but they require a two-stage operation and, nowadays, myocutaneous flaps based on muscles such as the pectoralis major, latissimus dorsi, or trapezius, are used in a one-stage operation. Early pedicle flaps replaced the skin only (and used skin to replace oral mucosa), but these myocutaneous flaps also contain muscle which can replace bone and give adequate bulk to repair the cosmetic defect.

2. *Free flaps.* Microvascular surgery now facilitates excellent cosmetic surgery at a single operation. Using forearm flaps based on the radial vessels or groin flaps based on the circumflex iliac vessels, bone as well as muscle and skin can be replaced.

3. *Bone grafts:* usually from the iliac crest or rib.

4. *Prostheses.* Maxillary defects are usually filled using obturators (Volumes 3 and 4).

Mandibular defects, if small and posterior, may not need replacement but if they do, stainless steel, titanium or other implants are sometimes used to maintain aesthetics and anatomy temporarily until the patient is shown to be tumour-free and a bone graft can be carried out.

Complications of surgery

Patients with oral cancer are often aged and have poor oral hygiene. Wound infection is not uncommon.

Specific complications in the surgery of oral cancer include infection and rupture of the carotid artery (rare but usually fatal), and salivary fistulae and chylorrhoea (leakage of lymph from a damaged thoracic lymph duct).

Chemotherapy

Theoretical advantages of cancer chemotherapy include the ability to some extent to:

(a) reduce tumour bulk;
(b) control micrometastases.

There could be major benefit if the chemotherapeutic agent used was selectively toxic (or cytocidal) to the tumour but not to host cells, when chemotherapy could be more effective than either radiotherapy or surgery. However, the main disadvantages of present chemotherapy include the following.

1. A low response rate: at present the very *best* figures for a *partial* response are of the order 85–90% with combination therapy, but most studies have given far worse figures and cure is not possible.

2. Survival is increased only by a few months at best.

3. Side-effects: especially gastrointestinal upset, bone marrow suppression, hair loss, and mouth ulcers (see Fig. 15.27). These have increased somewhat with newer drugs such as cisplatinum.

Therapy using combinations of two, three or sometimes four cytotoxic agents is more effective than with drugs used singly. Regimens simultaneously using two drugs, for example cisplatinum and fluorouracil, or those using three drugs, for example bleomycin, cisplatinum and vincristine, have given the best responses in oral cancer. Administration of several agents in sequence may give a good response with minimal adverse effects.

The use of agents given into a vessel feeding the tumour was developed in an attempt both to avoid adverse reactions and to concentrate the agent at the tumour site, but although this technique still has advocates, it is not substantially more effective than the usual intravenous systemic route, it may produce severe local toxic reactions, and it can itself be hazardous.

Oral complications of chemotherapy for oral cancer or for other malignant neoplasms

Many of the cancer chemotherapeutic agents, used especially in treating lymphoproliferative conditions, can cause oral complications, particularly if treatment is prolonged or in high dosage.

1. *Ulcers.* Oral ulceration is especially common and may be severe enough to preclude further chemotherapy. Ulceration often begins shortly after chemotherapy is started. The ulcers are shallow and painful, but usually heal within 2 weeks of cessation of cytotoxic therapy (Fig. 15.27).

It may be possible to reduce oral ulceration caused by methotrexate by using systemic or topical Leucovorin (folinic acid). Established mucositis or oral ulceration is managed by maintaining good oral hygiene with 0.2% aqueous chlorhexidine mouthwash. A viscous 2% lignocaine solution or 0.15% benzydamine hydrochloride solution helps to reduce discomfort.

2. *Bleeding.* Drug-induced thrombocytopenia may cause gingival bleeding, mucosal petechiae or ecchymoses and a bleeding tendency and therefore a careful oral assessment should be carried out to enable extractions and any other surgery to be completed before chemotherapy.

3. *Infections.* Cytotoxic agents predispose to oral

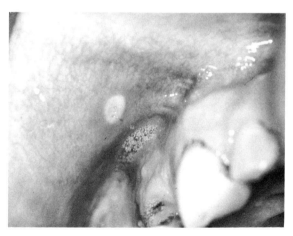

Fig. 15.27 *Ulcers induced by cytotoxic agents.*

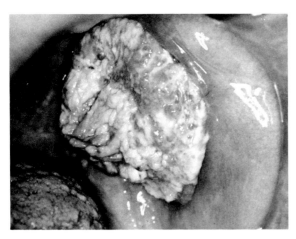

Fig. 15.28 Verrucous carcinoma.

infections with fungi, viruses and bacteria, and to postoperative infections. Many patients develop oral candidosis. Nystatin oral suspension, 100 000 u/ml as a mouthwash or miconazole gel four to six times daily are therefore usefully given as prophylactic antifungals. Dentures should be carefully cleaned and stored overnight in chlorhexidine 0.2% or 1% hypochlorite to reduce candidal carriage. Oral or labial herpetic infections may be prevented or treated with acyclovir.

Other treatment modalities

Cryosurgery and laser therapy are in their infancy, but there is some disquiet and uncertainty about cryosurgery since it may not reliably eliminate cancer. At present its use is deprecated. Lasers are expensive, found only in a minority of centres, and offer few if any advantages over conventional techniques.

Current treatment

This varies greatly between centres, but widely accepted guidelines and factors influencing choice are shown in Table 15.1 (p. 181).

VERRUCOUS CARCINOMA (see Chapter 19)

Verrucous carcinoma is an uncommon, slow-growing, locally invasive exophytic carcinoma typically seen in the buccal mucosa of elderly males. It metastasizes late and often responds well to surgery, not to radiotherapy (Fig. 15.28).

ORAL MALIGNANT NEOPLASMS OTHER THAN ORAL SQUAMOUS CELL CARCINOMA

Oral squamous carcinoma accounts for well over 90% of all oral malignant tumours. Other malignant neoplasms include the following.

1. Some salivary gland tumours (see Chapter 24).
2. Malignant melanoma (see Chapter 20).
3. Lymphomas (see Chapter 31).

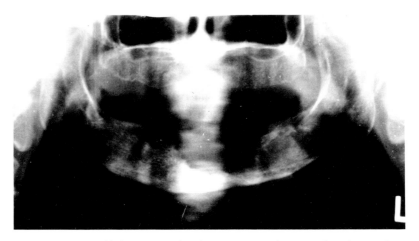

Fig. 15.29 Mandibular metastasis from breast carcinoma: this presented as a lump in the lower incisor–premolar region.

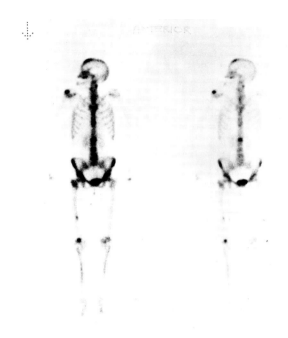

Fig. 15.30 *Technetium disphosphonate skeletal scan, showing widespread bone metastases in maxilla, skull, spine, humerus, pelvic girdle and femur.*

4. Rarely, other neoplasms such as Wegener's granulomatosis, a granulomatous neoplastic disease of the respiratory tract that eventually involves the kidneys (see Chapter 21).

5. Neoplasms of bone and connective tissue (see Chapter 7).

6. Some odontogenic tumours (see Chapter 6).

7. Maxillary antral carcinoma (or other neoplasms) (see Chapter 10).

8. Metastatic neoplasms (see Chapter 7 and below).

9. Histiocytoses (see Chapter 7).

10. Kaposi's sarcoma (Volume 1).

Metastatic neoplasms (see also Chapter 7)

Metastases to the oral tissues are rare, accounting for only 1% of all oral tumours. Most occur in bone, particularly the mandibular premolar or molar area or condyle, and may appear as an alveolar or gingival swelling or ulcer. Metastases may present with pain, paraesthesia, sensory loss, loosening of teeth, delayed healing of an extraction wound or pathological fracture. The usual sites of origin of oral metastases are carcinomas of:

(a) breast (Fig. 15.29),
(b) lung,
(c) kidney,
(d) stomach,
(e) liver.

A general history, physical examination and investigations, often including skeletal radiography or bone scan (Fig. 15.30) to reveal other lesions may well be indicated.

FURTHER READING

Beetham K. W., Williams R. G. (1980). The curative potential of surgery in the management of advanced mouth cancer. *Clin. Oncol.*, **6**: 337–341.

Carter R. L., Pittman M. R. (1980). Squamous carcinomas of the head and neck: some patterns of spread. *J. Roy. Soc. Med.*, **73**: 420–427.

Cawson R. A., Binnie W. H. (1982). Candida leukoplakia and carcinoma: a possible relationship. In *Oral premalignancy* (I. E. Mackenzie, E. Dabelsteen and C. A. Squier, Eds.). Iowa: University of Iowa Press.

Coleman J. J. (1986). Complications in head and neck surgery. *Surg. Clin. N. Amer.*, **66**: 149–169.

Henk J. M., Langdon J. D. (1985). *Malignant tumours of the oral cavity.* London: Edward Arnold.

Larson D. L. (1986). Management of complications of radiotherapy of the head and neck. *Surg. Clin. N. Amer.*, **66**: 169–183.

Lowe O. (1986). Oral concerns for the pediatric cancer patient. *J. Pedodont.*, **11**: 35–46.

McElroy T. H. (1984). Infection in the patient receiving chemotherapy for cancer: oral considerations. *JADA*, **109**: 454–456.

Morrish R. B. *et al.* (1981). Osteonecrosis in patients irradiated for head and neck carcinoma. *Cancer*, **47**: 1980–1983.

Murray C. G., Daly T. E., Zimmerman S. O. (1980). The relationship between dental disease and radiation necrosis of the mandible. *Oral Surg*, **49**: 99–104.

Palmer R. M. (1987). Tobacco smoking and oral health. *Health Education Authority* occasional Paper 6.

Pindborg J. J. (1980). *Oral cancer and precancer.* Bristol: John Wright & Son.

Scully C., Cox M., Maitland N., Prime S. Infective agents on the aetiology of oral cancer. *Oral Cancer.* Ed. Johnson N. J., Cambridge: Cambridge University Press (in press).

Scully C., Cawson R. A. (1988). *Colour aids to oral medicine.* Edinburgh and London: Churchill-Livingstone.

Scully C., Flint S. (1988). *An atlas of stomatology.* London: Martin Dunitz (in press).

Scully C., Malamos D., Levers B. G. H. *et al.* (1986). Sources and patterns of referrals of oral cancer: the role of general practitioners. *Br. med. J.*, **293**: 599–601.

Chapter
16

The sore mouth: 3. Ulcers in association with systemic disease

A wide range of systemic diseases, especially blood, gut and skin disorders, may cause oral lesions which, because of the moisture, trauma and infection in the mouth, tend to break down to leave ulcers or erosions. Oral ulceration is also frequently caused by infections and can be caused by drugs. Aphthae are occasionally associated with systemic disease; these and Behçet's syndrome are discussed in Chapter 14.

HAEMATOLOGICAL DISEASES

As outlined previously (Chapter 14), low iron, folate or vitamin B12 levels may be predisposing factors in a small percentage of patients with aphthae. A few of these patients have anaemia, sometimes with other oral features such as glossitis, or angular cheilitis—or general features (Figs. 16.1–16.3)—but many have a deficiency state with no established anaemia.

Disorders in which there are quantitative or qualitative deficiencies in polymorphonuclear leucocytes are often characterized by oral ulceration, and HIV infection may present with mouth ulcers (Chapter 14 and Volume 1). Only the more common of these disorders are included here.

Leucopenias and agranulocytosis

Oral ulceration may be a major symptom in patients with leucopenias, and may be the first sign of a drug-induced agranulocytosis or AIDS. Painful, deep, irregular ulcers occur anywhere in the oral cavity or pharynx. There is often only a minimal inflammatory halo visible, and such ulcers tend to extend and penetrate slowly. Patients may well suffer from recurrent infections else-

where. In the rare condition of cyclical neutropenia, ulcers appear episodically at 21-day intervals in association with the neutropenic episodes (Fig. 16.4).

Severe periodontitis is often also a feature of leucocyte defects (Chapter 13 and Volume 1).

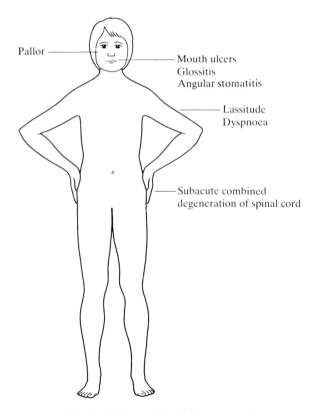

Fig. 16.1 *Features of iron deficiency anaemia.*

188

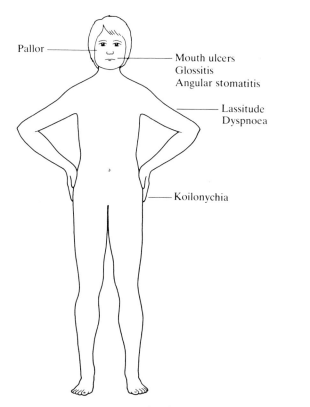

Pallor

Mouth ulcers
Glossitis
Angular stomatitis

Lassitude
Dyspnoea

Koilonychia

Fig. 16.2 *Features of folate deficiency anaemia.*

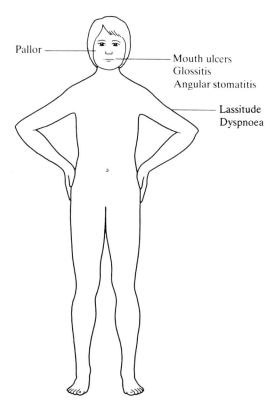

Pallor

Mouth ulcers
Glossitis
Angular stomatitis

Lassitude
Dyspnoea

Fig. 16.3 *Features of vitamin B12 deficiency anaemia.*

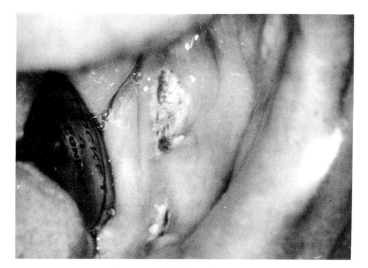

Fig. 16.4 *Oral ulcers in neutropenia.*

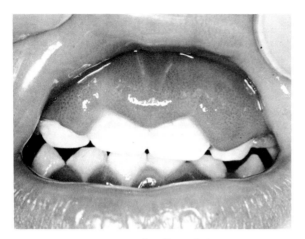

Fig. 16.5 Gingival swelling in leukaemia.

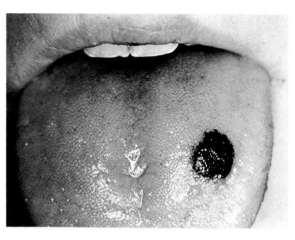

Fig. 16.6 Oral purpura because of thrombocytopenia in leukaemia.

Leukaemias

Similar oral ulceration may occur in leukaemia, especially in the acute leukaemias. Other oral manifestations of leukaemia include mucosal pallor, gingival haemorrhage, gingival swelling (Fig. 16.5), petechiae and ecchymoses (Fig. 16.6). Most patients have generalized lymph node enlargement. Oral infections with *Candida albicans* and Gram-negative bacteria including *Pseudomonas* species,

Escherichia coli, *Proteus*, *Klebsiella* and *Serratia* species, are common, especially in acute leukaemias (Fig. 16.7). Such oral lesions may act as a portal for septicaemia. Oral ulceration due to herpes simplex or herpes zoster–varicella viruses is also common (Figs. 16.7 and 32.9). Chemotherapeutic agents used in the treatment of leukaemia (see p. 185) complicate the situation since they themselves can produce oral ulceration.

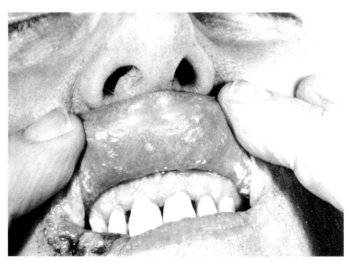

Fig. 16.7 Thrush inside the upper lip, with recurrent herpes labialis on the lower lip in leukaemia.

Coeliac disease

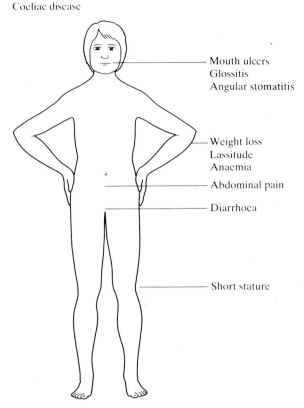

Mouth ulcers
Glossitis
Angular stomatitis

Weight loss
Lassitude
Anaemia

Abdominal pain

Diarrhoea

Short stature

Fig. 16.8 *Features of coeliac disease.*

Management

Since septicaemia may arise from oropharyngeal ulcerations, it is important to manage the lesions carefully. Antiseptic mouthwashes such as aqueous 0.2% chlorhexidine gluconate and careful oral hygiene measures should be used. If ulceration is severe and painful, a 2% lignocaine viscous solution is helpful but disturbs taste. Antivirals such as acyclovir may be indicated.

GASTROINTESTINAL DISEASES

Pernicious anaemia, coeliac disease, Crohn's disease and disorders in which there is gastrointestinal blood loss (e.g. peptic ulcer or cancer) may give rise to deficiency states predisposing to recurrent aphthous stomatitis. Oral ulceration is also sometimes found in ulcerative colitis.

Coeliac disease (gluten-sensitive enteropathy)

Coeliac disease is characterized by sensitivity of the mucosa of the small intestine to gluten in wheat and other cereals. The patient is well, unless exposed to gluten, when the mucosa loses villi (villous atrophy) with subsequent malabsorption and its sequelae (Fig. 16.8), including mouth ulcers (Fig. 16.9). The diagnosis is made from a history and examination suggesting malabsorption, haematological examination for deficiency states

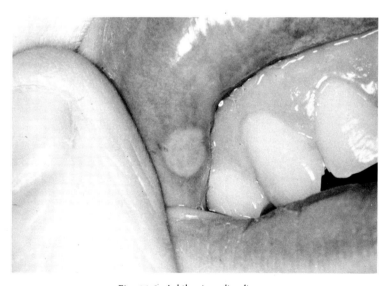

Fig. 16.9 *Aphthae in coeliac disease.*

Crohn's disease

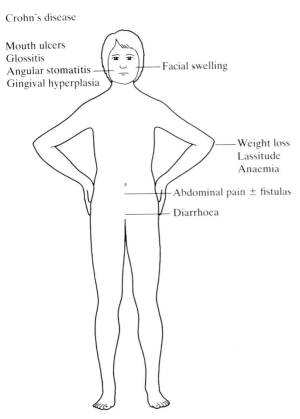

Mouth ulcers
Glossitis
Angular stomatitis —
Gingival hyperplasia

— Facial swelling

— Weight loss
  Lassitude
  Anaemia

— Abdominal pain ± fistulas

— Diarrhoea

Fig. 16.10 *Features of Crohn's disease.*

and anti-reticulin antibodies, and a small bowel biopsy showing villous atrophy. A gluten-free diet prevents symptoms.

Crohn's disease

Crohn's disease is a granulomatous disorder of unknown cause that affects mainly the ileum but can affect any part of the gastrointestinal tract (Fig. 16.10).

Oral ulceration in Crohn's disease may be due not only to malabsorption, but to primary Crohn's disease of the oral mucosa or to coincidental ulceration of other aetiology (Fig. 16.11). Ulcers classically involve the buccal sulcus where they appear as linear ulcers, often with granulomatous masses flanking them.

Mucosal lesions also include thickening and folding of the mucosa to produce a 'cobblestone' type of appearance and mucosal tags (Fig. 16.12). Purple granulomatous enlargements may appear on the gingiva. The lips or face may chronically swell (Figs. 16.13 and 32.15, and there may be splitting of the lips and angular stomatitis.

Management

Oral biopsy, haematological, gastrointestinal and other investigations may be required in suspected Crohn's disease (Fig. 16.14), especially to exclude sarcoidosis (Chapters 26 and 31). Topical or intralesional corticosteroids may effectively control the lesions but more

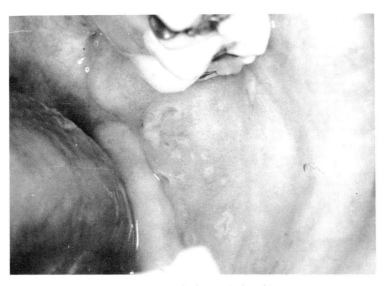

Fig. 16.11 *Mouth ulcers in Crohn's disease.*

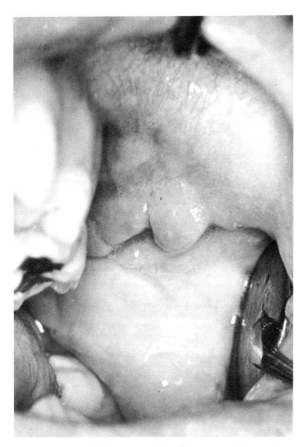

Fig. 16.12 Cobblestoning of buccal mucosa and mucosal tags overlying parotid duct in oral Crohn's disease.

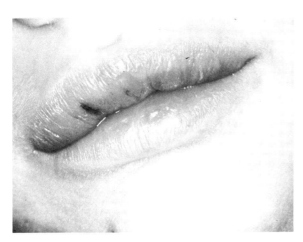

Fig. 16.13 Labial swelling in Crohn's disease.

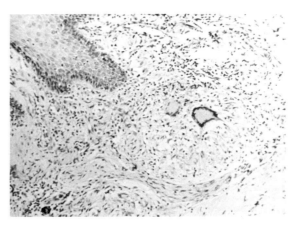

Fig. 16.14 Non-caseating granuloma containing giant cells in oral Crohn's disease.

frequently systemic corticosteroids, azathioprine or sala-zopyrine are required.

Some patients develop similar oral lesions because of an adverse reaction to various foodstuffs, and the term orofacial granulomatosis has come into vogue in some centres since it is unclear where in the spectrum of Crohn's disease/sarcoidosis these lesions lie.

DERMATOLOGICAL DISEASES

A range of dermatoses may be associated with oral erosions; lichen planus is the most common—pemphigus the most serious.

Lichen planus

Lichen planus is more fully discussed in Chapter 19 (White Lesions) since the common oral lesions are white lesions without erosion or ulceration, though they may cause soreness. A small number of patients suffer from atrophic or erosive forms of lichen planus which frequently affect the dorsum and lateral borders of the tongue, or the buccal mucosae on both sides. The erosions are often large, slightly depressed or raised with a yellow slough, and have an irregular outline (Fig. 16.15). They may not be quite as painful as might be imagined. The surrounding mucosa is often erythematous and glazed in appearance, with loss of filiform papillae of the tongue, and pathognomonic whitish Wickham's striae. Lichen planus may also produce a desquamative gingivitis (Volume 2) and lesions elsewhere (Fig. 16.16).

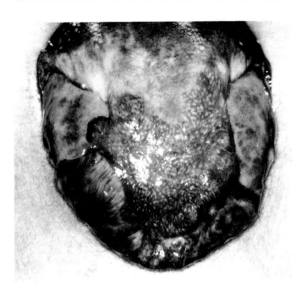

Fig. 16.15 *Erosive lichen planus of the tongue showing large erosions on each side, and multiple white lesions.*

Lichen planus

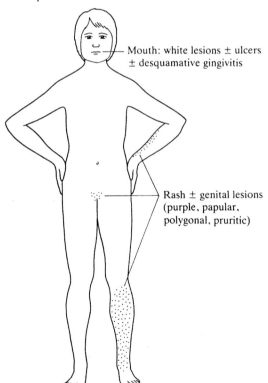

Mouth: white lesions ± ulcers
± desquamative gingivitis

Rash ± genital lesions
(purple, papular,
polygonal, pruritic)

Fig. 16.16 *Features of lichen planus.*

Management

Biopsy is usually necessary to confirm the diagnosis and exclude keratosis, lupus erythematosus and other disorders. Some lichenoid lesions may be drug-induced (e.g. by non-steroidal anti-inflammatory agents), in which case it may be beneficial to change these or related to restorations. Topical corticosteroids are useful in controlling oral lichen planus but secondary infection, especially with *Candida albicans,* is not uncommon. Agents such as etretinate and griseofulvin have not been reliably effective.

In view of the slight possibility of premalignancy, especially in erosive lichen planus (a risk of the order of 1%), patients should be regularly reviewed.

Pemphigus

Pemphigus is a potentially lethal autoimmune bullous disease of the stratified squamous epithelium which

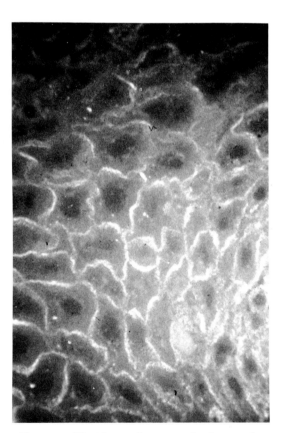

Fig. 16.17 *Direct immunofluorescence of oral mucosa from a patient with pemphigus showing IgG deposits. (Courtesy of Dr J. W. Eveson.)*

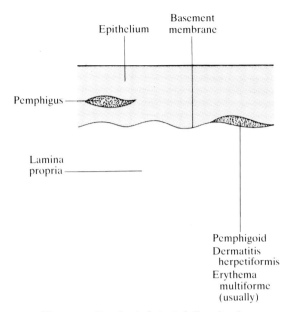

Fig. 16.18 labels:
- Epithelium
- Basement membrane
- Pemphigus
- Lamina propria
- Pemphigoid
  Dermatitis herpetiformis
  Erythema multiforme (usually)

Fig. 16.18 *Site of vesiculation in bullous disorders.*

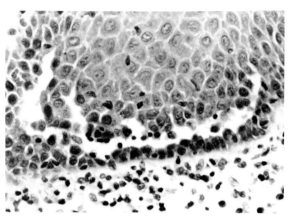

Fig. 16.20 *High-power histology of a lesion in pemphigus, showing separation of cells (acantholysis); rounding up of free cells (acantholytic or Tzanck cells); and a row of basal cells lining the basement membrane (tombstone cells).*

almost exclusively affects late-middle-aged or elderly adults, often of Jewish or Italian extraction. There is no sex predilection. There is an association with HLA-A10, HLA-DR4 and HLA-DQβ.

Serum IgG, IgM or sometimes IgA autoantibodies to intercellular substances of the suprabasal epithelium of skin and mucosa are found in 95% of cases of pemphigus and are diagnostically helpful, especially where biopsy examination is difficult. The autoantibody titre is some-

times correlated with the severity of pemphigus and antibody tends to disappear as the lesions heal. Direct immunofluorescence on biopsy demonstrates IgG antibodies and complement components bound to intercellular areas of epithelium in patients with pemphigus (Fig. 16.17). These autoantibodies are therefore probably the cause of the lesions, which manifest histologically as loss of adhesion of cells of the stratum spinosum such that they separate (acantholysis) and a bulla forms intra-epithelially (Figs. 16.18–16.21). Acantholysis is usually supra-basal and may be caused by an autoantibody-induced release of autolytic enzymes, particularly proteinases, from the epithelial cells (Fig. 16.21).

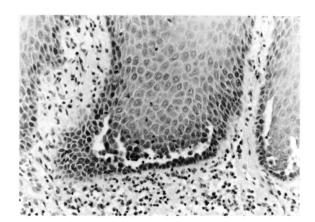

Fig. 16.19 *Acantholysis in the suprabasal layer of oral epithelium in pemphigus.*

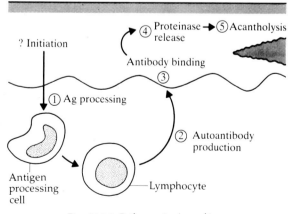

Fig. 16.21 labels:
- ? Initiation
- ④ Proteinase release → ⑤ Acantholysis
- Antibody binding ③
- ① Ag processing
- ② Autoantibody production
- Antigen processing cell
- Lymphocyte

Fig. 16.21 *Pathogenesis of pemphigus.*

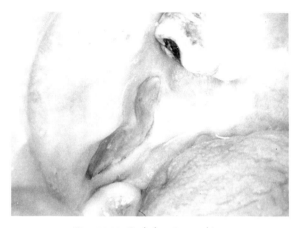

Fig. 16.22 *Oral ulcers in pemphigus.*

Pemphigus

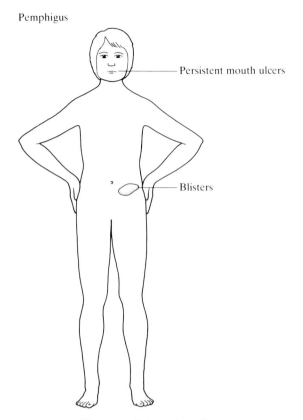

Persistent mouth ulcers

Blisters

Clinical features

The oral mucosa is almost invariably involved in pemphigus vulgaris and oral lesions are often the presenting feature (Fig. 16.22). Bullae appear on any part of the oral mucosa including the palate, but rapidly break down within hours to leave large, painful, irregular and persistent erosions. Other mucosae may be involved.

Flaccid blisters eventually appear on the skin, especially in response to trauma—Nikolsky sign (Figs. 16.23 and 16.24).

Fig. 16.24 *Features of pemphigus.*

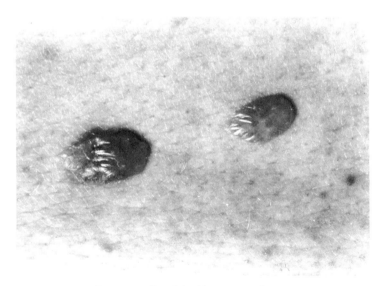

Fig. 16.23 *Flaccid skin blisters in pemphigus.*

Prognosis

Pemphigus is a life-threatening disorder. Untreated, patients inevitably die, usually from staphylococcal septicaemia.

Management

The oral lesions of pemphigus can sometimes be difficult to differentiate clinically from other erosive lesions such as pemphigoid, though the Nikolsky sign is more often positive in pemphigus. In view of the seriousness of a diagnosis of pemphigus, it is important to biopsy a lesion for conventional histology (see Fig. 16.20) and immunostaining (see Fig. 16.17). Intracellular intra-epithelial deposits of mainly IgG, and acantholysis occur in pemphigus. Serum should be taken and examined for autoantibodies to epithelial intercellular substance (Table 16.1). Smears for cytology are of little *practical* value.

Systemic corticosteroids or immunosuppressants are invariably required in the management of pemphigus.

Pemphigoid

Pemphigoid is a bullous disorder of less serious prognosis than pemphigus though it may affect the eyes. Pemphigoid is probably an autoimmune disease and serum autoantibodies directed against basement membranes of stratified squamous epithelia may be found, with tissue immune deposits at the epithelial basement membrane zone. However, the evidence that the autoantibodies cause the disease is less clear than is the case with pemphigus.

Table 16.1

Immunostaining in mucosal disorders

Disease	DIF*	Deposits mainly	Pattern of IF	IIF†	Autoantibodies against
Pemphigus	+	IgG C3	Epithelial, intercellular	+	Epithelial intercellular cement
Mucous membrane pemphigoid	+	C3 IgG	Linear–epithelial basement membrane	±	None or epithelial basement membrane
Bullous pemphigoid	+	IgG C3	Linear–epithelial basement membrane	+	Epithelial basement membrane
Dermatitis herpetiformis	+	IgA C3	Granular–epithelial basement membrane	−	Reticulin
Linear IgA disease	±	IgA C3	Linear–epithelial basement membrane	−	Reticulin
Erythema multiforme	+	C3 IgM	Vessel walls in lamina propria	−	−
Lichen planus	±	Fibrin‡ mainly IgM IgG IgA C3	Globular–epithelial or lamina propria and in Civatte bodies	−	−
Discoid lupus erythematosus	+	IgG IgA IgM C3	Granular–epithelial basement membrane	±	None, or antinuclear

* DIF = direct immunofluorescence (biopsy).
† IIF = indirect immunofluorescence (serology).
‡ Non-specific deposits.

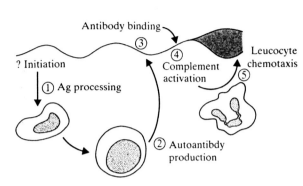

Fig. 16.25 *Pathogenesis of pemphigoid.*

Mucous membrane pemphigoid

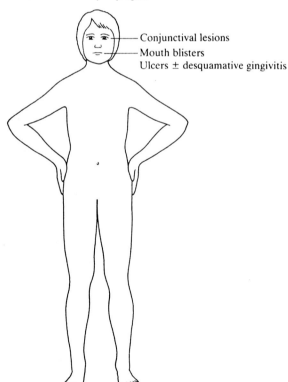

Fig. 16.26 *Features of mucous membrane pemphigoid.*

There are two main forms of pemphigoid.

1. *Bullous pemphigoid.* Bullous pemphigoid is a chronic bullous disease which involves mainly the skin rather than the mouth. It is clinically similar to pemphigus although less severe and it lacks the characteristic histopathological features of acantholysis and intra-epithelial vesiculation. Bullous pemphigoid is most common in elderly persons and there is no apparent sex predilection.

Serum IgG autoantibodies to epithelial basement membrane occur in 80% of cases (Table 16.1). The complement components C1q, C3, C4 and IgG (see Chapter 13) are deposited in the epithelial basement membrane region and vesiculation occurs subepithelially (Figs. 16.18, 16.25, and 16.27).

2. *Mucous membrane pemphigoid.* Mucous membrane pemphigoid (cicatricial or ocular pemphigoid) is a bullous lesion predominantly involving the mucous membranes rather than the skin (Fig. 16.26). Lesions characteristically heal with scarring. It occurs mainly in the fourth decade and is more frequent in females than in males. Histological examination of the lesion shows subepithelial vesiculation and deposition mainly of C3 and IgG in the epithelial basement membrane zone (Figs. 16.27–16.29). Serum autoantibodies to epithelial basement membrane are infrequently detected or are in low titre (Table 16.1).

Clinical features

The bullae in pemphigoid are subepithelial and tend to persist for longer than those of pemphigus. Mucous

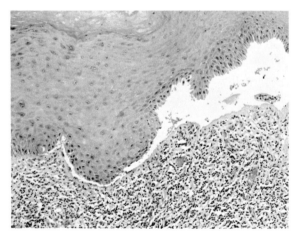

Fig. 16.27 *Mucous membrane pemphigoid: subepithelial vesiculation.*

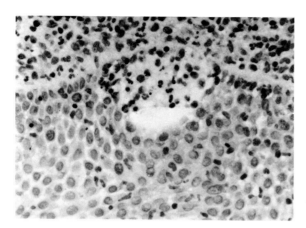

Fig. 16.28 *Mucous membrane pemphigoid: high power showing subepithelial vesiculation and infiltrate with large numbers of eosinophils.*

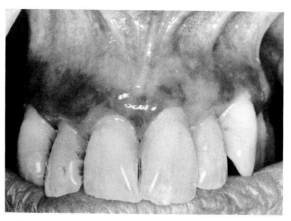

Fig. 16.30 *Desquamative gingivitis in pemphigoid (similar lesions may be seen in lichen planus).*

membrane pemphigoid commonly involves the oral mucosa. The usual lesion is desquamative gingivitis and is characterized by erythematous, glazed, sore gingiva (Fig. 16.30). Bullous lesions are also common (Fig. 16.31), particularly on the soft palate, and may rupture to form erosions (Fig. 16.32). The bullae may be blood filled or filled with serous fluid.

The skin is rarely involved in mucous membrane pemphigoid. Tense blisters form. Involvement of the eyes, and occasionally the larynx, is serious since there may be scarring (Fig. 16.33).

Management

A biopsy is required; subepithelial bullae occur and there are deposits of complement components and IgG at the epithelial basement membrane zone (see Figs. 16.27–16.29). Serum autoantibodies to epithelial basement membrane may be detected in a few patients. A very small minority of patients have an associated internal malignancy which should be excluded. An ophthalmological opinion is required.

Systemic corticosteroids may occasionally be required; topical steroids help if the lesions are restricted to the

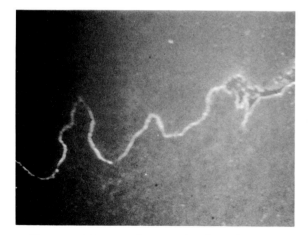

Fig. 16.29 *Mucous membrane pemphigoid: complement C3 deposits at basement membrane zone. (Courtesy of Dr J. W. Eveson.)*

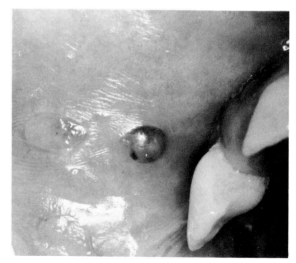

Fig. 16.31 *Vesicles in mucous membrane pemphigoid.*

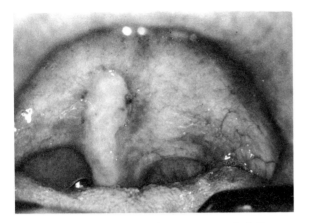

Fig. 16.32 *Erosion on soft palate after rupture of a bulla in mucous membrane pemphigoid.*

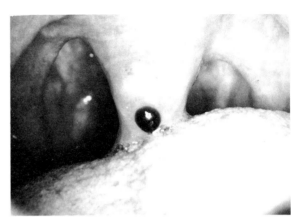

Fig. 16.34 *Palatal blood-filled vesicle and an ulcer just above it on the uvula, in angina bullosa haemorrhagica.*

oral mucosa. Dapsone may be useful in the treatment of desquamative gingivitis.

Angina bullosa haemorrhagica (localized oral purpura)

This is the term given to a benign condition of unknown aetiology that usually presents in the elderly with blood blisters in the palate that rupture to leave ulcers (Figs. 16.34 and 16.35). The patients appear well otherwise, with no immunological disease or disorder of haemostasis. Only symptomatic care is available.

Dermatitis herpetiformis and linear IgA disease

Dermatitis herpetiformis (Duhring's disease) is an uncommon, chronic, papulovesicular, itchy eruption which mainly involves the skin. It is more common in males and usually appears in middle-age. Serum IgA anti-basement membrane antibodies have occasionally been identified, but anti-reticulin antibodies are commonly seen, as in coeliac disease. There is an almost pathognomonic fixation of IgA at the dermo-epidermal junction at the tips of dermal papillae, especially in apparently unaffected skin. It has been postulated that immune complexes of IgA are deposited subepithelially and initiate the formation of microabsceses by activation of the alternate complement path and a polymorphonuclear leucocyte

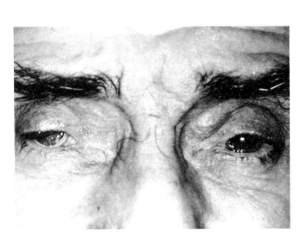

Fig. 16.33 *Conjunctival scarring and blindness as a result of pemphigoid.*

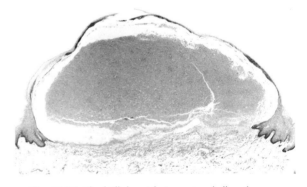

Fig. 16.35 *Blood-filled vesicle in angina bullosa haemorrhagica. (Courtesy of the Editor of* Oral Surgery, Oral Medicine *and* Oral Pathology.*)*

infiltration. Serum immune complexes have been demonstrated in 80% of patients, but in only 30% of those on a gluten-free diet, suggesting that gluten may be one component of the complexes.

The bullae are subepithelial in dermatitis herpetiformis, as in pemphigoid and erythema multiforme. Dermatitis herpetiformis is associated with HLA-B8 and even more frequently with HLA-DR3.

Linear IgA disease is a rare variant in which IgA is deposited along the epithelial basement membrane zone and not just at the tips of papillae.

Oral features

Oral lesions may occur in dermatitis herpetiformis and in linear IgA disease. Macules, papules, petechiae, vesicles, bullae and erosions are the usual manifestations.

Management

Biopsy in dermatitis herpetiformis is diagnostic, showing IgA deposits at the papillae and, in linear IgA disease, at the epithelial basement membrane zone (see Table 16.1). A jejunal biopsy is often indicated since there may be an associated gluten-sensitive enteropathy (coeliac disease). Dapsone and sulphapyridine are effective therapeutic agents.

Erythema multiforme

Erythema multiforme is a mucocutaneous disease characterized by skin lesions, with oral or ocular involvement in some cases, and with a marked tendency to recur (Fig. 16.36). The condition mainly affects young adult males, and has a seasonal incidence, being seen mainly in the spring or autumn.

The aetiology of erythema multiforme has not been established but many agents have been implicated though in most cases, however, no causal factor is found, and there is little evidence for an allergic cause. The most common identifiable factor associated with erythema multiforme is a preceding herpes simplex virus infection, but this is found only in up to about 15% of patients. A wide range of drugs, especially the barbiturates, sulphonamides, and anticonvulsant drugs of the hydantoin and succinimide groups, may be responsible but the mechanism is unclear. Other cases occur in relation to radiotherapy or pregnancy.

Histologically there are degenerative changes at the epithelial basement membrane zone and thickening of the prickle cell layer (acanthosis), with bullae either sub- or intra-epithelially: the degenerating oral epithelium is strikingly eosinophilic and there is a lymphohistiocytic infiltration in the lamina propria, especially around blood vessels (Fig. 16.37; Table 16.1).

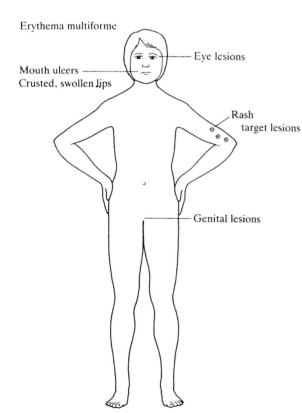

Erythema multiforme

Mouth ulcers
Crusted, swollen lips

Eye lesions

Rash
target lesions

Genital lesions

Fig. 16.36 *Features of erythema multiforme.*

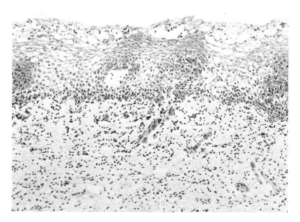

Fig. 16.37 *Perivascular leucocytic infiltrate in erythema multiforme.*

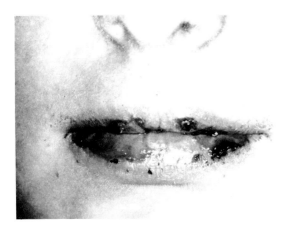

Fig. 16.38 *Serosanguinous exudate and swollen lips of localized oral erythema multiforme.*

No consistent abnormalities of immunoglobulin levels, lymphocyte transformation or delayed hypersensitivity have been reported, but it is possible that immune complexes activate the classical pathway of complement to initiate the bulla formation.

Clinical features

Erythema multiforme has an acute, explosive onset. The oral mucosa may be involved alone or in association with lesions on skin or other mucosae. Mucosal lesions commence as erythematous areas which vesiculate and form bullae that break down to leave irregular large, painful erosions with surrounding erythema extensively involving the mucosa. The labial mucosa is often involved, and a serosanguinous exudate leads to blood crusting of the swollen lips (Fig. 16.38). There may be pyrexia and the cervical lymph nodes are often enlarged and tender.

A variety of rashes (erythema *multiforme*) may be seen, particularly target or iris lesions (Fig. 16.39).

Genital and/or ocular mucosa may be involved— when the complex is termed the Stevens–Johnson syndrome.

Management

An attempt should be made to identify and avoid any precipitating factor, but often this is impossible. A biopsy may occasionally be required if the diagnosis is doubtful.

Oral hygiene should be maintained and, in severe cases, systemic corticosteroids may be needed.

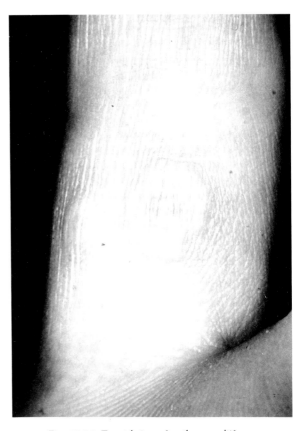

Fig. 16.39 *Target lesions of erythema multiforme.*

Epidermolysis bullosa

Genetic defects in a basal lamina protein appear to underlie this rare cause of mouth ulcers, which is discussed in Chapter 12.

CONNECTIVE TISSUE DISEASE

Lupus erythematosus

Systemic lupus erythematosus (SLE) is an uncommon multisystem disease, affecting particularly the skin, joints, kidney and brain (Fig. 16.40), characterized by exacerbations and remissions and showing a high morbidity. Females, especially blacks, are affected more frequently than males.

The aetiology of SLE involves immunogenetic factors but a few cases are drug-induced. Experimental work with NZB/NZW mice, which show a syndrome having all the features of the human disease, indicates a depression

Systemic lupus erythematosus

Major features

Psychoses; fits

Butterfly rash over nose and cheeks

Myalgia
Pleuritis
Pericarditis

Arthralgia

Minor features

Alopecia
Eye lesions
Sjögren's syndrome
Mouth ulcers

Hepatosplenomegaly
Anaemia, leucopenia, thrombocytopenia

Renal disease and hypertension

Raynaud's phenomenon

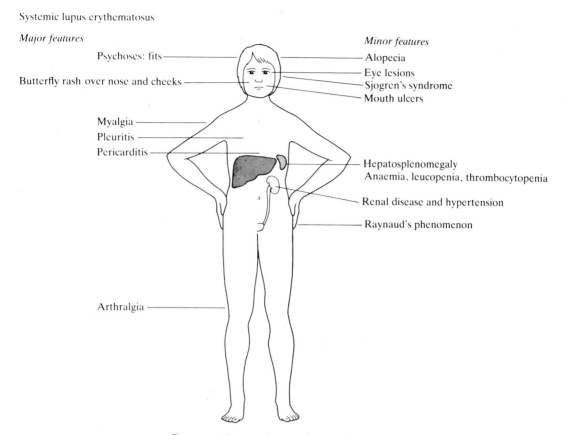

Fig. 16.40 *Features of systemic lupus erythematosus.*

of suppressor T-lymphocytes with a resultant hyperactive humoral response associated with multiple autoantibodies and complement-fixing immune complexes.

Antinuclear antibodies are found in most patients: anti-double-strand DNA seems to be most specific. The lupus erythematosus (LE) cell test (an IgG antibody to native DNA is often positive and there are autoantibodies to many other tissues. Serum immune complexes activate both classic and alternate complement pathways, leading to reduced serum complement levels. Biopsies from mucocutaneous lesions show granular deposits of IgG and sometimes IgM, IgA and complement at the dermo-epidermal junction, even in unchanged skin or mucosa (see Table 16.1). Immune complex deposition leading to lysosomal enzyme release from macrophages is probably responsible for the tissue damage.

Discoid lupus erythematosus (DLE) is a related condition in which lesions are restricted to skin and/or mucosa.

Clinical features

Almost half of the patients with SLE suffer from oral lesions, which begin as red patches which break down to irregular ulcers which often heal with scarring. Petechiae and herpetic infections are also common. Similar erosions, with a white border, occur in DLE (Fig. 16.41). Sjögren's syndrome may be seen in SLE (Chapter 25).

Diagnosis

Oral lesional biopsy is indicated and shows thickening and periodic acid-Schiff positivity of the epithelial basement membrane with a perivascular mononuclear cell infiltrate (Fig. 16.42). There may be linear deposits of C3 and immunoglobulin at the epithelial basement membrane zone.

Blood should be taken for haematological studies,

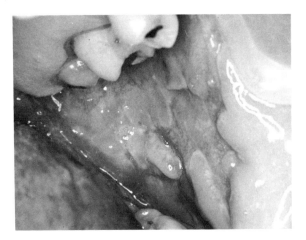

Fig. 16.41 *Lupus erythematosus: central red lesion with white speckling, and irradiating white striae as a brush border. Note close resemblance to lichen planus.*

since anaemia and leucopenia are common, for complement studies, and for autoantibodies, especially anti-nuclear antibodies. Urinalysis is needed to exclude proteinuria in SLE.

Management

Systemic corticosteroids, often with an immunosuppressant, are required, and referral to a rheumatologist.

Other connective tissue diseases

Dermatomyositis (a collagen disorder) may be associated with non-specific mucosal erosions.

Oral involvement in Reiter's syndrome may include red patches or superficial painless mucosal erosions (Fig. 16.43). Other lesions include conjunctivitis, arthritis and a peculiar thickening of the soles of the feet known as keratoderma blenorrhagica.

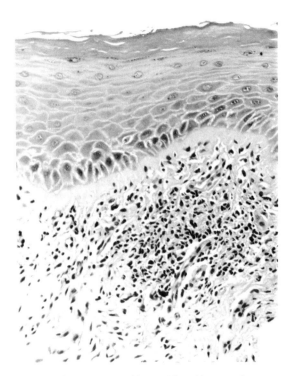

Fig. 16.42 *Biopsy of oral lesion of discoid lupus erythematosus showing perivascular mononuclear cell infiltrate, and thickened basement membrane.*

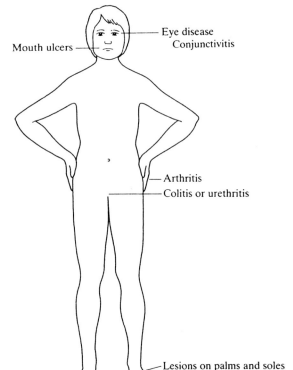

Fig. 16.43 *Features of Reiter's syndrome.*

INFECTIVE DISEASES

Oral ulceration is a feature of a number of bacterial diseases, notably acute ulcerative gingivitis, tuberculosis and syphilis, is common in many viral infections, but is rare in mycoses. Oral ulcers in the infectious diseases are usually acute and non-recurring, healing within 7–14 days, except in the cases of tuberculosis and syphilis.

Bacterial infections

Acute ulcerative gingivitis (acute necrotizing gingivitis; Vincent's disease; trench mouth)

Acute necrotizing gingivitis (ANG) is a not uncommon condition, and is discussed more fully in Volume 2. The ulceration is usually restricted to the gingiva, specifically the interdental papilla. The history is characteristic with an acute onset of soreness, bleeding and halitosis. Although ANG occurs usually in a previously healthy adolescent, it may follow a respiratory viral infection, presumably because this produces a transient immune defect. Oral examination reveals papillae which are ulcerated and blunted (Figs. 16.44 and 32.11). ANG occurs especially in the anterior part of the mouth. The gingiva are extremely tender to touch and readily bleed on minimal pressure. Halitosis may be marked. There is often enlargement of the cervical lymph nodes and there may be pyrexia and malaise. Occasionally the ulceration extends elsewhere on the gingiva, or onto the adjacent mucosa.

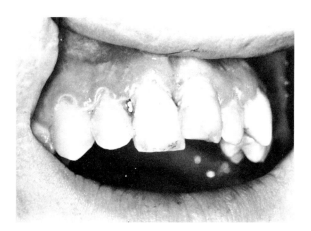

Fig. 16.44 *Acute necrotizing gingivitis showing papillary ulceration spreading to the gingival margins.*

Aetiology

There is no firm evidence of communicability of ANG although it may occur in epidemic form, especially in institutions or in the military (trench mouth). A mixed anaerobic flora (the fusospirochaetal complex), consisting mainly of *Fusobacterium nucleatum* and *Borrelia vincentii*, is associated with this infection. Viral respiratory infections, overwork and fatigue, smoking or immune defects may precede the onset of disease, suggesting depression of immunity as a predisposing cause.

A similar lesion may be a feature of AIDS and related diseases (Volume 1).

Management

Gentle cleansing with a soft toothbrush and a 5 volume strength hydrogen peroxide mouthwash is remarkably effective. Oral metronidazole 200 mg three times daily for 3–7 days is employed at an early stage to limit the amount of tissue destruction. Penicillin is equally effective. The patient should also be referred for periodontal advice (Volume 2).

Syphilis (see also Volume 1)

Oral ulcers may be seen at any stage of syphilis, but particularly in the secondary stage.

Though it is uncommon, there is a rising incidence of syphilis, which is one of the more serious sexually transmitted diseases as it may damage the cardiovascular and/or nervous systems and can be fatal if untreated.

Primary syphilis

Primary infection with *Treponema pallidum* causes a chancre (primary, hard or Hunterian chancre) which begins as a small, firm, pink macule usually on the glans penis or vulva. Primary chancres may also involve the lips, tongue or palate. The macule changes to a papule which ulcerates to form a painless, round ulcer with a raised margin and indurated base. Untreated chancres heal in 3–8 weeks but are highly infectious and are associated with enlarged, painless regional lymph nodes (Fig. 16.45).

Secondary syphilis

Secondary syphilis follows after 6–8 weeks, but a healing chancre may still be present. Oral lesions appear in about one-third of patients and are highly infectious.

Primary syphilis in mouth

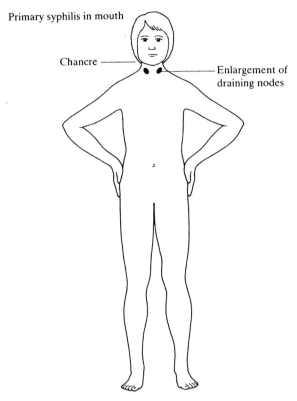

Chancre ———

——— Enlargement of draining nodes

Fig. 16.45 *Features of primary syphilis.*

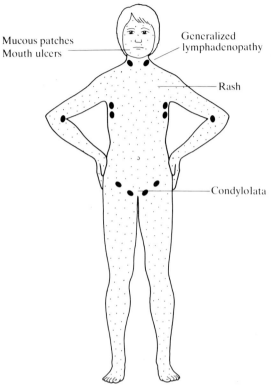

Mucous patches
Mouth ulcers

Generalized lymphadenopathy

Rash

Condylolata

Fig. 16.47 *Features of secondary syphilis.*

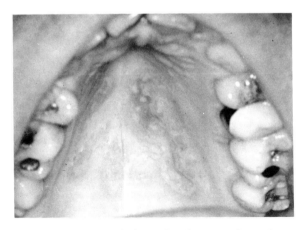

Fig. 16.46 *Snailtrack ulcers in the palate in secondary syphilis. (Courtesy of the Editor,* British Dental Journal.)

Painless oral ulcers (mucous patches and snailtrack ulcers) are the typical oral lesions at this stage (Fig. 16.46).

The typical general features of secondary syphilis are fever, headache, malaise, a rash (characteristically symmetrically distributed coppery maculopapules or lesions on the palms) and generalized, painless lymph node enlargement (Fig. 16.47).

Tertiary syphilis

Syphilis progresses to a tertiary stage 3–10 or more years after infection in about 30% of untreated patients. The remaining untreated patients are serologically reactive and said to have latent syphilis.

The characteristic lesion of tertiary syphilis is a localized granuloma varying in size from a pinhead to several centimetres, known as a *gumma*. Gummas break down to form deep punched-out ulcers which on the skin heal with depressed shiny scars (tissue-paper scars). Gummas

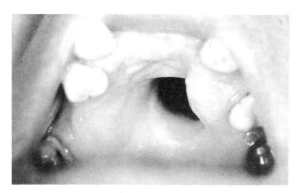

Fig. 16.48 Palatal gumma of tertiary syphilis.

may affect the long bones (especially the tibia) or skull, producing lytic lesions and periostitis with new bone formation. Gummas are not infectious.

Mucosal gummas affect particularly the palate, or the tongue (Fig. 16.48). The main oral manifestation of tertiary syphilis is, however, leukoplakia. This particularly affects the dorsum of the tongue and has a high potential for malignant change (Figs. 16.49 and 16.50; see also Chapter 19).

Cardiovascular syphilis, which affects only about 10% of patients, is a late complication and causes aortitis, coronary arterial stenosis or aortic aneurysms. A similar number of patients develop neurosyphilis which manifests often as general paralysis of the insane (GPI), or tabes dorsalis.

Congenital syphilis

Congenital syphilis is rare in the UK. Syphilis in the pregnant patient (after the fifth month) may result in infection of the fetus. Mental handicap, deafness and

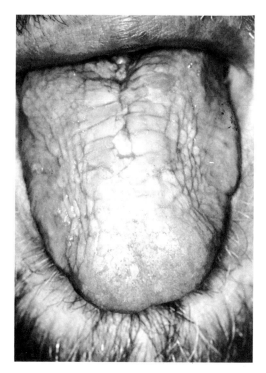

Fig. 16.49 Syphilitic leukoplakia.

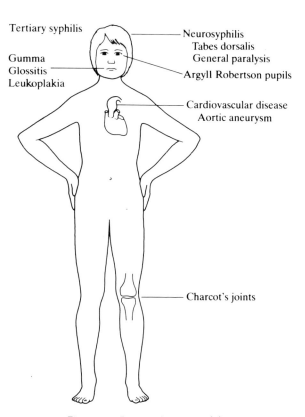

Fig. 16.50 Features of tertiary syphilis.

blindness are features and the child may have a collapsed nasal bridge (Fig. 16.51) and, when the permanent teeth erupt, dental anomalies such as Hutchinson's teeth are evident (Volume 3; Fig. 32.3, Chapter 33). Affected children are infectious for about 2 years. Oral ulcers are rare (Fig. 16.52).

Management

Syphilis should be considered as a possible cause in any unusual oral ulcer and, although no group is immune, should particularly be suspected in high-risk groups such as sexually promiscuous individuals, homosexuals, prostitutes, drug addicts, military service personnel and those who travel widely.

Exudate from a suspected lesion should be examined for treponemes by dark-ground microscopy since it is not possible to culture *T. pallidum*. In oral lesions, the diagnosis can be confused by oral commensal treponemes. Lesions should, therefore, be thoroughly swabbed with sterile gauze or cotton wool to remove as many contaminants as possible; gently but thoroughly scraped with a sterile spatula; and the scraping examined immediately by dark-ground microscopy. *T. pallidum* is characterized by large but slender, regular, helical forms with a leisurely rotational movement.

Serum antibodies to *T. pallidum* may not be detectable early on but serology is positive later. A non-specific test such as the Venereal Disease Research Laboratory (VDRL) test is useful for screening but, since there may be false positives, a more specific test such as the fluorescent treponemal antibody (FTA) test is required to confirm the diagnosis (see Table 16.2 and Volume 1).

Biopsy is not usually indicated, but lesions are characterized by a dense plasma-cell infiltrate (Fig. 16.53).

Other sexually transmitted diseases, including AIDS, should also be excluded.

Procaine penicillin 600 000 units intramuscularly, daily for at least 10 days (or tetracycline or erythromycin for 14 days), should be given. Patients must be followed up clinically and serologically for 2 years and contact tracing is required. In tertiary syphilis, systemic corticosteroids

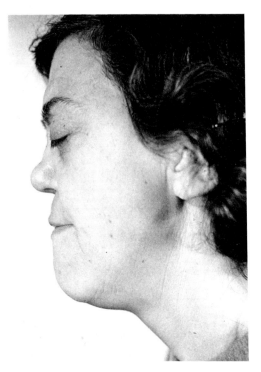

Fig. 16.51 *Collapsed nasal bridge and frontal bossing of congenital syphilis.*

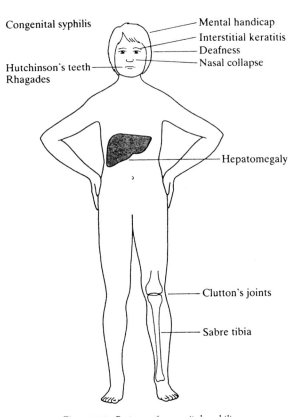

Fig. 16.52 *Features of congenital syphilis.*

Table 16.2
Serological tests for syphilis

| Test | Stage of disease | | | | | |
| | Primary | | Secondary | | Tertiary | |
	U	T	U	T	U	T
Non-specific test:						
VDRL	Becomes + ve late	− ve	+ ve	− ve	Usually + ve	+ ve
Specific test:						
FTA-Abs	Becomes + ve early	+ ve	+ ve	+ ve	+ ve	+ ve

U = untreated; T = treated.
VDRL = Venereal Disease Research Laboratory.
FTA-Abs = fluorescent treponemal antibody–absorbed, *see* Volume 1.

are given at the start of treatment with antibiotics in order to reduce the possibility of a Jarisch–Herxheimer reaction (febrile reaction often with exacerbation of the local syphilitic lesions).

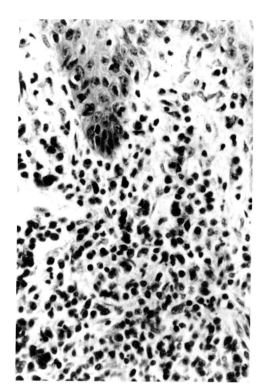

Fig. 16.53 *Dense plasma-cell infiltrate in a lesion of syphilis.*

Tuberculosis (see also Volume 1)

Oral lesions can develop in pulmonary tuberculosis but are uncommon. A chronic ulcer, usually of the dorsum of the tongue, is the main oral presentation and occasionally the diagnosis of pulmonary tuberculosis is made as a result of biopsy of an oral ulcer. Tuberculosis can also cause cervical lymph node enlargement or, rarely, lesions of the jaws.

Management

The diagnosis of tuberculosis is suggested by associated features such as a chronic cough, haemoptysis, loss of weight, night sweats and fever. It is confirmed by physical examination, chest radiography, sputum smears and culture, and tuberculin testing (Mantoux or Heaf test). Biopsies of oral ulcers should be sent for culture as well as histology. Histology shows caseating granulomas (Fig. 16.54) which arise as a consequence of a cell-mediated immune reaction (Fig. 16.55).

Though *Mycobacterium tuberculosis* is the classic cause of TB, it is nowadays frequently due to other mycobacteria: *M. avium* and *M. intercellulare* can cause pulmonary tuberculosis, while *M. scrofulaceum* is a cause of tuberculous lymphadenitis, for example. Mycobacterial ulcers have been reported as a complication of AIDS.

Treatment is started with three drugs in combination in order to avoid the emergence of bacterial resistance, and is then continued with two or more antibiotics, usually from the following: rifampicin, isoniazid, ethambutol or streptomycin.

Chemotherapy is usually effective but must be given

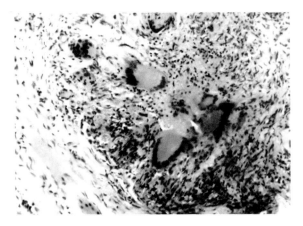

Fig. 16.54 *Granuloma containing Langerhan's giant cells, in tuberculous lesion.*

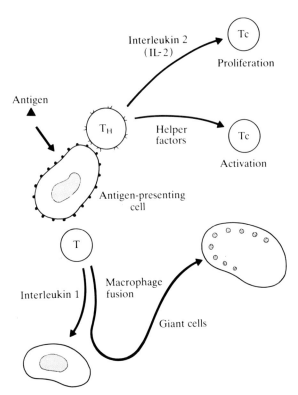

Activated macrophages

Fig. 16.55 *Granuloma formation (as in tuberculosis, sarcoidosis, Crohn's disease or foreign body reactions).*

for prolonged periods. Alcoholics, vagrants, the mentally handicapped or those with psychiatric disorders frequently default from treatment and, if chemotherapy is less than adequate, bacterial resistance readily develops.

Viral infections

Oral ulcers of infectious aetiology are usually caused by herpesviruses (chickenpox and zoster; primary herpetic stomatitis and recurrences), or enteroviruses (herpangina or hand–foot–mouth disease).

Herpesviruses

Four types of herpesvirus are known to affect humans and three can produce mouth ulcers:

(a) herpes simplex virus (HSV),
(b) Herpes varicella–zoster virus (VZV),
(c) Epstein–Barr virus (EBV: see Chapter 31).

Mouth ulcers are common in primary HSV infection and primary VZV infection but are not usually a major manifestation of EBV infection. The fourth herpesvirus—cytomegalovirus (CMV: Chapter 31)—is not known to cause mouth ulcers.

Herpesviruses are DNA viruses that usually cause a primary infection in childhood, adolescence or young adult life and are characterized by latency, i.e. following the primary infection the virus is not completely eliminated from the body but resides in certain cells from whence it can be reactivated and cause disease (Table 16.2). These recurrent diseases usually differ somewhat from the primary infections and are called secondary 'infections', even though they are *not* exogenous infections. It follows that a person with a primary infection can transmit primary infection to a non-immune contact but not to an immune contact. Furthermore, a person with a primary infection cannot immediately cause secondary 'infection' manifestations in a non-immune person (nor any other person). In contrast, a patient with secondary 'infection' can cause primary (but not secondary) disease in a non-immune but not in an immune individual.

All these viruses can cause severe widespread disease in immunocompromised persons including those with AIDS but, in those with an intact immune system, probably at least one-half of infections produce little or nothing in the way of symptoms, i.e. they are *subclinical*. Although symptoms may be absent, subclinical infections still elicit an immune response, are followed by latency, and reactivation may produce secondary 'infection'.

Since there is an immune response to herpesvirus infections, the question is often asked as to why secondary 'infection' is possible. The primary infection occurs in a non-immune person who subsequently develops a humoral and cellular immune response that results in resolution of the primary infection. The immune response (or at least the humoral response) can be measured by assay of the serum antibody titres, which rise, usually at least fourfold, between serum taken during the infection (acute serum) and that taken 2–3 weeks later (convalescent serum). The patient thereafter has persisting levels of serum antibodies to the virus and sensitized B- and T-lymphocytes (memory cells), and is thereby protected by mucosal and other defences against *re-infection* by the same virus. However, since virus is latent *intracellularly* (in the case of HSV and VZV, for example, in neurones), it is inaccessible to host immune defences. Serum antibodies are extracellular, and cell-mediated responses will not be initiated since the virus and viral antigens are 'hidden' within the neurones. If the virus is re-activated and replicates, releasing viral antigens extracellularly or altering host cell membranes, then the host immune mechanisms can come into play and again keep the infection under control. If there is, for any reason, an immune defect such as, for example, immunosuppression by drugs or AIDS, secondary 'infection' is more likely. Even a mild degree of immune defect such as may accompany a 'cold' can precipitate secondary herpes simplex 'infection'—hence the name *cold sore* (see below: herpes labialis).

Herpes simplex virus

Herpes simplex virus (HSV) infection is a common infection caused by one or other of the two types of HSV, termed HSV1 and HSV2. In general, HSV1 causes primary herpetic stomatitis (and the secondary 'infection' of recurrent herpes labialis) and other infections 'above the belt'. HSV2 causes genital lesions and other infections 'below the belt'. There are no precise distinctions, nowadays, presumably with more frequent orogenital and oro-anal sexual practices, and genital and anal infection with HSV1 and oral infection with HSV2 are also seen.

Primary herpetic stomatitis

Many infections with HSV occur in childhood and are subclinical. HSV is transmitted particularly in saliva. However, with improving socioeconomic circumstances and standards of hygiene, a larger number of children are not exposed to HSV and enter adult life with no immunity. Cases of primary herpetic stomatitis are, therefore, now seen occasionally in adults, and the manifestations can be severe.

1. *Clinical features.* The incubation period is 3–7 days. Primary herpetic stomatitis presents with the following features.

(a) General features: malaise, anorexia, irritability and fever.

(b) Anterior cervical lymph nodes are enlarged and tender.

(c) More specific features: diffuse, purple, boggy gingivitis, especially anteriorly, with multiple vesicles followed by round or ovoid ulcers 1–3 mm in diameter scattered across the oral mucosa and gingiva (Figs. 16.56–16.58; see also Fig. 32.8).

The disease varies greatly in severity and, in many, is trivial and passed off as 'teething'. Fever, however, is a feature of infection and not 'teething'.

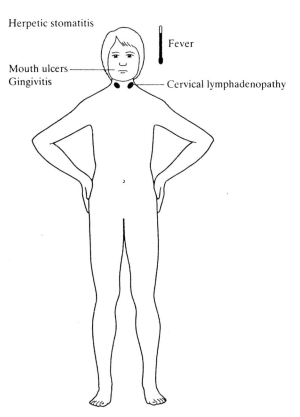

Fig. 16.56 *Features of herpetic stomatitis.*

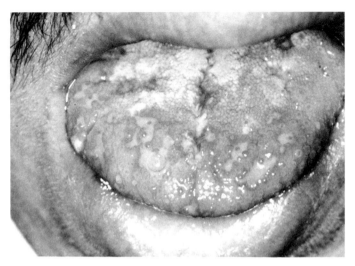

Fig. 16.57 *Multiple small mouth ulcers coalescing to form irregular lesions in herpetic stomatitis.*

The disease spontaneously resolves in 7–10 days but the virus remains latent in the trigeminal ganglion. The most obvious sequel is that about one-third of patients thereafter are predisposed throughout life to recurrent herpes labialis. Rarely, HSV causes more serious infections such as herpetic encephalitis.

2. *Transmission.* The saliva is teeming with HSV and infection easily spreads to the skin of the chin or anterior chest wall in infants who are drooling, or to the fingers if they are sucked, or elsewhere. Health care personnel, including the dentist, may contract an extremely painful herpetic whitlow if not wearing rubber gloves (Fig. 16.59).

3. *Diagnosis.* The main differential diagnoses are:

(a) chickenpox and other viral causes of mouth ulcers;

(b) acute leukaemia.

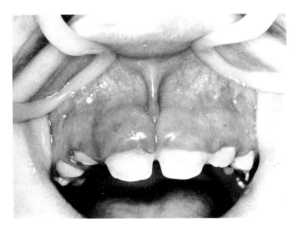

Fig. 16.58 *Purple boggy gingival swelling and ulceration in herpetic stomatitis.*

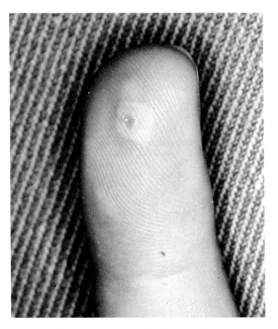

Fig. 16.59 *Herpetic whitlow in a dentist.*

The diagnosis is mainly clinical, based on the general features of infection (fever etc.) and the specific oral features of the fairly characteristic gingivitis together with mucosal ulcers. A history of contact with infectious diseases (especially chickenpox) should be sought. The patient should be examined generally to exclude a rash and to exclude the anaemia, bleeding tendency, generalized lymph node enlargement and hepatosplenomegaly suggestive of leukaemia.

The following investigations may be needed.

(a) Full blood picture, white cell count and differential—to exclude leukaemia or an immune defect.

(b) Viral studies:

    (i) viral culture—an oral swab placed in viral transport medium;

    (ii) serology—acute (and later the convalescent) sera;

    (iii) electron microscopy—rarely.

(c) Cytological smear from lesion, rarely (shows multinucleate giant cells: Fig. 16.60).

4. *Management.* Specific antiviral agents are slowly becoming available but need to be used in the very early stages of disease—before most patients present for treatment—and in general their use is restricted to immunocompromised patients who may otherwise suffer severe infection. Oral and intravenous preparations of acycloguanosine (acyclovir) appear to be effective; the drug is inactive until activated by a viral thymidine kinase enzyme and thus is selectively toxic to the virus and not the host. Vaccines to give prophylaxis against HSV (particularly HSV2) are also being developed.

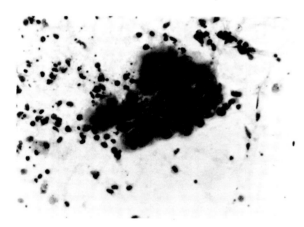

Fig. 16.60 *Smear from herpetic lesion showing epithelial cells clustered as giant cells.*

At present, however, management is 'supportive', i.e. symptoms are treated as they present and the patient kept generally comfortable. The most important aspects of this are as follows.

(a) To reduce the fever: since this not only makes the patient feel miserable and irritable but, in a young child, may precipitate convulsions (febrile convulsions). Antipyretic analgesics (paracetamol) and sponging with tepid water are most effective at reducing fever. The child should *not* be wrapped in an attempt to keep him warm.

(b) To maintain hydration: children easily become dehydrated, with serious consequences. A high fluid intake is needed. Food is not particularly important for a few days and it is best to give milk, soups, purées, scrambled egg and other bland, non-irritating foods.

(c) Analgesia: analgesics (as elixirs or syrups for children) and, in adults, lignocaine mouthbaths (lignocaine viscous gel) help ease discomfort.

(d) Reduce secondary infection: 0.2% aqueous chlorhexidine mouthbaths aid resolution.

(e) Rest: an antihistamine such as promethazine may help sedate an irritable child and allow him (and the parents) to sleep.

Recurrent herpes labialis (cold sores)

From time to time, HSV is reactivated and the virus moves down from the trigeminal ganglion along the nerve axons to be released, often asymptomatically, into the saliva. Sometimes it produces skin lesions, usually at, or very close to, a mucocutaneous junction. In most individuals, lesions appear on the lips, but in some they involve the anterior nares, eyelids or ears. Patients of all ages can be affected. The lesions begin with a prodromal burning sensation followed by vesicles which change to pustules before they scab and heal over 7–14 days (Fig. 16.61). Lesions vary in site and size but can be extremely widespread in immunocompromised or eczematous patients (Fig. 16.62). The lesions are infectious.

Immunocompromised patients may also develop intraoral secondary 'infection' and ulceration with HSV (Fig. 16.63) but this is very rare in healthy patients. Other factors that may trigger reactivation are shown in Figure 16.64.

Complications of herpes labialis are rare, although, if hygiene is not good, bacterial superinfection may lead to impetigo (Fig. 16.65).

1. *Diagnosis.* The diagnosis is usually obvious from

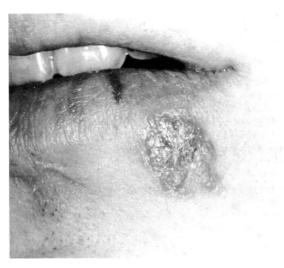

Fig. 16.61 *Recurrent herpes labialis: vesicles at the mucocutaneous junction.*

the clinical features but may be confusing if, for example, there is haemorrhage into the lesions because of a bleeding tendency such as in leukaemia. The only real and rare differential diagnoses are from:

(a) impetigo (Fig. 16.65),
(b) carcinoma (Fig. 16.66) and keratoacanthoma.

Vesicle fluid can be sent for culture and (occasionally) electron microscopy. Serology will show a high titre of antibodies to HSV in the *acute* serum with little or no rise in the convalescent serum if the lesion is herpes labialis, and therefore serology is of no true value in diagnosis.

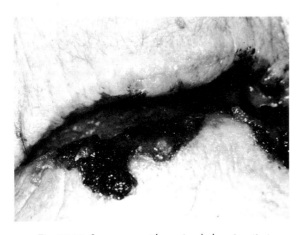

Fig. 16.62 *Severe recurrent herpes in a leukaemic patient.*

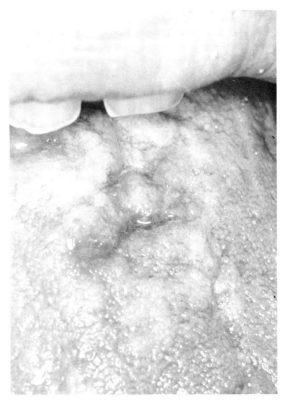

Fig. 16.63 *Recurrent intra-oral herpes simplex infection causing an irregular ulcer on the tongue in a patient with AIDS.*

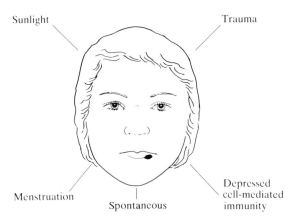

Sunlight

Trauma

Menstruation

Spontaneous

Depressed cell-mediated immunity

Fig. 16.64 *Factors that may reactivate herpes simplex virus.*

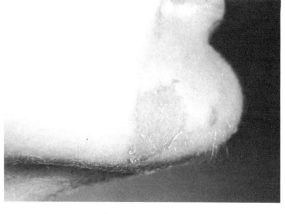

Fig. 16.65 Impetigo.

2. *Management.*

(a) *Prevention.* Avoidance of precipitating factors (see Fig. 16.64) that cause viral re-activation may reduce the recurrence rate to a limited extent. The use of barrier creams to protect against ultraviolet irradiation (e.g. Uvistat) may be a useful measure for those about to go to sunny climes. Most other precipitating factors are unavoidable.

(b) *Treatment.* A number of supposed therapies are available, from topical applications of ether or alcohol to various antiviral agents. Few have been tested in controlled double-blind trials; there is a significant placebo response; and again there is the difficulty that treatment may not be started soon enough.

Currently, the most effective antivirals are:

(i) acyclovir cream, and possibly
(ii) inosoprine, and
(iii) vidarabine.

Acyclovir as a 5% cream appears useful if applied as early as possible in the development of the lesion. Idoxuridine, in vogue for several years, has never been

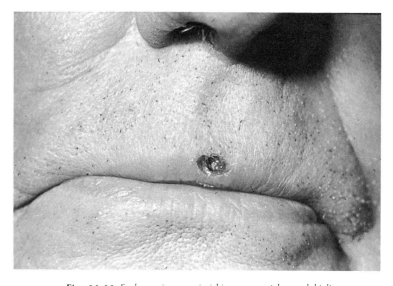

Fig. 16.66 *Early carcinoma mimicking recurrent herpes labialis.*

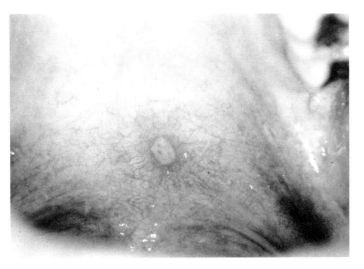

Fig. 16.67 Mouth ulcer in chickenpox.

conclusively shown to be effective, although some patients find it useful.

Herpes varicella (*chickenpox*)

Many primary infections with VZV virus are subclinical or produce so few lesions as to pass almost unnoticed. The incubation period is 14–21 days. Chickenpox affects children predominantly and may present with the following features.

(a) General features: malaise, anorexia, irritability and fever.

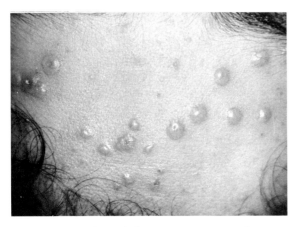

Fig. 16.68 Rash of chickenpox: crops appear and pass through macular, papular, vesicular and pustular stages before crusting.

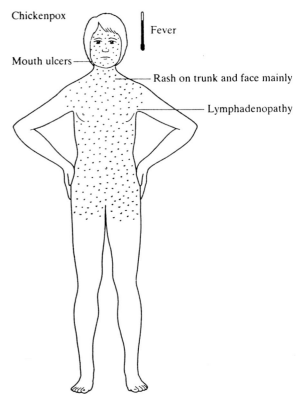

Fig. 16.69 Features of chickenpox.

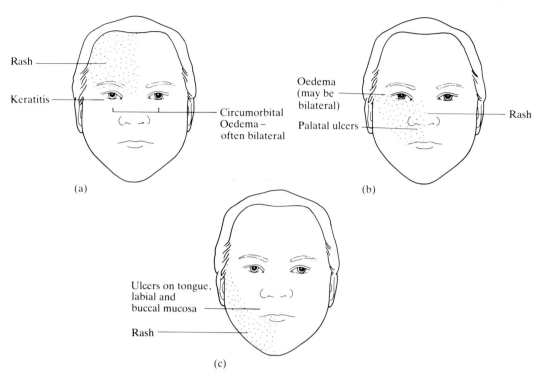

Fig. 16.70 *Trigeminal herpes zoster: (a) ophthalmic zoster; (b) maxillary zoster; (c) mandibular zoster.*

(b) More specific features:

(i) mouth ulcers: which resemble those of herpetic stomatitis (Fig. 16.67)—but there is no gingivitis.

(ii) rash: this is centripetal and crops, i.e. it affects the head, neck and trunk mainly and lesions are seen at all stages in development from itchy macules to papules, vesicles, pustules and scabs (Figs. 16.68 and 16.69).

Most patients recover spontaneously in 2–3 weeks but a few develop complications, such a pneumonia. Immunocompromised patients can develop widespread and severe disease.

The lesions are infectious until they have all scabbed. VZV remains latent, thereafter, mainly in dorsal root (sensory) nerve ganglia.

1. *Diagnosis.* Diagnosis is clinical and usually straightforward. Before smallpox was eradicated, that was the most important differential diagnosis but, nowadays, only the enterovirus infections (p. 218) and a few other viral infections need to be excluded.

2. *Management.* Management is supportive in most cases (see above), but antivirals such as acyclovir may be indicated if the patient is immunocompromised.

Herpes zoster (shingles)

Reactivation of VZV is not as common as reactivation of HSV, and usually occurs at a later age. However, the consequent lesions are usually far more painful and cause extreme distress. Most shingles affects elderly patients, and usually in the thoracic region. If the ophthalmic division of the trigeminal nerve is involved, corneal ulceration and even blindness can result. If the maxillary or mandibular divisions of the trigeminal nerve are involved, mouth ulceration is usually seen (Fig. 16.70).

1. *Clinical features.*

(a) *Pain.* Severe pain often precedes, accompanies and follows the rash (post-herpetic neuralgia), sometimes persisting for months or years. The pain may simulate toothache.

(b) *Rash.* The rash resembles that of chickenpox in its development but is restricted to a dermatome, i.e. the area of skin supplied by a sensory nerve. The rash is

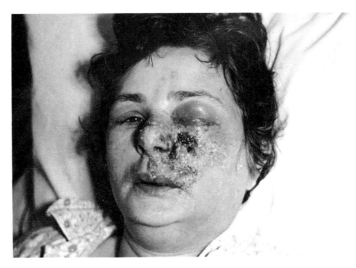

Fig. 16.71 *Maxillary zoster: the mouth (palate) is ulcerated but the eye is unaffected despite the circumorbital oedema. There are lesions of chickenpox on the forehead.*

unilateral but sometimes a few chickenpox-type lesions can be also found elsewhere (Fig. 16.71).

(c) *Mucosal ulcers*—in trigeminal zoster. These occur in the distribution of the involved division, i.e. there is ulceration of one side of the tongue, floor of mouth, lower labial and buccal mucosa if the mandibular division of the trigeminal nerve is involved (Fig. 16.72). In maxillary zoster the ulcers involve one side of the palate, the upper gingiva, and buccal sulcus.

A *rare* type of shingles occurs if the geniculate ganglion of the facial nerve is affected: there is unilateral facial palsy, with vesicles in the ipsilateral ear and ulcers in the soft palate ipsilaterally (Ramsay–Hunt syndrome).

2. *Diagnosis.* Diagnosis is usually clinical, but there may be a mis-diagnosis of toothache leading to extraction—the true diagnosis only becoming apparent when the rash appears. Usually, however, the diagnosis is obvious clinically from the unilateral rash restricted to a dermatome. Occasionally, cutaneous recurrent herpes simplex lesions occur in one dermatome and simulate zoster.

3. *Management.* An underlying immune defect, such as AIDS, or malignancy should be excluded.

Treatment is mainly supportive but, in ophthalmic zoster, it is important to refer the patient for a specialist opinion because of the danger to sight.

Antivirals such as acyclovir are most needed in ophthalmic zoster but can be useful elsewhere.

Analgesics are indicated in zoster, but the pain may prove refractory to even potent analgesics. Amantadine may be of value in controlling the pain of herpetic neuralgia.

Epstein–Barr virus (see Chapter 31)

Enteroviruses

Coxsackie, and sometimes echoviruses, can cause relatively minor illnesses, characterized by mouth ulcers. Small epidemics of these infections are not uncommon, particularly in schoolchildren.

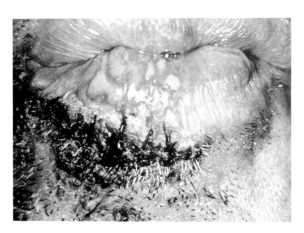

Fig. 16.72 *Mandibular zoster showing oral ulcers.*

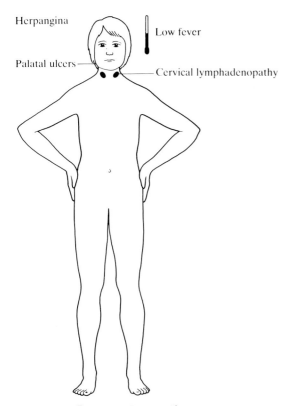

Fig. 16.73 *Features of herpangina.*

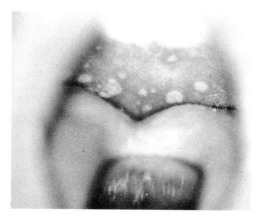

Fig. 16.74 *Mouth ulcers in herpangina.*

Herpangina

Herpangina is caused particularly by Coxsackie viruses. The incubation period is 3–7 days and young children are predominantly affected.

1. *Clinical features.* Many infections are subclinical but features of the clinical syndrome include (Fig. 16.73):

(a) general features: malaise, anorexia, irritability and low fever;
(b) anterior cervical lymph nodes may be slightly enlarged and tender;
(c) mouth ulcers: predominantly on the soft palate (Fig. 16.74).

Sequelae of any consequence are rare, the disease resolving spontaneously in 7–10 days.

2. *Diagnosis.* Diagnosis is usually clinical, but it is possible to culture Coxsackie viruses in suckling mice if absolutely necessary. There may be a contact history.

The main differential diagnosis is primary herpetic stomatitis, but in herpangina there is:

(a) less fever,
(b) no acute gingivitis,
(c) ulceration almost only on the soft palate.

3. *Management.* This is supportive only (see p. 213).

Hand, foot and mouth disease

Hand, foot and mouth disease is caused particularly by Coxsackie A viruses. It is a quite different condition from foot and mouth disease of cattle. The incubation period is 3–10 days and, though young children are predominantly infected, outbreaks not infrequently also affect adults. Many infections are subclinical but features of the clinical syndrome include (Fig. 16.75):

(a) general features: malaise, anorexia, irritability and fever may be present but only in severe cases;
(b) anterior cervical lymph nodes may be slightly enlarged and tender but this is not common;
(c) mouth ulcers are round or ovoid, usually sparse and affect any site;
(d) rash: painful, sometimes deep-seated vesicles may appear, usually on the hands and/or feet, particularly between digits or at the base of the phalanges (Fig. 16.76).

Diagnosis and management are as for herpangina.

HIV infection (see Volume 1)

Fungal infections

Oral ulcers are a rare complication of candidosis, but

Hand, foot and mouth disease

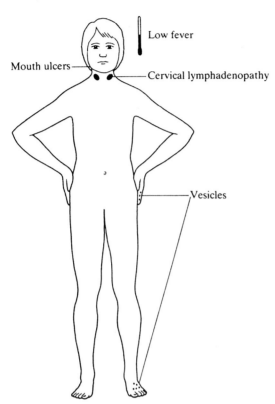

Fig. 16.75 Features of hand, foot and mouth disease.

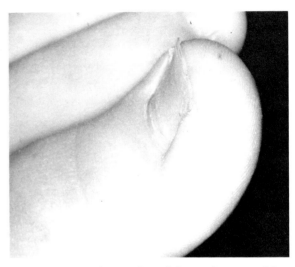

Fig. 16.76 Hand, foot and mouth disease, showing painful vesicle on side of great toe.

angular stomatitis (angular cheilitis or cheilosis) may ulcerate and be sore (Chapter 17).

Ulcers may be caused by other fungal infections but are rare in the UK, except in travellers from the Third World or in severely immunocompromised individuals. These include mucormycosis, aspergillosis, blastomycosis and histoplasmosis. Their presence should raise the suggestion of AIDS, leukaemia or diabetes mellitus.

Protozoal infestations

Leishmaniasis is rare except in travellers from outside Europe; it is not uncommon, however, in Crete and may cause ulcers on lips or mouth. Toxoplasmosis is discussed in Chapter 31.

FURTHER READING

Jones J. H., Mason D. K. (Eds.) (in press). *Oral manifestations of systemic disease*, 2nd edn. London: Balliere Tindall and Cox.

Lancet (1981). Acyclovir. *Lancet*, **ii:** 845–846.

Lancet (1981). Herpes simplex—changing patterns. *Lancet*, **ii:** 1025.

Scully C. (1988). Infectious diseases in oral medicine. In *Oral medicine* (D. Millard, D. K. Mason, eds.). Michigan: University of Michigan Press.

Scully C., Cawson R. A. (1988). *Colour aids to oral medicine.* Edinburgh and London: Churchill-Livingstone.

Scully C., Elkom M. (1985). Lichen planus: review and update on pathogenesis. *J. oral Pathol.*, **14:** 431–458.

Scully C., Porter S. R. (1988). The mouth and skin. In *Relationships in dermatology*, Vol. 8 (J. Verbov, Ed.) Lancaster: MTP Press.

Stephenson P., Lamey P.-J., Scully C., Prime S. S. (1987). Angina bullosa haemorrhagica: clinical and laboratory features in 30 patients. *Oral Surg.*, **63:** 560–565.

Chapter 17

The sore mouth: 4. Other causes

ERYTHEMA MIGRANS

A common cause of a sore tongue is the benign idiopathic condition of geographic tongue (erythema migrans, benign migratory glossitis).

This common oral condition can be seen at any age and a positive family history may be obtainable. However, only a tiny minority complain of soreness and these

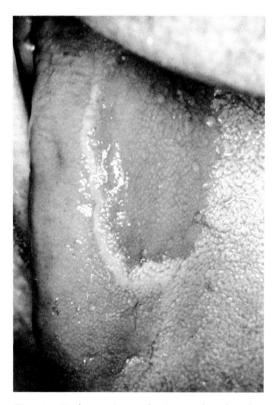

Fig. 17.1 *Erythema migrans, showing a red patch with a surrounding whitish border.*

patients are usually middle-aged. Why the condition should give rise to symptoms after it has presumably been present for decades is unclear, but it is possible that some have recently noticed and become alarmed by the appearance.

It is characterized by map-like red areas with increased thickness of the intervening filiform papillae. Alternatively, there are rounded, sometimes scalloped, reddish areas with a white margin (Fig. 17.1). These patterns change from day to day and even within a few hours (Fig. 17.2). Rarely, the lesion affects other sites, such as the labial or palatal mucosa. Many patients with a fissured tongue (scrotal tongue) also have erythema migrans.

Some have atopic allergies such as hay fever and a few relate the oral lesions to various foods, e.g. cheese. Similar lesions may be seen in Reiter's syndrome and in psoriasis.

Histologically there is epithelial thinning at the centre of the lesion with an inflammatory infiltrate mainly of polymorphonuclear leucocytes.

Management

Blood examination is necessary to exclude anaemia. In those with no systemic disorder, no treatments are available and reassurance remains the best that can be given.

INFLAMMATORY LESIONS

Any inflammatory lesion in the mouth may cause soreness. Pericoronitis—inflammation of the operculum or gingiva overlying a partially erupted tooth (usually a lower wisdom tooth)—is a particular cause, in which soreness is associated with halitosis, bad taste and trismus, and the operculum may be oedematous and

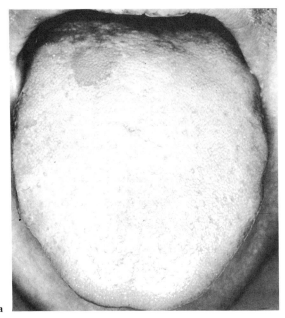

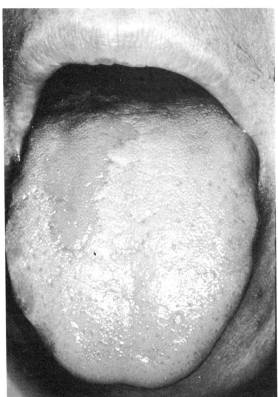

Fig. 17.2 *Erythema migrans: (a) an early lesion; (b) the same lesion 24 hours later.*

tender. Antibiotics and dental attention may well be indicated (Volume 3).

ACUTE CANDIDOSIS

A sore tongue may be caused by candidosis (antibiotic sore tongue: Chapter 18), when it is fiery red. Candidosis is also often the cause of soreness in patients with xerostomia (Fig. 17.3).

GLOSSITIS

A similar appearance with depapillation of the anterior two-thirds may be caused by deficiency states (of iron, folic acid or B vitamins). The different types of glossitis due to the various deficiency states may not be clinically distinguishable one from another (see Chapter 18).

ANGULAR STOMATITIS

This is a bilateral condition affecting adults and characterized by lesions at the commissures infected by *Candida* species, staphylococci and sometimes streptococci. Most

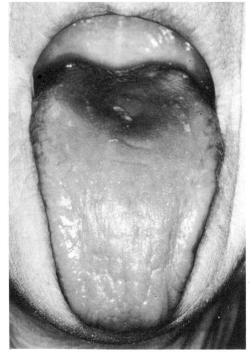

Fig. 17.3 *Sore tongue caused by candidosis in a patient with xerostomia.*

Angular stomatitis

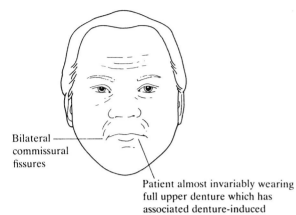

Bilateral commissural fissures

Patient almost invariably wearing full upper denture which has associated denture-induced stomatitis

Fig. 17.4 *Features of angular stomatitis.*

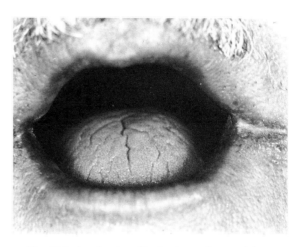

Fig. 17.5 *Angular stomatitis showing erythema and fissuring at both commissures.*

patients also have denture-induced stomatitis which acts as a source of persistent *Candida* infection (Chapter 18). Contributing factors occasionally include ill-fitting dentures, or deficiencies of iron, folate or vitamin B12—but not allergy to denture materials.

HIV infection is a rare cause of angular stomatitis.

Clinical features
Angular stomatitis usually presents as mere erythema at the commissures without soreness, but may cause moderate soreness with ulceration or fissuring (Figs. 17.4–17.6). Occasionally persistent lesions cause scarring.

Diagnosis
The diagnosis is clinical and there is rarely a need to undertake microbiological investigation.

Management
Any underlying deficiency state should be excluded and treated if present.

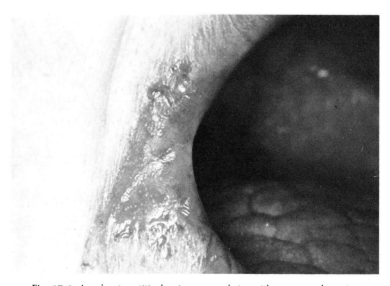

Fig. 17.6 *Angular stomatitis showing a severe lesion with soreness and weeping.*

Most patients have an associated denture-induced stomatitis which must be treated if the angular stomatitis is not to recur (Chapter 18). Staphylococci and streptococci, as well as *Candida* species, are found on the skin lesions and therefore miconazole, which has antifungal and antibacterial activity, is useful in the treatment of angular stomatitis. Nystatin or amphotericin is also suitable.

The most important facet of treatment, however, is to leave the dentures out at night (and as much as possible at other times) and to cleanse the dentures by scrubbing and storing them in a solution with antifungal activity, such as 0.2% chlorhexidine or 1% hypochlorite. The denture otherwise acts as a reservoir for *Candida* species and recurrence is common (see Chapter 18 and Volume 3).

CRACKED AND SORE LIPS (Fig. 17.7)

Cracks on both sides at the commissures are usually angular stomatitis, but sores are also caused at the angles by trauma (such as dental treatment), or infection such as recurrent herpes labialis.

In winter, especially where the patient is breathing through the mouth because of, for example, a cold, the lips may crack. Usually the lower lip is affected—often centrally (Fig. 17.8). Bland creams or petroleum jelly may help; rarely is surgery required.

Cheilitis may also be caused by trauma, burns (including sunlight), chemicals, candidosis, or allergies.

SORE BUT APPARENTLY NORMAL MOUTH

Soreness of the mouth without physical abnormalities does not exclude the possibility of a deficiency state, particularly vitamin B12 deficiency, or even anaemia, but the complaint is common at or near the menopause mainly because psychogenic complaints are more frequ-

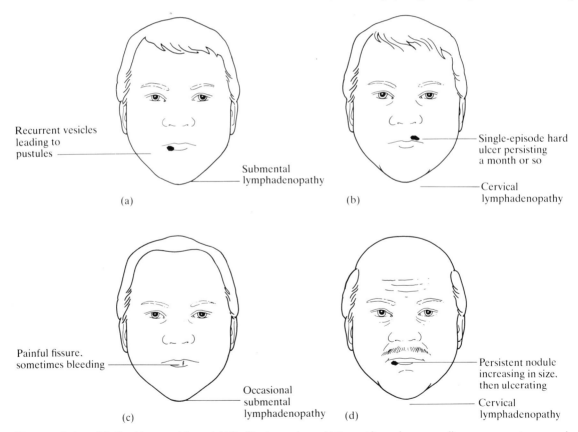

Fig. 17.7 *Lesions of the lips: (a) recurrent herpes labialis; (b) primary chance; (c) fissure; (d) neoplasm—usually squamous carcinoma, rarely keratoacanthoma or basal cell carcinoma.*

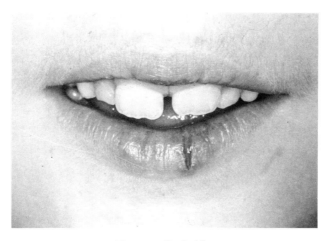

Fig. 17.8 *Cracked lip.*

ent then. A hormonal basis has *not* been confirmed though diabetes mellitus is occasionally found.

The suggestion that soreness of the tongue or other parts of the oral mucosa is a symptom of such diverse diseases as gastric 'hyperactivity' or hypothyroidism has never been substantiated.

A sore tongue or sore mouth (often described as a burning sensation) can be a manifestation of a psychogenic disorder (psychosomatic disease) and is sometimes known as oral dyaesthesia (Chapter 27; Volume 1). A psychogenic basis may be suggested by a history of recent adverse life events, depression, the presence of recognizable depressive or delusional features, migratory symptoms, or rejection and resistance to treatment.

FURTHER READING

Scully C. (1982). The sore mouth. *Dermatology in Practice,* **i**: 19–29.

Scully C., Cawson R. A. (1988). *Colour aids to oral medicine.* Edinburgh and London: Churchill-Livingstone.

Scully C., Flint S. (1988). *An atlas of stomatology.* London: Martin Dunitz (in press).

Wray D., Scully C. (1986). The sore mouth. *Med. Int.,* **2**: 1134–1137.

Chapter
18   *Red lesions*

Whereas most red lesions are inflammatory in origin, some are due to mucosal atrophy or to premalignancy. Red mucosal patches with a velvety surface (erythroplasia) are frequently premalignant or malignant, and Kaposi's sarcoma may present as a red, purplish or bluish lesion.

GEOGRAPHICAL TONGUE (Chapter 17)

Geographical tongue (erythema migrans, migratory glossitis) manifests with irregular depapillated areas, which change in size and shape, usually in the dorsum of the tongue. No treatment is needed or available.

CANDIDOSIS

Denture-induced stomatitis (denture sore mouth)

This common form of mild chronic atrophic candidosis consists of inflammation of the mucosa beneath a denture—usually a complete upper denture—and is *not* sore. Dentures worn throughout the night, or a dry mouth, favour development of this infection with *Candida* species. It is *not* caused by allergy to the denture material.

However, it is still not clear why only some denture-wearers develop denture stomatitis; it is a disease mainly of the middle-aged or elderly and is more prevalent in women than men but patients appear otherwise healthy. The erythema is limited to the denture-bearing area (Fig. 18.1), is usually asymptomatic and, although it may be associated with angular stomatitis (Chapter 17), has no other serious complications. Occasionally small nodules appear (papillary hyperplasia) in the vault of the palate.

Dentures should be left at night in 0.2% chlorhexidine

or 1% hypochlorite since the fitting surface is infested, usually with *Candida albicans*. The mucosal infection is eradicated with miconazole gel, nystatin pastilles or

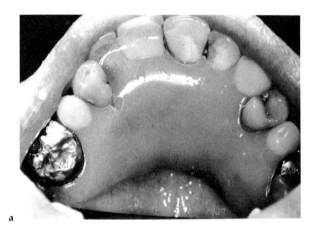

a

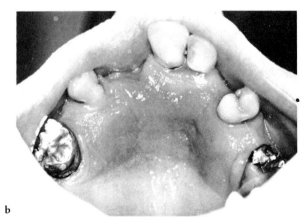

b

Fig. 18.1 (a) *'Gum-stripper' acrylic upper denture in situ.* (b) *Diffuse erythema, indicative of denture-induced stomatitis limited to the denture-bearing area (note also cervical caries).*

226

amphotericin. The immediate improvement, however, only lasts until the denture is recolonized by the fungus, unless the dentures are left out at night. The dentures may need attention (Volume 3).

Antibiotic or steroid-induced stomatitis

Acute oral candidosis may complicate corticosteroid or antibiotic therapy, particularly with long-term broad-spectrum antimicrobials, and cause widespread erythema and soreness of the oral mucosa, sometimes with thrush (see Chapter 17 and 19).

GLOSSITIS

Antibiotic sore tongue (see p. 222)

This is discussed above.

Median rhomboid glossitis

This is a depapillated rhomboidal area in the centre line of the dorsum of the tongue, just anterior to the sulcus terminalis (Fig. 18.2). Formerly thought to be caused by persistence of the tuberculum impar, this lesion is now thought to be associated with candidosis. *Candida* species, even in the healthy, colonize mainly the posterior dorsum of the tongue, and smoking and denture-wearing predispose to this lesion.

There is rarely soreness from median rhomboid glossitis. It is usually detected by the patient or dentist as a persistent red, rhomboidal depapillated area.

Histology shows irregular epithelial hyperplasia which resembles a carcinoma (because of pseudo-epitheliomatous hyperplasia) but it is not malignant or pre-malignant.

Median rhomboid glossitis may respond to cessation of smoking (presumably because smoking has predisposed to candidal proliferation), and the use of anti-fungals such as nystatin or amphotericin.

Anaemic glossitis

In anaemic glossitis the tongue is red, sore and smooth (Fig. 18.3). Occasionally pernicious anaemia can also produce red areas or patterns of red lines. In others, the tongue can become sore but appear completely normal—such patients' complaints are liable to be mislabelled as psychogenic. Glossitis may be related to deficiency of iron, folate or vitamin B12, and then may be associated with angular stomatitis and/or mouth ulcers. Deficiencies of vitamins of the B group other than B12 are an occasional cause of glossitis, mainly seen in chronic alcoholics or in those with malabsorption.

A full blood picture is essential in management, as sore tongue can be the initial symptom of a deficiency of iron, folate or vitamin B12 and can precede any fall in the haemoglobin level. The cause of the deficiency should be sought before treatment is completed (see p. 224).

HAEMORRHAGIC LESIONS

Oral petechiae are commonplace and are often seen as one or two inconsequential lesions at the occlusal line,

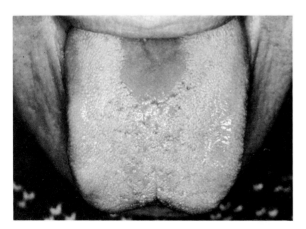

Fig. 18.2 *Median rhomboid glossitis.*

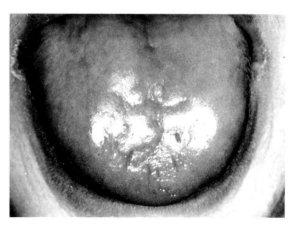

Fig. 18.3 *Anaemic glossitis: smooth, sore red tongue with almost complete depapillation.*

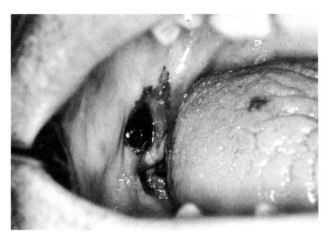

Fig. 18.4 Purpura in thrombocytopenia.

caused by cheek-biting. Occasionally patients develop blood blisters or oral purpura secondary to minimal or unnoticed trauma, but no haemostatic defect is found on investigation (angina bullosa haemorrhagica: Chapter 16).

More obvious or widespread lesions are usually of more serious significance (Fig. 18.4). Minor trauma such as at the occlusal line or post-dam area of a denture tends to precipitate lesions in patients with purpura (Fig. 18.5). Major trauma, including jaw fractures, may lead to extensive petechiae or ecchymoses but, in the absence of major trauma, these signs should lead one to suspect a bleeding tendency, particularly purpura (see Fig. 32.13). In such patients there may be skin petechiae, an

obvious bleeding tendency or spontaneous gingival haemorrhage. A full blood picture, white count and differential, and platelet count are indicated (Volume 1).

Amyloidosis may present with oral purpura or blood blisters as well as a chronically swollen tongue (Chapter 21).

VASCULAR LESIONS

Telangiectases (dilated capillaries) may be seen after irradiation of the mouth and in various systemic disorders such as hereditary haemorrhagic telangiectasia and systemic sclerosis. What appear to be haemangiomas (dilated blood vessels) are usually small, isolated hamartomas (tumour-like new growths of blood vessels; see Chapter 21) but may be part of the Sturge–Weber syndrome of facial and oral haemangioma with an intracranial haemangiomatous extension that calcifies and may be associated with epilepsy and hemiplegia (Chapter 12).

Lingual veins (varices) may be conspicuous in the elderly in the ventrum of the tongue and may cause unnecessary alarm.

Kaposi's sarcoma—a common neoplasm in AIDS—appears in the mouth as purplish red areas or nodules, especially on the palate (see Chapter 20 and Volume 1).

Hereditary haemorrhagic telangiectasia (Osler–Rendu–Weber syndrome)

Hereditary haemorrhagic telangiectasia (HHT) is a rare

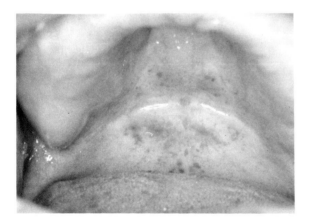

Fig. 18.5 Purpura at the post-dam region beneath a denture, localized by pressure and suction.

genetic disorder, inherited as an autosomal dominant condition.

Clinical features

The characteristic feature is multiple telangiectasia. Typically, telangiectases are seen on the lips, perioral skin, and in the mouth (Fig. 18.6), but they may affect the palms and the gastrointestinal or upper respiratory tract.

Apart from the aesthetic problem, the most important complications are severe repeated nose bleeds (epistaxes) or bleeds from the gastrointestinal tract, leading to iron deficiency anaemia.

Diagnosis

The family history and clinical features are usually obvious.

Management

Bleeding oral telangiectases may need treatment by cautery or cryosurgery. Anaemia should be treated.

ERYTHROPLASIA (ERYTHROPLAKIA)

Erythroplasia is a rare, red and often velvety lesion. It affects patients of either sex in their sixth and seventh decades and typically involves the floor of the mouth, the ventrum of the tongue, or the soft palate. Unlike leukoplakias (see Chapter 19), erythroplasia does not form a plaque but is level with, or depressed below, the surrounding mucosa.

The importance of erythroplasia is that some 75–90% prove to be carcinoma or carcinoma-in-situ or show severe dysplasia (Fig. 18.7). Red oral lesions are generally more dangerous than white.

Management

The incidence of malignant change in erythroplasia is 17 times higher than in leukoplakia, and virtually all the lesions show dysplasia, carcinoma-in-situ, or invasive carcinoma. Therefore, areas of erythroplasia should be excised and sent for histological examination.

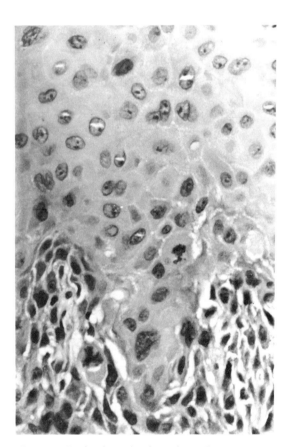

Fig. 18.7 *Erythroplasia: histology shows the severe epithelial dysplasia of carcinoma-in-situ; there is just about to be invasion through the basal lamina.*

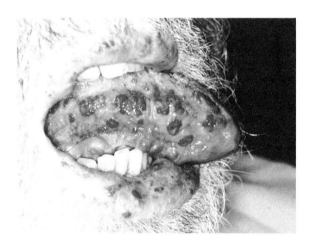

Fig. 18.6 *Hereditary haemorrhagic telangiectasia affecting tongue and lips.*

REDNESS OF THE GINGIVA

Redness is usually inflammatory in origin (gingivitis) and then seen mainly at the gingival margins (Volume 3). Generalized erythema is a feature in herpetic gingivo-stomatitis and also in desquamative gingivitis (Chapter 16) which is almost invariably caused by lichen planus or mucous membrane pemphigoid.

Various other red gingival lesions, including a variety of benign epulides and Wegener's granulomatosis, are discussed in Chapters 14 and 21.

FURTHER READING

Eveson J. W. (1983). Oral premalignancy. *Cancer Surveys*, **2**: 403–424.

Scully C. (1986). Chronic atrophic candidosis (Leading Article). *Lancet*, **ii**: 437–438.

Scully C., Cawson R. A. (1988). Colour aids to oral medicine Edinburgh and London: Churchill-Livingstone.

Scully C., Flint S. (1988). *An atlas of stomatology*. London: Martin Dunitz.

Chapter
19
White lesions

There are many causes of oral mucosal white patches (Table 19.1). When persistent they are usually due to increased keratinization (for example in keratosis or lichen planus), or chronic candidosis. However, oral carcinoma may appear initially as a white patch and patients infected with human immunodeficiency viruses (HIV) may present with a 'hairy leukoplakia'. In many patients the diagnosis is unclear until a biopsy has been carried out, and the term leukoplakia is now usually restricted to those white patches for which a cause cannot be found, and therefore implies a diagnosis by exclusion (e.g. exclusion of lichen planus, candidosis, etc.). The term is also used irrespective of the presence or absence of epithelial dysplasia, though there is a premalignant potential to some keratoses.

Table 19.1
Causes of oral white lesions

Local causes
Frictional keratosis
Smoker's keratosis
Idiopathic keratosis
Papillomas
Carcinomas
Burns
Skin grafts

Systemic causes
White sponge naevus
Candidosis
Lichen planus
Lupus erythematosus
Hairy leukoplakia (AIDS)
Syphilitic keratosis
Candidal leukoplakia
Chronic renal failure
Measles (Koplik's spots)

KERATOSIS (LEUKOPLAKIA)

Leukoplakia is a clinical term for a persistent adherent white patch; it has no histological connotation and does not necessarily imply any premalignant potential, though there is a small premalignant potential in some. The cause of most keratoses is unknown (idiopathic keratoses) but some are caused by chronic irritation, infective agents or other aetiologies.

The prevalence of keratosis is less than 3–4%. It is of interest to note that, while there is clear evidence of the premalignant potential of some oral leukoplakia, with a malignant transformation of 3–6% over 10 years, a greater percentage of leukoplakias (about 15%) regress clinically.

Clinically, keratoses fall into one of two main groups. The most common are uniformly white plaques (homogeneous leukoplakias), prevalent in the buccal (cheek) mucosa and usually of low premalignant potential (Fig. 19.1). Far more serious are nodular and, especially, speckled leukoplakias—which consist of white patches or nodules in a red, often eroded, area of mucosa (Fig. 19.2). Chronic candidal infection is common in speckled leukoplakias and may be associated with an increased risk of malignant change. Candidal leukoplakias are often found at the commissures (Fig. 19.3).

Syphilitic leukoplakia (Fig. 19.4), seen in tertiary syphilis, though of little more than historical interest, may have had a high malignant potential.

Leukoplakia of the anterior floor of the mouth and undersurface of the tongue (sublingual keratosis) may have a particularly high risk of malignant change (Fig. 19.5). The cause of this lesion is unknown but it is more common in women than men and has a typical 'ebbing-tide' appearance clinically.

Though years of pipe smoking can lead to a characteristic type of benign keratosis of the palate—stomatitis nicotina (smoker's keratosis: Fig. 19.6)—there are no

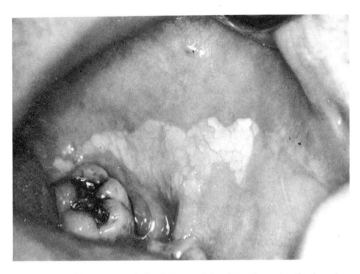

Fig. 19.1 *Homogeneous leukoplakia: a flat white plaque in the buccal mucosa—usually benign.*

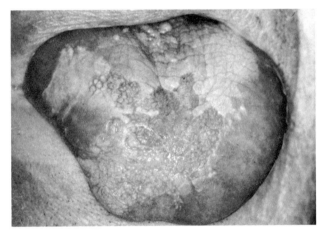

Fig. 19.2 *Mixed red and white lesions and speckled leukoplakia: biopsy showed carcinoma in the red area on the right side of the tongue.*

comparable lesions attributable to cigarette smoking. The diffuse palatal keratosis in stomatitis nicotina is covered by red dots which are the openings of the inflammed palatal mucous glands. However, tobacco smoking is the most important identifiable factor in the aetiology of leukoplakia, especially of the buccal mucosa and commissures and floor of mouth. Paradoxically, malignant change is more likely in non-smokers than smokers

with leukoplakia. Nevertheless, stopping smoking reduces the chances of malignant change in smokers with keratosis.

Trauma occasionally causes keratosis, usually at the buccal mucosal occlusal line (Fig. 19.7) or on edentulous ridges when the patient does not wear a denture (Fig. 19.8).

A recently described white lesion that affects predominantly the tongue is the so-called hairy leukoplakia seen in

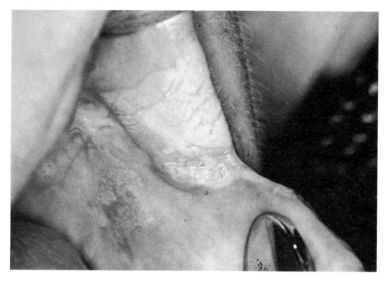

Fig. 19.3 *Candidal leukoplakia: white lesion and a speckled lesion more posteriorly.*

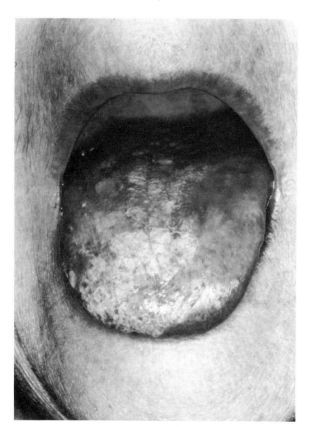

Fig. 19.4 *Syphilitic leukoplakia on the tongue.*

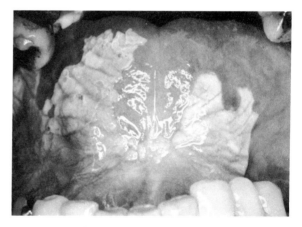

Fig. 19.5 *Sublingual keratosis: there may be a high risk of malignant transformation in this lesion.*

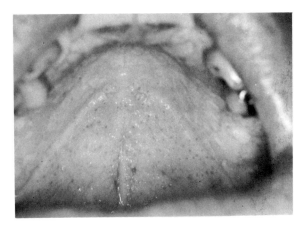

Fig. 19.6 *Smoker's keratosis: a benign lesion in pipe smokers.*

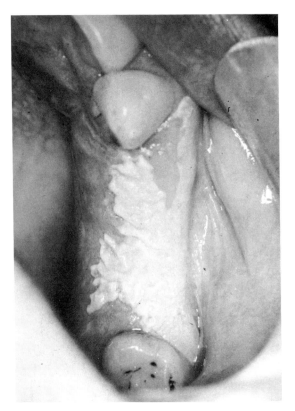

Fig. 19.8 *Frictional keratosis over the edentulous alveolus (an extreme example).*

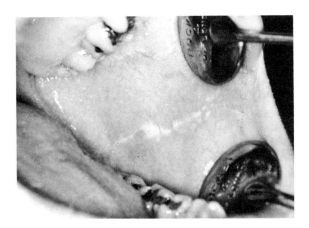

Fig. 19.7 *Occlusal keratosis: a benign lesion caused by occlusal friction.*

AIDS and related syndromes. This is not known to be premalignant (p. 249).

Chronic renal failure may also be associated with oral keratosis.

It is often difficult to be certain of the precise diagnosis of a white patch on clinical examination as even carcinoma can present as a white lesion (Fig. 19.9). Biopsy is therefore indicated.

Histology

Leukoplakias show, to a varying degree, three main microscopic features (Figs. 19.10 and 19.11): increased

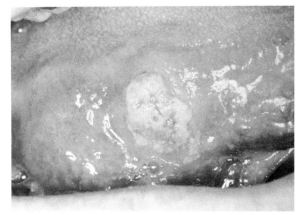

Fig. 19.9 *Carcinoma of the tongue presenting as a white lesion.*

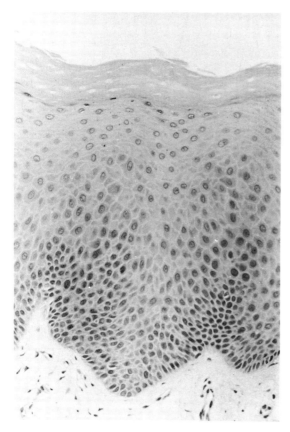

Fig. 19.10 *Keratosis: hyperorthokeratosis with a prominent stratum granulosum and thickening of the epithelium but only minimal disturbance of epithelial organization.*

keratin production, change in epithelial thickness, and disordered epithelial maturation. The last-mentioned is the feature most suggestive of premalignancy. The presence of severe epithelial dysplasia indicates a considerable risk of malignant development but mild dysplasia is not usually of serious significance.

Increased keratin production

Increased keratin produces the white clinical appearance of keratoses. If nuclei persist into the superficial cell layers, the term hyper*para*keratosis is used, whereas if there is excessive mature keratin, with a prominent granular cell layer, the term hyper*ortho*keratosis is applied. Any leukoplakia can show either or both types of change, neither of which is an index of premalignancy.

Change in epithelial thickness

Thinning (hypoplasia) or thickening (hyperplasia) may be present and, although neither are indices of premalignancy, malignant change is more likely in a hypoplastic epithelium.

Disordered epithelial maturation

Although clinical features such as the admixture of red lesions may suggest the degree of premalignant potential of a keratotic lesion (whether the lesion is leukoplakia or lichen planus) histological assessment of the degree of disordered proliferation, maturation and organization of the epithelium (i.e. the degree of *dysplasia*) continues to provide the best guide. However, not all dysplastic lesions are premalignant, though many are. Furthermore, some lesions that often do become malignant (such as some sublingual ketatoses) do not always show a great deal of dysplasia.

Dysplasia (dyskeratosis; atypia)

The features of dysplasia are discussed in Chapters 14 and 18. Where few of the features of dysplasia are present and the epithelium is reasonably well organized, the lesion is classified as mild atypia, while if organization is disrupted and many cellular abnormalities are present, the term severe dysplasia is used—the connotation being that malignant change is likely. The pathologist attempts to guide the surgeon as to the management of the patient, but the best that can be achieved is a subjective (or at very best semi-objective) assessment of prognosis. Much research effort is directed toward identifying membrane and other cellular changes that might assist this decision but, for the present, the best the clinician can do is to take adequate and

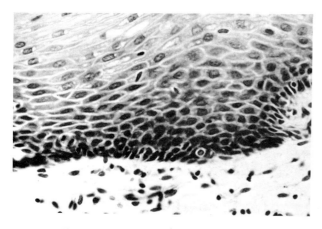

Fig. 19.11 *Keratosis: early features of dysplasia.*

appropriate biopsies to give the pathologist the opportunity to give a true diagnosis, and prognosis, for the patient. To this end the following guidelines are suggested.

1. Always biopsy ulcers that fail to heal within 3 weeks of the removal of any obvious cause; isolated red mucosal lesions; suspicious white lesions; lumps; and any other suspect lesion.
2. Select a *red* area for biopsy where possible and always take an adequately sized biopsy (*at least* an oval 1 × 0.5 cm in an adult).
3. Seriously consider taking two or even more biopsies if the clinical suspicion is of frank malignancy.
4. If there is a high clinical suspicion of malignancy but the histology fails to confirm this, seriously consider taking another biopsy.

The pathologist can only give an opinion on the sample you supply, which should, but may not, be representative of the nature of the lesion.

Carcinoma-in-situ

This is the term applied to a lesion which shows extreme dysplasia throughout the thickness of the epithelium, but in which the basement membrane is intact and invasion has not occurred. Malignant change appears to be imminent. Clinical erythroplasia often proves to be carcinoma-in-situ on biopsy examination (Chapter 18).

Management of leukoplakia

Management of leukoplakia can be difficult, not least because of the wide extent of some lesions; their not infrequent admixture with areas of erythroplasia (speckled leukoplakias); and controversy as to the long-term effects of various therapies.

Management generally includes the following (Table 19.2).

1. *Biopsy and other investigations.* Incisional biopsy to exclude malignant change of dysplasia should be carried out, selecting for biopsy indurated, red, erosive or ulcerated areas rather than the more obvious whiter areas (see above). Candidal leukoplakia, lichen planus, lupus erythematosus and hairy leukoplakia can all be clinically difficult to differentiate from idiopathic keratosis.

There may be evidence suggesting syphilis, HIV infection, renal failure or an underlying anaemia in some patients, in which case suitable investigations should be arranged.

2. *Reduce predisposing factors.* Obvious factors to be reduced include sharp tooth edges, alcohol consumption, smoking or similar habits (e.g. betel chewing). Some studies have shown regression of leukoplakia in over one-half of patients who stopped smoking for 1 year.

Other less common predisposing factors which may require treatment include:

(a) chronic candidosis,
(b) tertiary syphilis,
(c) chronic renal failure,
(d) AIDS.

Table 19.2
Treatment of the patient with keratosis

Treatment	Advantages	Disadvantages	Comments
Remove predisposing factors	Non-invasive; easy; may produce resolution	—	Advised
Surgical excision	Effective; specimen available for histological examination	Invasive; may need to be fairly major procedure in widespread lesions; skin graft may be required	Advised where there is severe dysplasia or in any small keratosis
Observation only	Non-invasive; some leukoplakias resolve spontaneously and only a small percentage turn malignant	Original biopsy may have missed a severely dysplastic area; feeling of therapeutic inactivity	Advised where there is mild or only moderate dysplasia in extensive lesions; photographs should be taken regularly

3. *Definitive management.*

(a) If the lesion is severely dysplastic, it should be excised (large lesions will require skin grafting of the surgical defect). The patient should then be followed up regularly, as in (b) below.

(b) If the lesion is only mildly or moderately dysplastic, the patient should be followed up at regular 3–6-monthly intervals, recording the clinical appearance photographically and rebiopsying if there are changes suggesting malignancy. Some clinicians advocate removal of these lesions with the cryoprobe (Volume 1).

4. Other measures sometimes used are summarized in Table 19.3.

LICHEN PLANUS

Lichen planus is a fairly common, distinctive mucocutaneous disease, of uncertain aetiology but of unique histopathological features.

The prevalence of lichen planus is of the order of 1%. It is predominantly a disease of the middle-aged and elderly; children are only occasionally affected. It afflicts both sexes but there is a slight female predominance.

Immunocytochemical findings in lichen planus suggest an immunopathogenesis (p. 243). In most cases no cause can be identified, but in a minority of patients various drugs (Fig. 19.12) or dental filling materials can be

Table 19.3
Alternative methods for treatment of idiopathic keratoses used in some centres

Treatment	Advantages	Disadvantages	Comments
Electrosurgery	Apparently effective and with little operative bleeding	As for surgical excision, plus the unpleasant smell of electrosurgery under LA; lack of evidence of long-term results; margins not available for histological examination	Very infrequently used
Laser treatment	As for electrosurgery	As for electrosurgery, plus unavailability of tissue for histological examination; expensive equipment	Very infrequently used
Cryosurgery	Apparently effective and with little operative bleeding; more pleasant for patient at operation under LA; equipment inexpensive	As for surgical excision, plus unavailability of tissue for histological examination, fairly extensive postoperative swelling and lack of evidence of long-term results; some workers have shown a 33% recurrence rate; suggested increased likelihood of malignant change after cryosurgery is controversial	Infrequently used although there are some advocates
Vitamin A analogues (retinoids)	Non-invasive systemic treatment aimed at treating lesion at cellular level; some resolution in up to 60%	?Uncertain mode of action in 'treating' a lesion of uncertain pathogenesis; tendency to recurrence; may be severe systemic adverse effects (e.g. on liver)	Rarely used now
Bleomycin	Non-invasive topical treatment; apparent resolution in some cases	Uncertain mode of action, long-term results and sequelae of this new type of therapy are unclear	Rarely used at present

Lichen planus—occasional associations

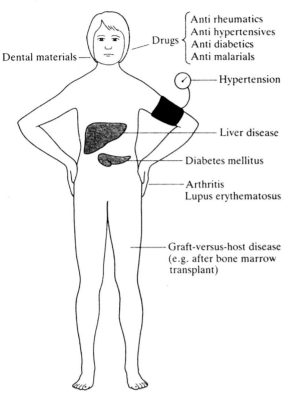

Dental materials ———

Drugs {
Anti rheumatics
Anti hypertensives
Anti diabetics
Anti malarials
}

——— Hypertension

——— Liver disease

——— Diabetes mellitus

——— Arthritis
Lupus erythematosus

——— Graft-versus-host disease
(e.g. after bone marrow
transplant)

Fig. 19.12 *Occasional associations of drugs and diseases with lichen planus.*

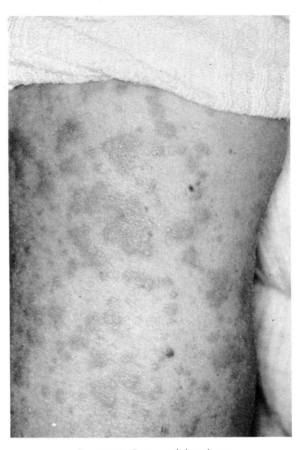

Fig. 19.13 *Cutaneous lichen planus.*

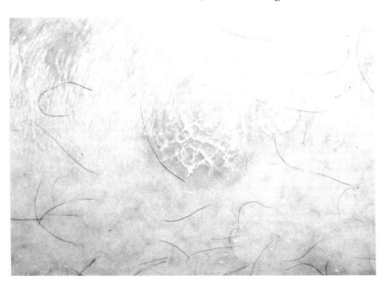

Fig. 19.14 *Wickham's striae on a skin lesion of lichen planus.*

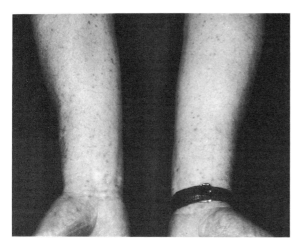

Fig. 19.15 Rash of lichen planus on a typical site—the flexor surfaces of the wrists.

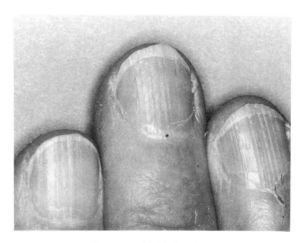

Fig. 19.17 Nail lichen planus.

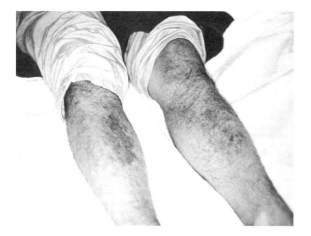

Fig. 19.16 Rash of lichen planus on the anterior surface of the lower legs (another classic site), showing the hyperpigmentation that may result as the lesions heal.

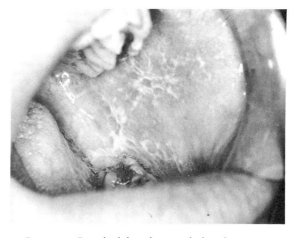

Fig. 19.18 Reticular lichen planus in the buccal mucosa—the usual site for lichen planus.

implicated, but the mechanisms involved are unknown. Similar lesions are also a feature of chronic graft-versus-host disease, seen in bone marrow transplant patients. Lichen planus may occasionally be associated with a variety of systemic disorders such as diabetes (Fig. 19.12). *However, most patients with oral lichen planus are otherwise well, with no definable systemic disease.*

Clinical features

Lichen planus involves the skin and appendages, oral mucosa and other mucous membranes in any combina-

tion. Cutaneous lichen planus may precede or follow involvement of other tissues. The characteristic cutaneous lesion is a flat-topped, violaceous papule about 2–4 mm in diameter (Fig. 19.13). The papule is polygonal and can be pruritic (itchy) or asymptomatic. It may have whitish striae (Wickham's striae) on the surface (Fig. 19.14). Cutaneous lesions affect predominantly the lumbar region, genitalia, flexor surfaces of the wrists and the anterior surface of the lower legs (Figs. 19.15 and 19.16). Cutaneous lichen planus usually resolves spontaneously within 2 years.

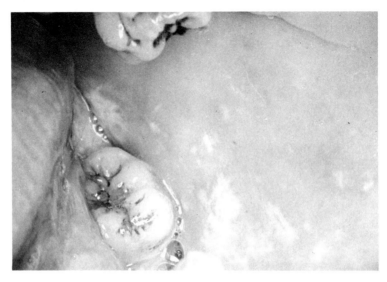

a

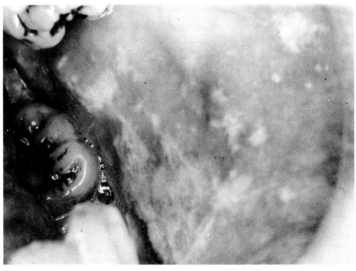

b

Fig. 19.19 (a) Papular oral lichen planus at presentation. (b) The same patient 6 months later showing spread of lesions.

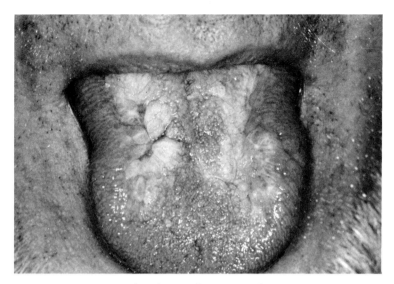

Fig. 19.20 *Lichen planus on the tongue, another common site.*

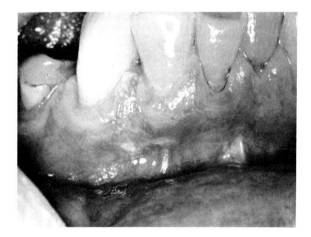

Fig. 19.21 *Gingival lichen planus is quite unusual.*

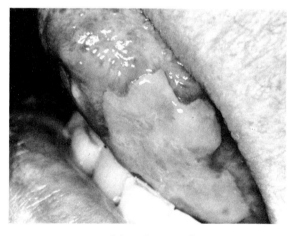

Fig. 19.22 *Erosive lichen planus on the ventrum of the tongue.*

Alopecia occurs in some patients with lichen planus. Nail changes, particularly longitudinal ridging and grooving, are seen in up to 10% of patients (Fig. 19.17).

Oral lichen planus may precede, accompany, or follow lesions of other mucosae or skin, or may appear in isolation. The distribution is characteristically in the posterior buccal mucosa bilaterally (Figs. 19.18 and 19.19), the dorsum of the tongue (Fig. 19.20), occasionally the gingiva (Fig. 19.21) or lips and, rarely, the palate.

The white lesions are most often reticular but may be papular or plaque-like and associated with atrophic areas. Often asymptomatic, there may be soreness from atrophic areas of thin, red mucosa, usually with peripheral striae. More painful still are erosions (Fig. 19.22; Chapter 16), which can also occasionally be widespread or, rarely, the first major manifestation of the disease. A desquamative gingivitis may also develop (Fig. 19.23).

Lichen planus has a small premalignant potential—

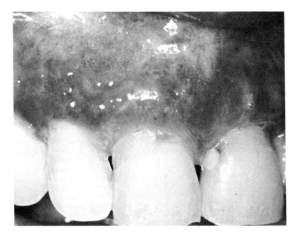

Fig. 19.23 *Desquamative gingivitis caused by lichen planus.*

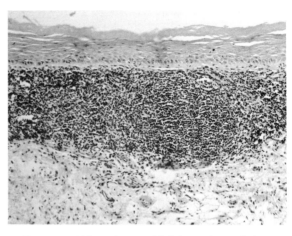

Fig. 19.25 *Lichen planus: epithelial atrophy, and dense inflammatory cell infiltrate in upper lamina propria.*

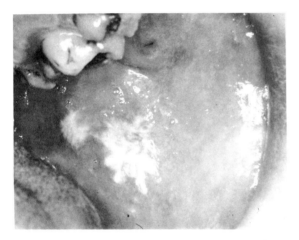

Fig. 19.24 *Plaque-type lichen planus can be difficult to differentiate from keratosis.*

probably of the order of 1%—which is predominantly associated with the atrophic or erosive forms.

Lichen planus less commonly involves mucous membranes other than the oral mucosa.

Diagnosis

Lichen planus is often fairly obviously diagnosed from the clinical features, but it can closely simulate lupus erythematosus, especially DLE (Chapter 16), or keratosis (Fig. 19.24) and biopsy may therefore be indicated.

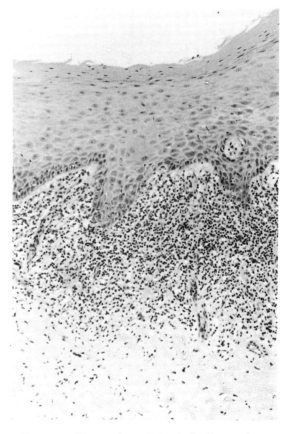

Fig. 19.26 *Hyperparakeratosis: basal cell infiltrate and saw-tooth rete ridge in oral lichen planus.*

The classical histopathological features (Figs. 19.25 and 19.26) include:

(a) hyperorthokeratosis or hyperparakeratosis;
(b) acanthosis (less common in mouth lesions);
(c) thickening of the granular cell layer;
(d) basal cell liquefaction;
(e) 'saw tooth' configuration of the rete ridges (uncommon in mouth lesions);
(f) band-like, dense inflammatory cellular infiltrate in the upper lamina propria.

The earliest features of lichen planus are changes in, and close to, the basal epithelium. The basal cells of the epithelium undergo flattening and hydropic changes and intercellular spaces appear, with splitting of epithelium away from the basement membrane.

Colloid bodies (also termed cytoid, globular, hyaline, Civatte and Sabouraud's bodies) may be seen in the epithelial Malpighian layer and in the lamina propria. These are usually round or ovoid bodies caused by degeneration and premature cell death of basal keratinocytes, and are often infiltrated with serum proteins (see below).

Characteristically there is a dense mononuclear inflammatory cell infiltrate in the upper lamina propria (mainly T-cells), suggesting a cell-mediated immune response, the location of which makes a relationship to the basal epithelial changes highly likely. One of the first observable changes is the appearance of Langerhans' cells, which are antigen-processing cells (Chapters 11 and 13). The antigen(s) that may be responsible is/are un-

known, but preliminary studies have revealed a lichen-planus-specific epidermal antigen in some epithelial cells.

Although immune deposits are seen in tissues in lichen planus they have no specific type or pattern of deposition. There tend to be deposits of fibrin and sometimes IgM at the basement membrane zone and in colloid bodies, which probably represent non-specific exudation and *not* autoantibodies (Fig. 19.27).

Often the histological and immunological findings are no more than 'consistent with lichen planus', but at least serve to exclude more dangerous conditions.

Management of lichen planus

Any causal drugs should be changed. Topical corticosteroids (Chapter 14) are often effective in the control of lesions. Rarely, for intractable cases, intralesional or systemic corticosteroids may be needed. Etretinate, griseofulvin and levamisole are of questionable value and their side-effects can be severe.

CANDIDOSIS (CANDIDIASIS)

Candida albicans is the only common cause of oral fungal infection in the UK. It resides particularly on the posterior dorsum of the tongue. Some 50% of the apparently healthy population harbour *C. albicans* as a normal oral commensal and this is more common in cigarrette smokers.

Infection is likely to result from xerostomia, local disturbances in salivary flora, or depressed immune responses. There are several clinical presentations of candidosis (Table 19.4) but only thrush, candidal leukoplakia and chronic mucocutaneous candidosis present as white lesions.

Thrush

Neonates, who have yet to develop immunity to *Candida* species, may develop thrush. In most other patients it is related to antibiotic or corticosteroid use, or xerostomia. However, if these local factors cannot be identified, systemic disease should be suspected. Thrush is a 'disease of the diseased' (Fig. 19.28), and although a well-recognized feature of primary T-cell immunodeficiencies, is far more common after the severe T-cell immunosuppression necessary for organ transplantation and in other secondary immunodeficiencies, such as leukaemia, diabetes or AIDS. It is a common and early feature of AIDS and

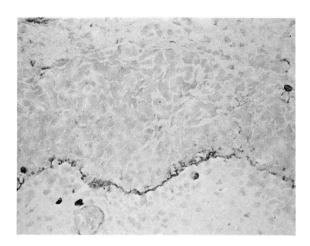

Fig. 19.27 *Fibrin deposits predominantly at epithelial basement membrane zone in lichen planus. (Courtesy of Dr J. W. Eveson.)*

Table 19.4
Oral candidosis

Type of candidosis	Age at onset	Associated factors
Acute pseudomembranous candidosis (thrush)*	Any age	Local or general
Acute atrophic candidosis ('antibiotic mouth'; antibiotic sore mouth)	Any age	Broad-spectrum antibiotics or steroids
Chronic atrophic candidosis (denture-induced stomatitis)	Adults	Denture wearing
Chronic hyperplastic candidosis (candidal leukoplakia)*	Usually middle aged or elderly	Tobacco smoking, denture wearing
Median rhomboid glossitis	Third or later decades	Tobacco smoking, denture wearing
Chronic mucocutaneous candidosis*	Usually first decade	Often immune defect; rarely endocrinopathy

* White lesions.

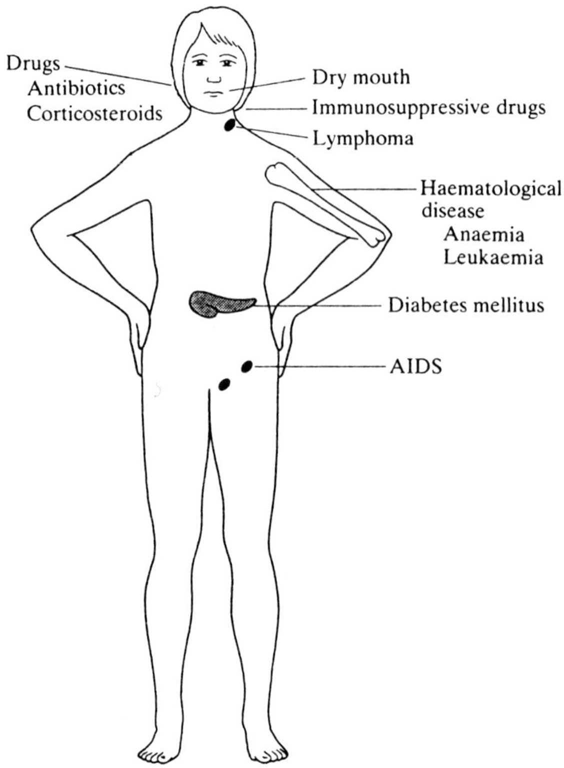

Causes of oral thrush*

*The neonate is also predisposed—through lack of immunity

Fig. 19.28 *Factors predisposing to oral thrush.*

related syndromes and may be a portent of full-blown AIDS.

The soft, creamy patches of thrush, which resemble milk curds, can be wiped off the mucosa with gauze and leave no more than an area of erythema (Figs. 19.29 and 32.14).

Chronic candidosis

Very long-standing candidosis produces tough, adherent white patches (chronic hyperplastic candidosis or candidal leukoplakias) which can be indistinguishable from other leukoplakias except by biopsy, when candidal hyphae can be seen after staining with periodic acid-Schiff (PAS). Candidal leukoplakias may, however, be speckled and, not infrequently, have a premalignant potential.

Chronic mucocutaneous candidosis syndromes are *rare* (Fig. 19.30); several are familial and present early in life, and one type is associated with autoimmune endocrinopathies, especially hypoparathyroidism, and hypoadrenocorticism (polyendocrinopathy syndrome type I) (Figs. 19.31 and 19.32, Table 19.5).

Nevertheless, in many patients with persistent oral candidosis no local cause or underlying defect can be identified though nutritional and immune defects should be excluded.

Diagnosis of candidosis

The diagnosis of thrush is usually clinical and straightforward but it has been overdiagnosed in the past. In

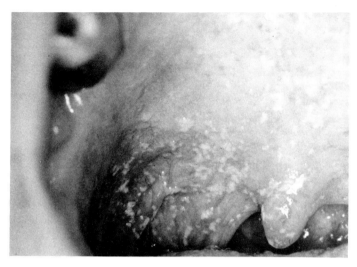

Fig. 19.29 *Oral thrush: scattered whitish papules. (These can be wiped off with gauze.)*

Chronic mucocutaneous candidosis

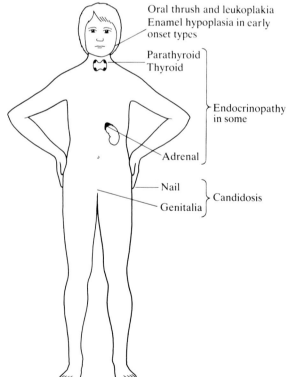

Fig. 19.30 *Features of chronic mucocutaneous candidosis.*

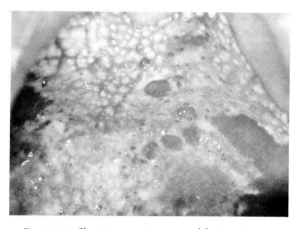

Fig. 19.31 *Chronic mucocutaneous candidosis causing a speckled candidal leukoplakia in the palate.*

immunosuppressed patients, a Gram-stained smear should be taken to distinguish it from the thrush-like plaques produced by opportunistic bacteria. Hyphae seem to indicate that the *Candida* are acting as pathogens (Fig. 19.33).

Chronic leukoplakia-like candidosis should be biopsied, both to distinguish it from other non-candidal plaques and also because of the possible presence of dysplasia. Although candidal hyphae and a neutrophil infiltrate may be seen on haematoxylin and eosin

Table 19.5
Chronic mucocutaneous candidosis

Type	Main lesions	Other features
Familial chronic mucocutaneous candidosis	Mouth, nails, skin	—
Diffuse mucocutaneous candidosis	Mouth, nails, skin and occasionally eyes, pharynx and larynx	
Candidosis–endrocrinopathy syndrome	Mouth, nails, skin; larynx or vagina sometimes	Hypoadrenocorticism, hypoparathyroidism, occasionally diabetes mellitus or hypothyroidism

(H & E) staining, it is usual to search for hyphae using the periodic acid-Schiff (PAS) reagent to demonstrate purple staining of the hyphae.

Management of candidosis

Except in healthy neonates, possible predisposing causes should be looked for and dealt with, if possible. Topical polyenes such as nystatin or amphotericin, or imidazoles such as miconazole are often indicated for acute candidosis.

The oral lesions of chronic candidosis, however, may

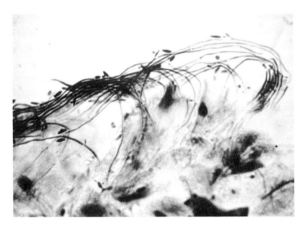

Fig. 19.33 *Candidal hyphae rather than yeast forms in a smear suggest the* Candida *are behaving as opportunistic pathogens.*

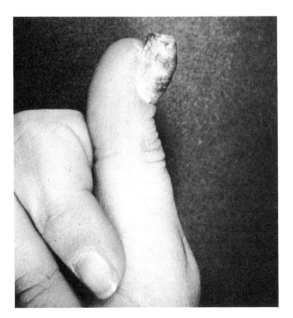

Fig. 19.32 *Chronic mucocutaneous candidosis affecting the nails.*

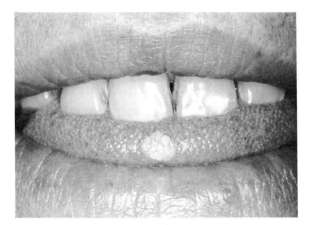

Fig. 19.34 *Papilloma on tip of tongue.*

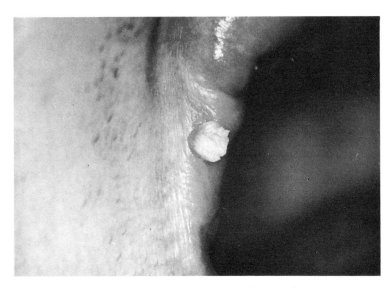

Fig. 19.35 *A common wart (verruca vulgaris) on the lip.*

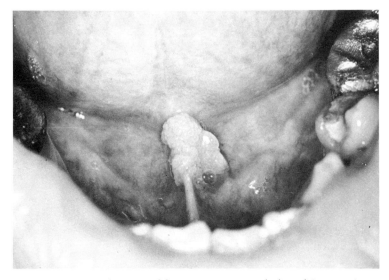

Fig. 19.36 *Genital wart (condyloma acuminatum) on the lingual fraenum of an HIV-positive male bisexual patient.*

prove poorly responsive to the polyene antifungal drugs and, in some cases of chronic mucocutaneous candidosis, oral lesions respond only to intravenous amphotericin with or without fluocytosine, or to ketoconazole.

PAPILLOMAS

Only keratinized variants of papillomas appear as white nodules. Oral papillomas are common, particularly on the soft palate, and often have an appearance like an anemone or cauliflower (Fig. 19.34). The finger-like papillae may make the diagnosis obvious, but papillomas should be excised and their nature confirmed by microscopy. Common warts (verrucae) and venereal warts (condyloma acuminatum) are rare in the mouth (Figs. 19.35 and 19.36) but readily recognizable microscopically.

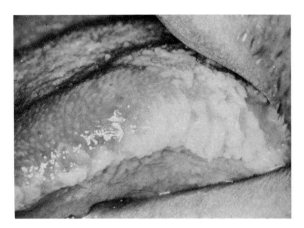

Fig. 19.37 *Hairy leukoplakia of HIV infection (patient diagnosed by Dr S. R. Porter).*

They are more common in AIDS. The lesions are all caused by various human papilloma viruses (HPV). None is known to be premalignant; most can be removed by excision, cryosurgery or laser.

SQUAMOUS CELL CARCINOMAS

Apart from malignant change in oral leukoplakias, a few carcinomas appear from the start as white lesions (see Fig. 19.9; Chapter 15). *The need for biopsy of all oral white lesions which have no obvious cause cannot therefore be emphasized too strongly.*

VERRUCOUS CARCINOMA (see Chapter 15)

Verrucous carcinoma is an uncommon variant of carcinoma which is extensive, warty and white (Fig. 15.9). Some appear to develop as a result of the local use of snuff or tobacco. Confirmation of diagnosis by biopsy is particularly important as verrucous carcinoma responds well to surgical excision but may undergo anaplastic change, with subsequent acceleration of growth and invasiveness, if irradiated.

LUPUS ERYTHEMATOSUS

Oral lesions of lupus erythematosus can be difficult to differentiate from lichen planus (Chapter 16).

WHITE SPONGE NAEVUS

White sponge naevus (familial white folded gingivostomatosis) is a benign hereditary mucosal condition of no consequence that involves the oral and sometimes other mucous membranes (Chapter 12).

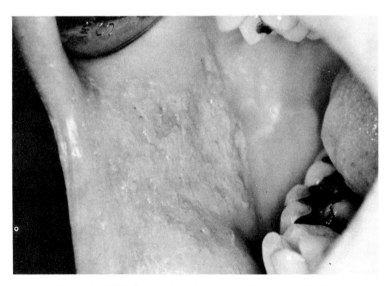

Fig. 19.38 *White lesion on buccal mucosa resulting from cheek biting.*

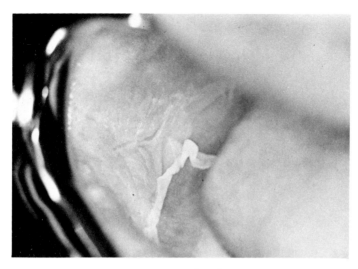

Fig. 19.39 *Burn of buccal mucosa.*

HAIRY LEUKOPLAKIA

Patients infected with HIV may develop white oral lesions with a corrugated or 'hairy' surface—hence termed hairy leukoplakia. This usually affects the lateral margins or dorsum of the tongue (Fig. 19.37). There is evidence that Epstein–Barr virus may be found in this lesion, though the precise cause is unclear.

The majority of affected patients appear eventually to develop full-blown AIDS (Volume 1).

CHEEK BITING

Cheek biting causes a whitish, shredded appearance, usually of the buccal or lower labial mucosa at the occlusal line (Fig. 19.38). The habit is most common in tense or anxious individuals and there may also be bruxism, mandibular pain-dysfunction or other features of psychogenic disorders.

BURNS

Thermal or chemical burns (due, for example to holding drugs such as aspirin in the buccal mucosa) can cause white sloughing lesions of the mucosa (Fig. 19.39).

FURTHER READING

Banoczy J. (1982). *Oral leukoplakia.* Budapest: Akademiai Kiado.

Eversole L. R., Jacobsen P., Stone C. E., Freckleton V. (1986). Oral condyloma planus (hairy leukoplakia) among homosexual men: a clinicopathological study of thirty six cases. *Oral Surg.*, **61**: 249–255.

Eveson J. W. (1983). Oral premalignancy. *Cancer Surveys*, **2**: 403–424.

Pindborg J. J. (1980). *Oral cancer and precancer.* Bristol: Wright.

Scully C., Cawson R. A. (1988). *Colour aids to oral medicine.* Edinburgh and London: Churchill-Livingstone.

Scully C., Elkom M. (1985). Lichen planus: review and update on pathogenesis. *J. oral Pathol.*, **14**: 431–458.

Scully C., Flint S. (1988). *An atlas of stomatology.* London: Martin Dunitz.

Silverman S., Gorsky M., Lozada F. (1984). Oral leukoplakia and malignant transformation. *Cancer,* **53**: 563–568.

Chapter
20
Oral pigmentation and staining

DISCOLORATION OF TEETH

This is reviewed in Volume 3.

Poor oral hygiene is often responsible for superficial tooth-staining, especially for the green stain in children and brownish stains in adults (Volume 3).

Superficial brown discoloration of the teeth (and soft tissues—often the dorsum of the tongue) may be caused by cigarette smoking, some drugs (such as iron salts), some foods and beverages (such as coffee and tea) and chlorhexidine. Such discoloration is easily removed and is of little consequence.

Intrinsic discoloration of the teeth may be of more consequence and sometimes signifies underlying serious disease (Volume 3). There are no conditions that cause intrinsic discoloration of both dental hard and soft tissues.

DISCOLORATION OF ORAL MUCOSA

Brown or black lesions

Superficial brown staining

Several causes of superficial staining are noted above, but a common problem is that of a furred tongue or the more extreme form—black hairy tongue (Fig. 20.1).

Furred tongue

A child's tongue is rarely furred in health but may be coated with off-white debris in many illnesses, particularly febrile diseases (Fig. 16.57). Coating of the tongue is quite commonly seen in healthy adults, particularly in edentulous patients, those who are on a soft non-abrasive

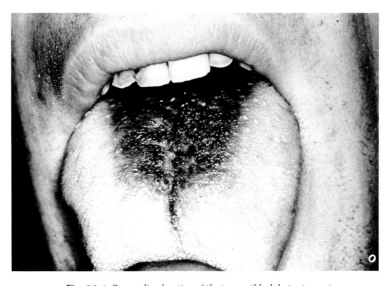

Fig. 20.1 *Brown discoloration of the tongue (black hairy tongue).*

diet, those with poor oral hygiene, or in those who are fasting. The coating in these instances appears to be of epithelial, food and microbial debris which collects since it is not mechanically removed. Indeed, the tongue is the main reservoir of some micro-organisms such as *Candida albicans* and some streptococci.

The coating appears more obvious in xerostomia and in ill patients, especially those with poor oral hygiene or who are dehydrated.

Black hairy tongue

Black hairy tongue (Fig. 20.1) affects the posterior dorsum of the tongue; the filiform papillae are excessively long and stained. Black and brown hairy tongue appears to be caused by the accumulation of epithelial squames and the proliferation of chromogenic micro-organisms. Patients with black hairy tongue may find the condition to be improved by increasing their standard of oral hygiene, brushing the tongue with a toothbrush, using sodium bicarbonate mouthwashes, or sucking a peach stone.

Occasionally, a brown hairy tongue may be caused by antimicrobial therapy, especially with broad-spectrum drugs such as tetracyclines. The latter condition is related to overgrowth of *Candida* species and may respond to withdrawal of the drug.

Intrinsic brown staining (Table 20.1)

Racial

The most usual cause of brown oral mucosal pigmentation is ethnic: it occurs in Blacks and Asians and also in

Table 20.1
Causes of mucosal pigmented lesions

Localized
Amalgam tattoo
Ephelis (freckle)
Naevus
Malignant melanoma
Kaposi's sarcoma
Peutz–Jegher's syndrome
Pigmentary incontinence

Generalized
Racial
Localized irritation, e.g. smoking
Drugs, e.g. phenothiazines or antimalarials
Addison's disease
Albright's syndrome
Other rare causes, e.g. haemochromatosis, von Recklinghausen's disease (Chapter 11), incontinentia pigmentii, heavy metals

patients of Mediterranean descent. The pigmentation is usually symmetrically distributed over the gingiva and palatal mucosa (Figs. 20.2 and 32.10). Patches may be seen elsewhere. Pigmentation may be first noted by the patient in adult life and then incorrectly assumed to be acquired rather than congenital in origin.

Addison's disease (Volume 1)

Addison's disease (adrenocortical hypofunction) is usually autoimmune (idiopathic) in the UK. Rare causes include carcinomatosis, tuberculosis and histoplasmosis. The pathophysiology is shown in Figure 20.3.

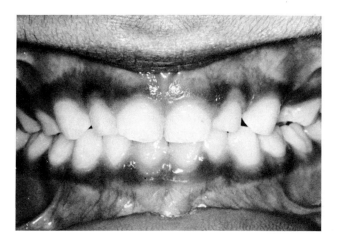

Fig. 20.2 *Racial pigmentation of the gingiva.*

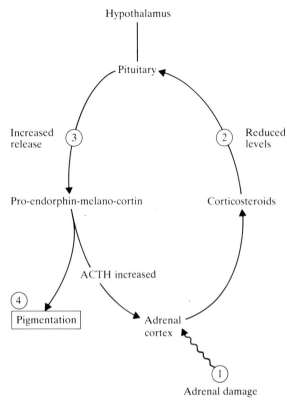

Fig. 20.3 *Pathophysiology of Addison's disease.*

1. *Clinical features.* Weakness, apathy, anorexia, weight loss, abdominal pain and oligomenorrhoea (infrequent menstruation) are common features, though there are many other causes of these.

Hyperpigmentation is generalized but most obvious in areas normally pigmented (e.g. the areolae of nipples, genitalia), skin flexures, and sites of trauma. The oral mucosa may show patchy hyperpigmentation (Fig. 20.4).

Other features include, especially, postural hypotension and, occasionally, associated autoimmune diseases (Fig. 20.5).

2. *Diagnosis.* Low blood pressure, high blood potassium with low sodium, high levels of adrenocorticotrophic hormone (ACTH), low cortisol levels, and impaired ACTH stimulation (Synacthen test) are found.

3. *Management.* This involves the replacement of mineralocorticoids, with cover during operations being provided by the use of additional systemic steroids (Volume 1).

Haemochromatosis

Haemochromatosis, an inborn error of iron metabolism which may cause diabetes and cardiomyopathy, is a rare cause of mucocutaneous brown pigmentation.

Albright's syndrome

Oral brown pigmentation may rarely be seen in

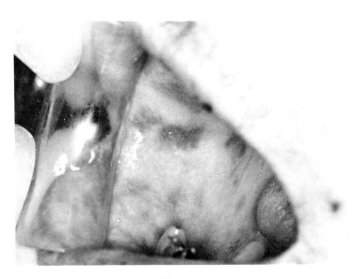

Fig. 20.4 *Addisonian pigmentation.*

Addison's hypoadrenalism

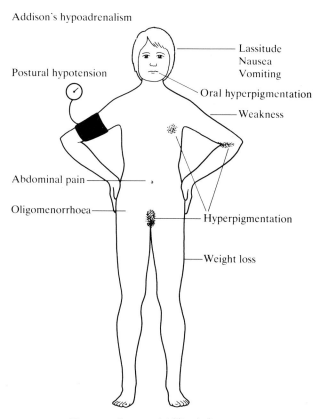

Fig. 20.5 *Features of Addison's disease.*

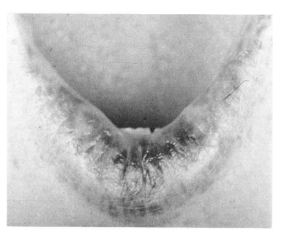

Fig. 20.6 *Peutz–Jegher's syndrome showing oral melanosis.*

therapeutically. Antimalarials produce a variety of colours in the mucosa, ranging from yellow with mepacrine to blue-black with amodiaquine. ACTH therapy may produce brown pigmentation, as may busulphan and some other cytotoxic drugs. Oral contraceptives, phenothiazines and anticonvulsants may also occasionally produce brown pigmentation.

ACTH-producing tumours

Brown pigmentation, particularly of the soft palate, may be an oral manifestation of an ACTH-producing neoplasm such as a bronchogenic carcinoma.

Albright's syndrome of polyostotic fibrous dysplasia and precocious puberty (Chapter 8).

Incontinentia pigmentii

This is a rare genetic disease causing mucocutaneous brown pigmentation, mental handicap and dental anomalies.

Drug-induced pigmentation

Many of the heavy metals formerly implicated in producing oral pigmentation are not used therapeutically now, although industrial exposure still occurs in some places.

Purplish gingival discoloration has been rarely reported after exposure to gold salts occupationally or

Peutz–Jegher's syndrome

Oral and circumoral patchy brown pigmentation is seen with small-intestinal polyps in the Peutz–Jegher's syndrome. Pigmentation may also be seen on the extremities and abdomen. Oral brown or black macules appear in infancy and affect especially the lips (Fig. 20.6) and buccal mucosa. They do not fade after puberty, although the cutaneous lesions tend to. The gut polyps may cause intussusception and intestinal obstruction.

Amalgam tattoo

Amalgam tattoos are common causes of blue–black pigmentation. Usually seen in the mandibular gingiva, or

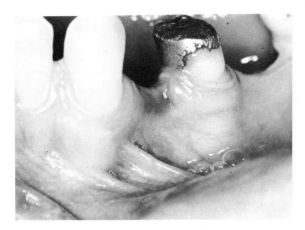

Fig. 20.7 Amalgam tattoo on the lower ridge.

at least close to the teeth (Fig. 20.7), or in the scar of an apicectomy where there has been a retrograde root-filling, amalgam incorporated into a wound causes a tattoo. Radio-opacities may or may not be seen on radiography.

Biopsy may be indicated to exclude a naevus or melanoma but otherwise these lesions are innocuous.

Pigmented naevi

Pigmented naevi are seen particularly on the vermilion border of the lip and on the palate (Figs. 20.8 and 20.9).

These lesions are usually brown, macular, do not change rapidly in size or colour, and are painless. Excision biopsy is recommended for cosmetic reasons, to exclude malignancy, and because of the premalignant potential of some—particularly the junctional naevus (Table 20.2).

Malignant melanoma

Malignant melanoma may arise in apparently normal mucosa or in a pre-existent pigmented naevus, usually in the palate (Figs. 20.10 and 20.11). Features suggestive of malignancy include a rapid increase in size, change in colour, ulceration, pain, the occurrence of satellite pigmented spots or regional lymph node enlargement.

The consensus of opinion is that lesions suspected of being malignant melanomas should not be biopsied until the time of definitive operation.

Pigmented neuro-ectodermal tumour of infancy

This is a very rare pigmented lesion of the anterior maxilla which is benign despite a histological appearance not unlike that of melanoma.

Jaundice

The oral mucosa, especially of the soft palate, may be yellow in jaundice of any cause.

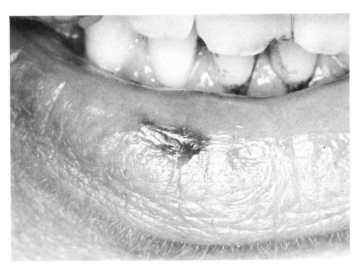

Fig. 20.8 Freckle on the lower lip, a common site. Ultraviolet irradiation in sunlight stimulates these lesions.

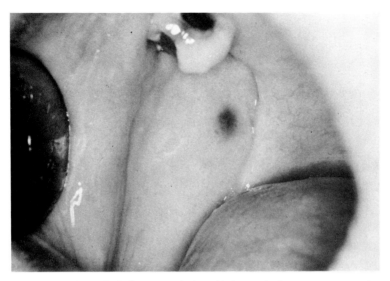

Fig. 20.9 *A small, fairly innocent-looking black macule that was a junctional naevus.*

Table 20.2

Terminology related to melanocytic naevi

Melanocyte	A pigment-producing cell characterized by its ability to synthesize melanosomes. Contains the enzyme dihydroxyphenylalanine (DOPA).
Theque	A group of melanocytes (generally 4 or more) in contact with the basal layer of the epithelium but budding downwards into the lamina propria
Junctional activity	The presence at the dermo-epidermal junction of theques of melanocytes. It may represent a premalignant state.
Junctional naevus	A pigmented or cellular naevus in which the main histological feature is that of junctional activity
Compound naevus	A pigmented or cellular naevus in which the histological features include both junctional activity and the presence of naevus cells in the lamina propria
Intradermal naevus	A cellular naevus in which there is little or no abnormality of melanocytes in the epithelium. The main feature is the presence of packets of naevus cells in the lamina propria. Such naevi may be clinically non-pigmented
Freckle	An area of increased melanin pigmentation. Result of functionally overactive melanocytes: no other histological changes. Lesions are stimulated by ultraviolet irradiation
Lentigo	An area of increased melanin pigmentation which shows histologically a linear replacement of keratinocytes in the basal layer of the epidermis by melanocytes. This replacement does not reach the level of theque formation.

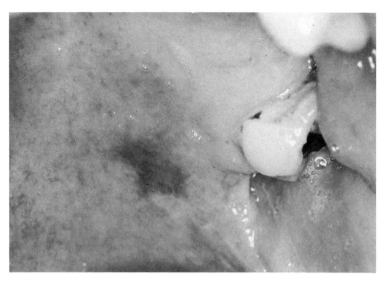

Fig. 20.10 *Malignant melanoma in the most common oral site—the palate.*

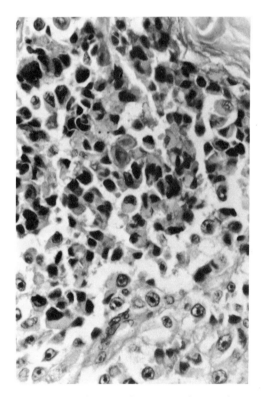

Fig. 20.11 *Histology of the excision biopsy showing obviously malignant pleomorphic cells with hyperchromatic nuclei in malignant melanoma.*

Red lesions (see Chapter 18)

Generalized mucosal erythema may be caused by polycythaemia, any inflammatory lesion or mucosal atrophy. Central cyanosis produces a blue–red discoloration.

Isolated red lesions of the oral mucosa may be telangiectasia (after irradiation; in hereditary haemorrhagic telangiectasia; or scleroderma), haemangiomas, purpura, inflammatory lesions, neoplasms, or associated with mucosal atrophy. Erythroplasia is one of the more important red lesions to be considered (see Chapter 18).

Bluish lesions

Severe central cyanosis may cause a bluish discoloration of the oral mucosa. Haemangiomas and some cysts may present a bluish appearance, as may some drug-induced pigmentation.

Kaposi's sarcoma (a malignant endothelial tumour) typically produces a bluish or purple macule or nodule, often in the palate, in AIDS or related syndromes, or in other immunocompromised patients (Fig. 20.12). Usually the oral lesions are part of more widespread disease, but in AIDS, Kaposi's sarcoma occurs primarily in the skin and mucosa in the head and neck.

Occasionally, in elderly Jews and those of Mediterranean or Middle Eastern origin, Kaposi's sarcoma appears in the absence of an identified immune defect.

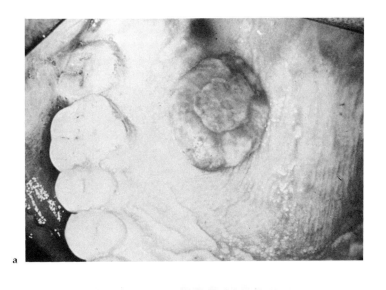

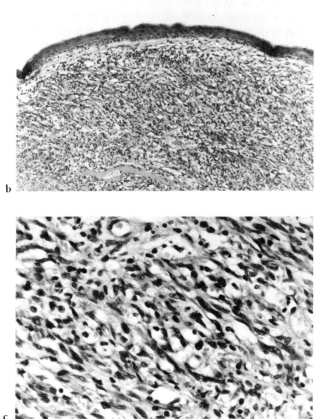

Fig. 20.12 *Kaposi's sarcoma: (a) clinical appearance (reproduced by kind permission of the Editor of* British Dental Journal, *C. Scully, R. A. Cawson and S. Porter); (b) and (c) photomicrographs.*

FURTHER READING

Batsakis J. G., Regezi J. A., Solomon A. R., Rice D. H. (1982). The pathology of head and neck tumours: mucosal melanomas. *Head & Neck Surg.*, **4**: 404–418.

Dummett C. O. (1985). Pertinent consideration in oral pigmentation. *Br. dent., J.* **158**: 9–12.

Lamey P. J., Carmichael F., Scully C. (1985). Oral pigmentation, Addison's disease and results of screening. *Br. dent. J.,* **158**: 297–305.

Scully C., Cawson R. A. (1986). White, red and pigmented patches. *Med. Int.,* **2**: 1120–1142.

Scully C., Cawson R. A. (1988). *Colour aids to oral medicine.* Edinburgh and London: Churchill-Livingstone.

Scully C., Flint S. (1988). *An atlas of stomatology.* London: Martin Dunitz (in press).

Chapter
21   *Lumps and swellings*

Numerous different lesions may present as oral lumps or swellings (Tables 21.1–21.3), many of which are discussed in detail in preceding chapters. Swellings of salivary glands are discussed in Chapter 24; swellings in the neck in Chapter 31. This chapter presents an overall review.

History

When patients refer to a lump in the mouth it is important to establish when it was first noticed. The tongue often detects even very small swellings and patients may also notice a lump because it is sore. Most people have only a passing interest in their mouths but some examine their mouths out of idle curiosity, some through fear (perhaps after hearing of someone with 'mouth cancer'). Indeed, it is not unknown for some individuals to discover and worry about the parotid papilla, foliate papillae on the tongue, or the pterygoid hamulus!

Other features of a lump which can be diagnostically useful are:

(a) the number of lesions—particularly with regard to whether the lesion is bilaterally symmetrical and thus possibly anatomical;
(b) alteration in size;
(c) any discharge from the lesion (clear fluid, pus, blood).

The medical history should be fully reviewed as systemic disorders may be associated with intra-oral or facial swellings (Tables 21.1–21.3 and Section VI).

Examination

Carefully note the site of the lump, whether it is in the midline or lateral, and consider what anatomical structures are present. For example, many midline lesions tend to be developmental in origin (e.g. torus palatinus:

Table 21.1
Lesions which may present as lumps or swellings in the mouth

Normal	Pterygoid hamulus
	Parotid papillae
	Foliate papillae
	Unerupted teeth
Developmental	Haemangioma
	Lymphangioma
	Maxillary and mandibular tori
	Hereditary gingival fibromatosis
	Von Recklinghausen's neurofibromatosis
Inflammatory	Abscess
	Oral Crohn's disease
	Wegener's granulomatosis
	Pyogenic granuloma
	Sarcoidosis
	Others
Traumatic	Epulis
	Fibroepithelial polyp
	Denture granulomata
Cystic	Eruption cysts
	Developmental cysts
	Cysts of infective origin
Hormonal	Pubertal gingivitis
	Pregnancy epulis/gingivitis
Drug therapy	Oral contraceptive (pill gingivitis)
	Phenytoin
	Nifedipine
	Cyclosporin
	Diltiazem
Blood dyscrasias	Leukaemia and lymphoma
Benign neoplasms	Various
Malignant neoplasms	Primary and secondary
Others	Angioedema
	Amyloidosis

Table 21.2

Lumps and swellings of gingiva

Localized	Localized inflammatory hyperplasia
	Abscess
	Pyogenic granuloma
	Epulis
	fibrous
	giant cell
	pregnancy
	Angioma
	Tumour
	Crohn's disease
	Sarcoidosis
Generalized	Developmental—hereditary gingival
	fibromatosis
	Generalized plaque-related hyperplasia
	'Reactionary' hyperplasia
	Hyperplasia associated with mouth-breathing
	Pubertal gingivitis
	Pregnancy gingivitis
	Drug-related enlargement
	oral contraceptive
	phenytoin
	nifedipine
	cyclosporin
	diltiazem
	Blood dyscrasias (chiefly leukaemia)
	Scurvy

Table 21.3

Causes of facial swelling

Inflammatory
Cutaneous infections
Insect bites
Crohn's disease (orofacial granulomatosis)
Melkersson–Rosenthal syndrome
Sarcoidosis

Traumatic
Traumatic oedema or haematoma
Postoperative oedema or haematoma
Surgical emphysema

Immunologically mediated (non-inflammatory)
Allergic angioedema
Hereditary angioedema

Endocrine and metabolic
Obesity
Systemic corticosteroid therapy
Cushing's syndrome
Myxoedema
Acromegaly
Nephrotic syndrome
Superior vena cava (SVC) syndrome (obstruction to SVC, e.g. by bronchial carcinoma)
Cysts
Hamartomas
Neoplasms
Foreign bodies

Chapter 1). If a lesion is lateral, determine whether it is bilateral since few neoplastic lumps are bilateral.

The site, shape, size (in millimetres) and colour of the lump should be noted. Is the lump pale in colour (suggesting underlying fibrosis, or soft tissues stretched over bony enlargement); red (suggesting inflammation); or deep red (suggesting haemangioma or giant-cell epulis)? Any variations in colour within the lump (e.g. a 'pointing' abscess) should be observed. The surface characteristics should be noted: papillomas have an obvious anemone-like appearance; carcinomas and other malignant lesions tend to ulcerate. Abnormal blood vessels suggest a neoplasm.

The proximity of the lump to other structures (e.g. teeth, dentures) should be noted. Does the swelling have an orifice, or sinus? If fluid is draining from the opening, is it clear, cloudy or purulent? Other similar or relevant changes elsewhere in the oral cavity should be noted.

After a thorough inspection, carefully palpate the lump. A rough assessment of its contents can be made and these can be put into such categories as fluid (fluctuant because of cyst fluid, mucus, pus or blood); soft; firm; or hard like a carcinoma (indurated). Palpation may cause the release of fluid (e.g. pus from an abscess) or cause the lesion to blanch (vascular). Sometimes palpation causes the patient pain (suggesting an inflammatory lesion). The swelling overlying a bony cyst may crackle (like an egg-shell) when palpated. Palpation may disclose an underlying structure (e.g. the crown of a tooth under an eruption cyst) or show that the actual swelling is in deeper structures (e.g. submandibular calculus in Wharton's duct). Bimanual palpation should be used when investigating lesions in the floor of the mouth, cheek, and occasionally the tongue.

Suitable categories for a provisional diagnosis are normal structure, developmental, inflammatory, traumatic, vesiculobullous, fibro-osseous, and neoplastic. Systemic factors in the development of intra-oral lumps may be hormonal, blood dyscrasias, drug therapy, gastrointestinal disease and respiratory disease. Occasionally the jaws are sites of metastatic malignant disease, which may present as epulides or lumps.

The provisional diagnosis will help in arranging further investigations or appropriate referrals in order to reach a definite diagnosis and to plan treatment.

Investigations

The nature of many lumps cannot be established without further investigation, especially radiography and biopsy. A summary of appropriate investigations is given in Table 21.4 and Volume 1. Note particularly that any teeth adjacent to a lump involving the jaw should be tested for vitality, and any caries or suspect restorations investigated. The periodontal status of any involved teeth should also be determined. Radiographs are required whenever lumps involve the jaws, and should show the full extent of the lesion and possibly other areas. Special radiographs (e.g. of the skull, sinuses, salivary gland function) may, on occasions, be indicated. Photographs may be useful for future comparison. Blood tests may be needed if there is suspicion that a blood dyscrasia or endocrinopathy may underlie the development of the lump. Special blood tests (e.g. for autoantibodies) may be indicated for suspected vesiculobullous lesions (Volume 1).

CAUSES OF LUMPS AND SWELLINGS ACCORDING TO SITE

Gingiva

A list of possible swellings of the gingiva is given in Table 21.2. Rapidly developing localized lumps, usually associated with discomfort, are most likely to be abscesses. Other localized swellings are usually inflammatory or neoplastic. Most generalized gingival swellings are related to plaque deposits, the effect of which, in many individuals, is increased by plaque-retentive factors (e.g. carious cavities, subgingival margins of restorations, appliances, partial dentures, drying due to mouth breathing) or exacerbated by hormonal changes (puberty, pregnancy) or drugs. Such changes often develop slowly— over weeks rather than days—and are usually without discomfort.

There are very few serious causes of generalized enlargements of gingiva appearing spontaneously or rapidly: leukaemia is a prime suspect but it is uncommon and not all patients with leukaemia develop gingival swelling.

Table 21.4
Investigations that may be needed for diagnosis in relation to a lump in the mouth

Visual examination

Palpation

Radiography

Blood tests (e.g. white cell count or HIV antibody test in AIDS)

Urinalysis (e.g. for protein in suspected myelomatosis)

Aspiration (plus protein analysis in investigation of cysts)

Incision, drainage, culture

Biopsy
  H & E or special stains
  Frozen section for direct immunofluorescence

Several of of these tests may necessitate referral of the patient to a specialist unit.

Palate

Lumps of the hard palate may develop from structures within the palate (intrinsic) or beyond it (extrinsic). Thus, for example, torus palatinus is an intrinsic bone lesion, whereas a dental abscess pointing on the palate (usually from the palatal roots of the first and second maxillary molars, or from upper lateral incisors) is extrinsic. Palatal swellings, apart from torus palatinus and those of dental origin (unerupted teeth, especially permanent canines, or second premolars and abscesses) are not common. However, it should be remembered that the palate is the second most common site (after the parotid) for development of pleomorphic adenomas and other salivary neoplasms. Developing unilateral hard palatal swellings, characteristically disturbing the fit of an upper denture in older patients, may denote Paget's disease. Invasive carcinoma from the maxillary sinus may produce a palatal swelling (Chapter 10). A gumma (tertiary syphilis) may present initially as a lump in the palate (Chapter 16). Kaposi's sarcoma, typical of AIDS (Chapter 20), may also present as a lump in the palate, or elsewhere.

Floor of mouth

Swellings in the floor of the mouth are more likely to arise from structures above the mylohyoid muscle than below. Patients occasionally worry about the normal sublingual fold and sublingual varices. However, the commonest swellings in the floor of the mouth are denture-induced hyperplasia and a salivary calculus in Wharton's duct. Other lesions producing swellings in this area are mucocele (known as ranula because of the resemblance to a frog's belly) and neoplasms of the sublingual salivary gland (usually malignant), but these are uncommon. Patients occasionally describe as a lump what proves to be a lesion in the floor of the mouth producing mucosal thickening (e.g. carcinoma) or swelling of the lingual aspect of the mandible (more characteristic of ameloblastoma than of dental abscesses or cysts). Swellings of the submandibular salivary gland and adjacent lymph nodes may occasionally be described by patients as being in the floor of the mouth. However, only very large swellings below the mylohyoid muscle are likely to produce a bulge in the mouth. Swellings in the floor of the mouth may inhibit swallowing and talking. Fixation or deviation of the tongue is a late sign in carcinoma of the tongue

Mandibular tori produce bony hard swellings lingual to the lower premolars.

Tongue

The tongue may be congenitally enlarged (macroglossia) in, for example Down's syndrome, or may enlarge in angioedema, gigantism, acromegaly or amyloidosis. Discrete lumps may be of various causes—congenital, inflammatory, traumatic or neoplastic.

Buccal and labial mucosa

Causes of swellings in the lips and cheeks include haematomas from trauma (such as occasional biting), infections, insect bites, fibro-epithelial polyps, fibrous lumps, mucoceles (which may burst and refill), vesiculobullous lesions, and carcinoma. Oral Crohn's disease and occasionally sarcoid may produce widespread irregular thickening (cobblestoning) of cheek mucosa. Some 'lumps' become ulcers, as in various bullous lesions, in primary and tertiary syphilis and in malignant neoplasms.

The flange of a denture impinging on the vestibular mucosa may stimulate a reactive irregular hyperplasia—the so-called denture granuloma or denture-induced hyperplasia. Salivary neoplasms in the lip may simulate, but are usually harder than, mucous cysts. Mucoceles are uncommon in the upper lip; discrete swellings there may well be salivary neoplasms.

ENLARGEMENTS OF DEVELOPMENTAL ORIGIN

Torus palatinus and mandibularis (Chapter 1)

These are developmental benign exostoses with a smooth or nodular surface. Torus palatinus occurs in the centre of the hard palate; torus mandibularis is lingual to the lower premolars and usually bilateral. Tori are common conditions of no consequence, apart from occasionally interfering with denture construction.

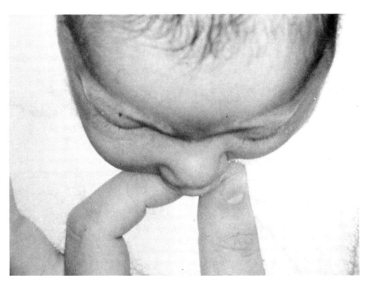

Fig. 21.1 *Haemangioma causing facial deformity in a neonate.*

Cysts (see Chapter 5)

Haemangioma

Haemangioma is a lesion of blood vessels generally regarded as a developmental lesion (hamartoma) and is usually present from birth (Fig. 21.1). It may affect any part of the oral mucosa. It rarely alters in size, though it may swell if traumatized and there is internal bleeding. A haemangioma is usually deep-red (even blue-purple) in colour, blanches on pressure, and is fluctuant to palpation (Fig. 21.2). It may have a lobulated or raised surface.

Haemangiomas are at risk from trauma and prone to excessive bleeding if damaged (e.g. during tooth extraction). Lesions suspected of being haemangiomatous should *not* be routinely biopsied; aspiration is far safer.

The lesion has a thin surface epithelium overlying numerous thin-walled vessels separated by sparse bands of collagenous tissue. The connective tissue component of a cavernous haemangioma has large, thin-walled spaces, lined with endothelium. These spaces, which probably communicate widely, contain numerous red blood cells. There is no capsule (Fig. 21.3).

Lymphangioma

Lymphangioma is uncommon in the mouth. It is of similar structure to a haemangioma, but contains lymph rather than blood. It often has a 'frogspawn' appearance (Fig. 21.4).

Hereditary gingival fibromatosis

Hereditary gingival fibromatosis is an uncommon condition which occurs in both sexes. The disorder is trans-

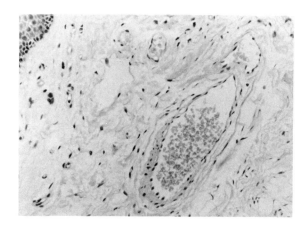

Fig. 21.3 *Histology of haemangioma showing dilated blood vessels.*

mitted by an autosomal dominant gene. It presents as generalized gingival enlargement, especially obvious during the transition from deciduous to permanent dentition. If the enlargement is gross, it may move or cover the teeth and bulge out of the mouth. The affected gingiva is usually of normal colour but firm in consistency, and the surface, although initially smooth, becomes coarsely stippled. The changes involve the papillae and later the attached gingiva (Fig. 21.5). Patients may also complain of hirsutism (excess hair).

The tissue is covered with stratified squamous, ortho-

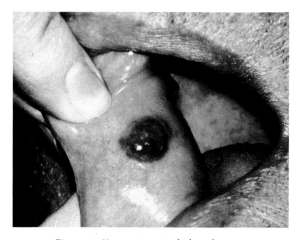

Fig. 21.2 *Haemangioma in the buccal mucosa.*

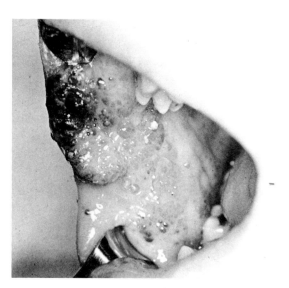

Fig. 21.4 *Lymphangioma.*

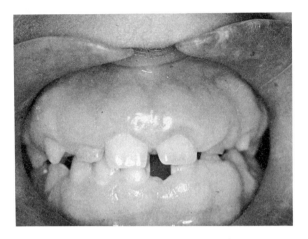

Fig. 21.5 *Hereditary gingival fibromatosis showing gross enlargement of the gingiva.*

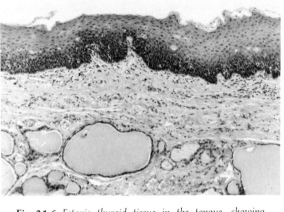

Fig. 21.6 *Ectopic thyroid tissue in the tongue, showing thyroid follicles filled with colloid.*

keratinized epithelium. The sulcular epithelium is thickened, usually with a smooth basal layer, but with acanthosis where there is underlying inflammation. The connective tissue is mainly composed of thick, interlacing collagen fibres forming, in the main, a dense almost avascular mass; in these areas any fibrocytes have dark, shrunken nuclei. Around blood vessels the collagen fibres form a looser network in which fibrocytes have plumper, more active nuclei. Mucoid material and some giant cells may be found.

Surgery is often indicated (Volume 3).

Other rare developmental swellings

Midline lumps in the posterior tongue rarely prove to be due to a lingual thyroid. The neck should be examined and a scan performed to ensure there is a normal thyroid before such a lump is excised (Fig. 21.6).

Gingival hyperplasia is found in mucopolysaccharidoses such as Hurler's syndrome.

ENLARGEMENTS OF INFECTIVE ORIGIN

Dental abscesses

The most common cause of an acquired lump in the mouth is a dental abscess. Acute periapical infection, a consequence usually of caries-induced pulpitis, often appears as a 'gum boil' apical to the mucogingival line (Volumes 1 and 3). The site at which such abscesses 'point' is governed by

the position of the root apex in relation to the bone surface, the density of the bone, and the position of muscle insertions. Thus abscesses from the mandibular molars usually break through the cortical plate below (inferior to) the buccinator and mylohyoid muscles and are likely to point extra-orally, whereas abscesses from the buccal roots of the maxillary molars are likely to point intra-orally. Because palatal mucosa is firmly bound to bone, abscesses from palatal roots of maxillary molars may track widely under the soft tissues, and may even sometimes extend beyond the midline of the palate. Abscesses arising from palatally inclined roots of maxillary lateral incisors point palatally and may occasionally track posteriorly as far as the junction of the hard and soft palates. Most but not all dental abscesses cause severe pain.

Thorough clinical examination and vitality testing of teeth in the vicinity of abscesses should reveal the tooth responsible. Periapical radiographs of the tooth may reveal a periapical radiolucency.

The old axiom of 'where there is pus, let it out' applies to dental abscesses in general, though having an abscess incised can be an unpleasant experience for the patient (Volume 1). No local analgesics should be injected near an abscess, partly because of the risk of disseminating pus, and partly because they rarely work effectively in such sites though *regional* local analgesia may be feasible. *Topical* anaesthesia may be partially achieved using an ethyl chloride spray. Intra-oral abscesses should be incised at their most dependent point by an incision moving at right-angles to the long axis of the teeth. Closed forceps can be introduced into the abscess and opened carefully, to facilitate better drainage. An ellipse of tissue should be excised from palatal abscesses which otherwise tend not to drain.

A swab of pus should be sent for culture, particularly where there may be problems over sensitivity of organisms to available antibiotics. The majority of dental abscesses seem to be a 'mixed infection' including anaerobes and viridans streptococci. However, the cultivable organisms may not be the infecting organisms, and there is evidence that Gram-negative bacteria are the most important (Volume 1).

If an abscessed tooth is to be retained by means of eventual endodontic therapy, then incision, drainage, and possibly antibiotic therapy may be feasible. These may also be indicated when a patient has lymphadenitis, malaise, and/or pyrexia or is immunocompromised. However, removal of the offending tooth may prove to be the quickest way of achieving drainage as well as of removing the cause of the abscess.

Lateral periodontal (parodontal) abscesses, arising in association with deep true periodontal pockets (Volume I), tend to be less common and also less painful than acute periapical abscesses. They generally point coronally to the mucogingival junction, and extra-oral spread is very uncommon. Alteration of the bacterial flora in a pocket, retention of bacterial products, invasion of the pocket wall by bacteria, and damage to the pocket wall by scaling may all be contributory factors. Lateral periodontal abscesses are most prevalent adjacent to molars, presumably because their inter-radicular surfaces are inaccessible to scalers, and tend to develop plaque of greater potential virulence.

The initial management of lateral periodontal abscesses is as for periapical abscesses. The decision as to whether to try to retain affected teeth depends mainly on the amount of alveolar bone remaining and the accessibility of involved root surfaces to treatment. Where an abscess involves only one root of a molar, it may be feasible to remove that root, if the remaining support of the tooth is adequate (Volume 3).

Syphilis

Lesions caused by syphilis are uncommon in the mouth, but are by no means unknown. Any bizarre lesions should be treated with caution; syphilis is well known as 'the great mimic' (Chapter 16).

A primary chancre may present as a painless indurated swelling, with a dark-red, glassy appearance.

The gumma of tertiary syphilis is often found on the palate, initially as a solid granulomatous lump, at which time it might resemble a pleomorphic adenoma. It later breaks down to form an ulcer which may progress to perforate the palate.

Viral lesions

The majority of viral infections in the mouth initially produce vesicles which may seem like small lumps to the patient.

Verruca vulgaris occasionally appears in the mouth, presumably by transfer of papilloma virus from warts on the hands. The lesion is a discrete, sessile, papillomatous lump, often resembling a minute cauliflower. It may be mistaken for a true papilloma or for condyloma acuminatum, a cauliflower-like growth resulting from orogenital or oroanal contact. These lesions are also a recognized complication of AIDS.

LUMPS RELATED TO TRAUMA

Fibrous lump (fibroepithelial polyp)

When oral tissues are traumatized, healing is usually rapid and complete, with negligible scar formation. Sometimes a more vigorous and extensive healing process ensues, producing a localized tissue overgrowth which generally takes the form of a smooth, sessile or pedunculated polyp (Figs. 21.7 and 21.8). Such fibrous lumps are common. They may attain their full size (which rarely exceeds 2.5 cm diameter) quite rapidly, and then stop growing. They may become ulcerated if traumatized but otherwise are usually asymptomatic and some patients tolerate such polyps for months or years. They occur equally in males and females but are rarely seen before 20 years of age.

Fibrous lumps should be excised with their entire base and examined histologically. Usually, a well-keratinized stratified squamous epithelium is found, overlying a connective tissue exhibiting criss-crossing thick collagenous bundles. Some avascular and acellular portions with hyaline changes may be present. Signs of inflammation may be minimal and there is no capsule. The lesion appears to be purely reparative in nature.

Fibrous lumps should not be confused with the true fibroma, a benign neoplasm derived from fibroblasts, which is *rare* in the mouth (see p. 271).

Fibrous epulis

The term epulis is applied nowadays to any lump arising from gingival tissue. In that it shows evidence of a

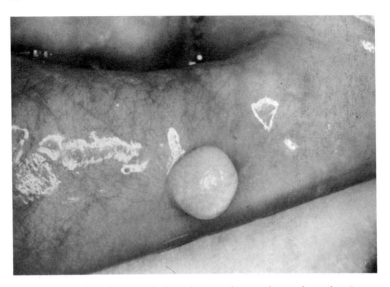

Fig. 21.7 Fibrous lump on the lower lip: note the smooth non-ulcerated surface and sessile nature.

reparative response, the fibrous epulis resembles a fibro-epithelial polyp, but the epulis also usually has an inflammatory component of varying extent. The variable inflammatory changes account for the different clinical presentations of fibrous epulides from red, shiny, and soft lumps to those which are pale, stippled and firm. Commonly, they are round, pedunculated swellings arising from the marginal or papillary gingiva, sometimes adjacent to sites of irritation (e.g. a carious cavity); they rarely involve attached gingiva, and rarely exceed 2 cm in diameter (Fig. 21.9). They are four times more common in females than males, and are most frequent in individuals in the 20–45-year age range. They are usually painless.

Fibrous epulides should be removed down to the periosteum, which should be curetted thoroughly. Such exci-

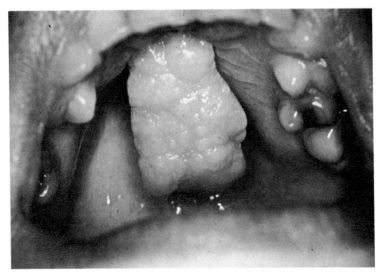

Fig. 21.8 Fibrous lump in the palate: for obvious reasons this is sometimes called a leaf fibroma.

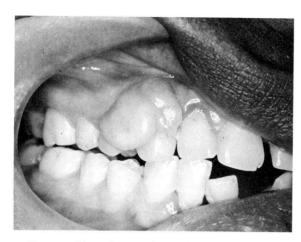

Fig. 21.9 Fibrous lump (epulis) on the gingiva: again the surface is smooth and non-ulcerated and the overlying mucosa is of normal clinical appearance.

sion will create an open wound which should be dressed. Removal of a large epulis from the labial aspect of the maxillary gingiva may create an unsightly gingival defect, about which patients should be warned in advance.

Histologically there are variations commensurate with the different clinical features. The overlying stratified squamous epithelium may exhibit inflammatory hyperplasia. The lesion consists of granulation tissue heavily infiltrated with plasma cells and lymphocytes, or polymorphonuclear leucocytes. There are dilated blood vessels in loose oedematous connective tissue, or vessels may be sparse. Immature bone formation may occur in some epulides.

A melanotic component in fibrous epulides is uncommon, but such lesions should be regarded with particular suspicion since they may be malignant melanomas.

Denture-induced hyperplasia (denture granuloma; epulis fissuratum)

Where a denture flange irritates the vestibular mucosa, a linear reparative process may be initiated. In time, an elongated fibroepithelial enlargement may develop (Fig. 21.10). Several leaflets with a fairly firm consistency may develop. Such a lesion (a denture granuloma) is little different in structure from a fibroepithelial polyp.

Although rarely symptomatic, a denture granuloma should be excised and examined histologically, particularly if modification of the denture does not induce the lesion to regress. *Rarely*, a denture granuloma arises because a lesion develops beneath a denture, e.g. antral carcinoma (see Volume 3).

Giant-cell epulis (Chapter 7)

The giant-cell epulis characteristically arises interdentally, adjacent to permanent teeth which have had deciduous predecessors. Classically, the most notable feature is the deep-red colour, although older lesions tend to be paler (Fig. 21.11).

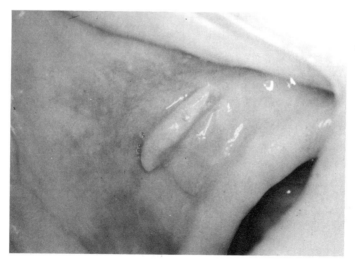

Fig. 21.10 Denture-induced hyperplasia in the labial sulcus.

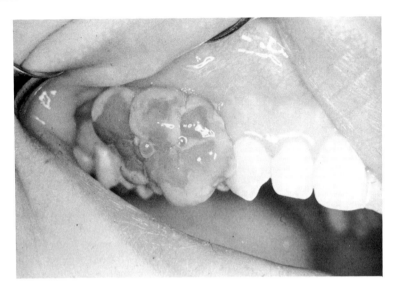

Fig. 21.11 Giant-cell epulis.

Histology shows many multinucleated giant cells distributed widely throughout the lesion or gathered into clumps. Older lesions have fewer giant cells. Considerable vascularity, with numerous blood vessels, is a feature mainly of younger lesions. Sheets of stromal cells in the younger lesion give way to greater numbers of collagen fibres and well-differentiated fibroblasts in the older lesion. The older lesion may also contain some woven bone, emphasizing the osteogenic potential of granula-

tion tissue. The lesion is covered with stratified squamous epithelium. There is no capsule (Chapter 7).

The resorption of deciduous teeth and remodelling of the alveolus at the mixed dentition stage indicate the osteoclastic potential of the area from which giant-cell epulides arise. The lesion probably arises because chronic irritation triggers a reactionary hyperplasia of mucoperiosteum and excessive production of granulation tissue.

Giant-cell granulomas are also a feature of hyperpara-

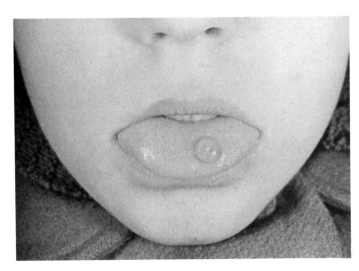

Fig. 21.12 Pyogenic granuloma on the tongue—a typical site.

thyroidism, and levels of plasma calcium, phosphate, and alkaline phosphatase should be assayed and the area examined radiographically (Chapters 2 and 7).

Pyogenic granuloma

The pyogenic granuloma usually affects the lip or tongue, and appears to represent an excessive reaction to trauma or infection (Fig. 21.12).

The lesion may grow to 1 cm or more in diameter. Basically red in colour, with a thin or ulcerated epithelium, it may bleed readily if traumatized. Clinically, a pyogenic granuloma may occasionally resemble a capillary haemangioma.

These lesions should be excised but will readily recur if excision is not adequate.

The pyogenic granuloma is composed of granulation tissue, with marked endothelial proliferation forming small vascular channels. The connective tissue is densely infiltrated with polymorphonuclear leucocytes, especially beneath areas of ulceration. In the deeper portions of larger lesions, connective tissue may be more mature than superficially (Fig. 21.13). Epithelium tends to proliferate inwards at the edges of the lesion.

A major point of difference between the pyogenic granuloma and capillary haemangioma is that the latter usually contains few inflammatory cells.

The histological features of the so-called pregnancy epulis are identical to those of pyogenic granuloma (see below).

Mucous cyst (mucocele) (see Chapters 5 and 24)

LUMPS RELATED TO HORMONAL CHANGES

Pregnancy gingivitis and pregnancy epulis

Pregnancy gingivitis is characterized by soft, reddish enlargements, usually of the gingival papillae. The lumps vary from small smooth enlargements to more extensive, ragged, granular lumps which sometimes resemble the surface of a strawberry (Volume 3). A similar appearance may complicate the use of the oral contraceptive. Sometimes there is a localized epulis—a pregnancy epulis (Fig. 21.14). Poor oral hygiene predisposes to these changes.

Changes of pregnancy gingivitis usually appear about the second month of pregnancy, and reach a peak at the eighth month. They may revert soon after parturition to the previous level of gingival health. Therefore, conservative treatment is indicated unless an epulis interferes with occlusion or is extremely unsightly—when it can be excised.

The patient's chief concern is usually of gingival bleeding, particularly on eating or toothbrushing. This tendency to bleed is an indication of the considerable vascularity of the affected tissues.

Histologically, a pregnancy epulis is a pyogenic granuloma with numerous immature vascular channels in a loosely arranged connective tissue stroma. Despite the vascularity, the immaturity of the vessels may lead to superficial ischaemia so that, clinically and histologically, there may be evidence of ulceration of the overlying epithelium. Larger lesions are also prone to trauma, which may contribute to the ulceration of the surface.

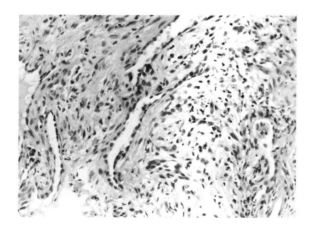

Fig. 21.13 *Pyogenic granuloma: high power showing multiple new blood vessels, fibroblasts and inflammatory cells.*

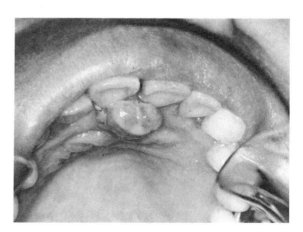

Fig. 21.14 *Pregnancy epulis.*

LUMPS AND SWELLINGS RELATED TO DRUG THERAPY

Oral contraceptives

Enlargements related to oral contraceptives are referred to in the previous section.

Phenytoin (see also Volume 3)

The anticonvulsant phenytoin (Epanutin; Dilantin), used mainly for the control of grand mal epilepsy, can produce a variable extent of gingival enlargement, which characteristically affects the interstitial tissues first but which may later involve the marginal and even attached gingiva. The palatal and lingual gingiva are usually involved less than the buccal and labial gingiva. The enlargement rarely affects edentulous sites. It is characteristically firm, pale and tough, with coarse stippling, but these features may take several years to develop, and the earlier lesions may be softer and redder, sometimes giving the impression of 'bubbling up' behind the existing papillae. Older lesions may become red if inflamed (Fig. 21.15). Phenytoin, like cyclosporin and nifedipine (see below), may also cause hirsutism.

Despite earlier reports that the degree of enlargement is related mainly to the dose of phenytoin, it has been shown that there is a positive correlation between the severity of overgrowth and gingival inflammation, plaque score, calculus accumulation, and pocket depths. There is *no* correlation between the extent of overgrowth and the dose of phenytoin, its serum level, or the age and sex of the patient.

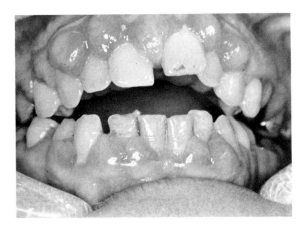

Fig. 21.15 *Phenytoin-induced gingival hyperplasia showing enlargement mainly of interdental papillae with resulting pseudoclefts between the enlarged papillae.*

Histology shows marked thickening of epithelium with long overgrowths into the connective tissue. Fibroblasts show increased mitotic activity but are not increased in number, and the collagen fibre component is not increased.

Treatment poses some problems. The physician may be willing to substitute another drug but, in any event, the patient's level of plaque control often needs considerable improvement and a chlorhexidine mouthwash may be helpful.

Excision of enlarged tissue may be indicated, but is difficult if the tissue is very firm and fibrous. Healing may be slow, possibly hampered by infection of the large wound, and packs may require changing. Unfortunately, the gingival enlargement readily recurs, although this is less likely with meticulous oral hygiene, particularly if phenytoin has been stopped.

Nifedipine

Nifedipine (an antihypertensive agent) causes, in some individuals, gingival hyperplasia typically affecting the papillae which become red and puffy and tend to bleed.

Increased numbers of fibroblasts containing strongly sulphated mucopolysaccharides may be demonstrated histochemically; their cytoplasm contains numerous secretory granules, suggesting an increased production of acid mucopolysaccharides.

Improved oral hygiene may achieve some reduction in the degree of nifedipine-induced hyperplasia. Excision of the enlarged tissue may be followed by recurrence, and patients should be warned accordingly. Again, it may be feasible for the physician to change medication.

Diltiazem

Diltiazem is an anti-anginal agent that may also cause gingival hyperplasia.

Cyclosporin

This immunosuppressive drug is particularly used to suppress the cell-mediated response after organ transplants.

Side-effects are uncommon below serum concentrations of 200 ng/ml. One side-effect of cyclosporin is gingival hyperplasia, initially of papillae, but only a third of patients may be affected, more commonly children, and this change may be lessened by meticulous removal of plaque before the drug is introduced.

Cyclosporin, like other immunosuppressive agents, predisposes to the development of lymphomas.

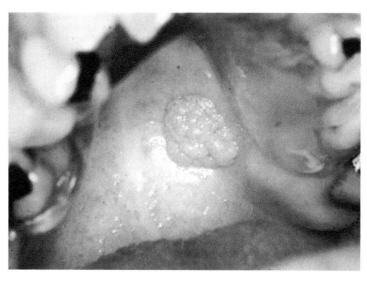

Fig. 21.16 Papilloma.

NEOPLASMS

Papilloma

This benign neoplasm of epithelium, caused by papillomaviruses, appears most often at the junction of the hard and soft palate (Fig. 21.16).

The papilloma is a cauliflower-like lesion with a whitish colour, and may resemble a wart. Papillomas of normal colour may be confused with the commoner fibroepithelial polyps, although the latter are commonest at sites of potential trauma.

Unlike papillomas of the larynx or bowel, which may undergo malignant transformation, papillomas in the oral cavity appear to remain benign. However, oral papillomas should be removed and examined histologically to establish a correct diagnosis. Excision must be total, deep and wide enough to include any abnormal cells beyond the zone of the pedicle.

Papillomas are discussed in Chapter 19.

Fibroma

The true fibroma—a benign neoplasm of fibroblastic origin—is rare in the oral cavity. It is probable that many lesions in the past called fibromas were fibroepithelial polyps (p. 265).

The true fibroma is a continuously enlarging new growth, not necessarily arising at a site of potential trauma. It is a pedunculated growth with a smooth non-ulcerated pink surface.

Removal should be total, deep, and wide. Histology shows marked proliferation of fibroblasts, with nuclei of uniform shape and size and of uniform staining characteristics, unlike the fibrosarcoma.

Lipoma

This benign neoplasm presents as a slow-growing, spherical, smooth and soft semifluctuant lump with a characteristic yellowish colour caused by the fat which makes up the bulk of the lesion (Fig. 21.17). Histology shows adult fat cells gathered into lobules by vascular septa of fibrous connective tissue. The fat cells themselves appear as clear, circular structures with nuclei compressed against the cell membrane; those cells cut in the plane of their nucleus thus resemble signet rings.

Osteoma

This lesion—a benign neoplasm of bone which grows by the continuous formation of lamellar bone—should be distinguished from an exostosis. Osteomas are usually unilateral, painless swellings covered by normal oral mucosa. They are usually smooth and (not surprisingly) very hard (see Chapter 7).

Multiple osteomas and polyposis coli are features of

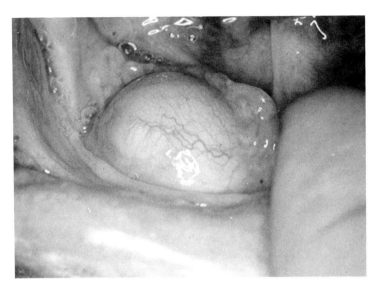

Fig. 21.17 *Lipoma.*

Gardner's syndrome; the polyps in the large bowel may become malignant (Chapters 7 and 33).

Myxoma

This is rare in the oral cavity. It can arise in bone or soft tissue and, although benign, is aggressive and difficult to eradicate because of its tendency to infiltrate normal tissue.

Histologically, it exhibits delicate and loosely arranged fibres and stellate cells widely separated by stroma. Occasionally the lesion may be multilocular.

Neurofibroma

Neurofibroma is an uncommon lesion and typically affects the tongue. It represents a benign overgrowth of all elements of a peripheral nerve (axon cylinder, Schwann cells, and fibrous connective tissue), arranged in a variety of patterns.

Neurofibromas may occur multiply as a feature of neurofibromatosis (von Recklinghausen's disease: Chapter 12) and rarely may undergo sarcomatous change.

Leiomyoma

This benign tumour of smooth muscle is rare in the oral cavity.

Leukaemia

Rapid gingival enlargement in the absence of any other known precipitating causes should always arouse a suspicion of malignancy such as leukaemia, especially if there is pallor, lethargy and gingival bleeding or petechiae. In its early stages, the oral manifestation of leukaemia may masquerade as acute necrotizing gingivitis (Vincent's disease: Chapters 16 and Volume 3).

Lymphoma (Chapter 31)

Carcinoma (Chapter 15)

Wegener's granulomatosis (Chapter 15)

Disseminated malignant granuloma (otherwise known as Wegener's granulomatosis) is a rare, lethal disorder in which there is necrotizing granulomatosis initially of the respiratory tract, followed by widespread arteritis of small vessels and renal damage.

A painless, progressive swelling of the gingiva in a previously healthy mouth, particularly associated with swollen, inflamed papillae, should arouse suspicion of this condition. The gingival enlargement may have a fairly characteristic 'strawberry-like' appearance.

Histology may show a non-specific but dense inflammatory reaction with groups of giant cells characteristic of this disorder.

Metastatic tumours (Chapter 15)

Kaposi's sarcoma (Chapter 20)

Myeloma (Chapter 7)

Salivary gland neoplasms (Chapter 24)

OTHER CAUSES OF LUMPS OR SWELLINGS

Crohn's disease (orofacial granulomatosis)

Crohn's disease is a chronic, inflammatory granulomatous disorder that may produce oral lesions in the presence or absence of any identifiable gut involvement. Only about 10% of patients with Crohn's disease of the bowel have oral lesions (Chapter 16).

Reddish, raised lesions on the gingiva, and hyperplastic folds of the oral mucosa, are features of Crohn's disease. Regional lymph node enlargement may be seen.

Histologically, the epithelium is intact but thickened, with epithelioid cells and giant cells surrounded by a lymphocytic infiltration.

Melkersson–Rosenthal syndrome is the rare association of facial swelling of similar pathogenesis, with facial palsy and fissured tongue.

Sarcoidosis

Sarcoidosis is an unusual cause of gingival enlargement which may resemble Wegener's granulomatosis or Crohn's disease. The swollen gingiva may be painful, with a pebbly erythematous appearance (Chapters 26 and 31).

Scurvy

Scurvy (vitamin C deficiency) is a very rare cause of gingival swelling and purpura.

Fibro-osseous lesions (Chapter 7)

Angioedema

Oral or facial swelling may be a feature of allergic angioedema (a type 1 hypersensitivity response: Chapter 13) or of hereditary angioedema (caused by a deficiency of the inhibitor of C1 esterase).

The swelling is of acute onset and is often only mild and transient (Fig. 21.18), but there is always the potential of obstruction of the airway.

Allergic angioedema is treated with intramuscular adrenaline, and with corticosteroids or antihistamines. Hereditary angioedema is discussed in Volume 1.

Amyloidosis

Amyloidosis (amyloid disease) is the deposition in tissue of an eosinophilic hyaline material. It is a term used to cover deposits of several different proteins, mainly either immunoglobulin light chains or a protein of uncertain nature known as amyloid A (AA) protein.

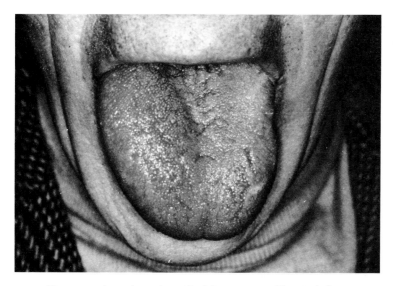

Fig. 21.18 *Angioedema of one side of the tongue caused by a food allergy.*

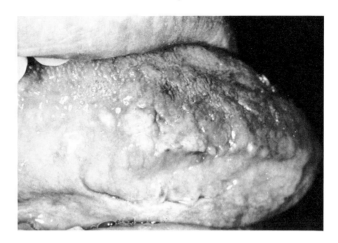

Fig. 21.19 *Amyloidosis showing macroglossia.*

Primary amyloidosis is a disorder characterized by deposits of immunoglobulin light chains in heart, skeletal muscle, oral tissues and gastrointestinal tract. The tongue becomes enlarged and indurated (Fig. 21.19) and there may also be yellowish submucosal nodules, lumps or petechiae.

Secondary amyloidosis can complicate chronic inflammatory disorders such as chronic sepsis or rheumatoid arthritis. Deposits of AA protein are found in the spleen, liver, kidney and adrenals.

Multiple myeloma (Chapter 7) may be complicated by amyloid but the deposits are of immunoglobulin light chains.

Management

Congo red or thioflavine T staining of a biopsy usually confirms the diagnosis, though, in extreme cases, the deposits are seen on conventional haematoxylin and eosin

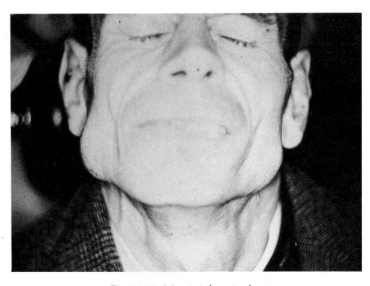

Fig. 21.20 *Masseteric hypertrophy.*

staining. Management is of the underlying disease, where present, and requires specialist care.

Masseteric hypertrophy

Continual clenching of the jaws (bruxism) may lead to hypertrophy of the masseters (Fig. 21.20).

FURTHER READING

Abbey L. M., Page D. G., Sawyer, D. R. (1980). The clinical and histopathologic features of a series of 464 oral squamous cell papillomas. *Oral Surg.*, **49**: 429.

Anneroth G., Sigurdson A. (1983). Hyperplastic lesions of the gingiva and alveolar mucosa. A study of 175 cases. *Acta. odont. Scand.*, **41**: 75–86.

Bouquot J. E., Gundlach K. K. H. (1986). Oral exophytic lesions in 23,616 white Americans over 35 years of age. *Oral Surg.*, **62**: 284–291.

Enzinger F. M., Weiss S. W. (1983). *Soft tissue tumours.* St Louis, Missouri: C. V. Mosby.

Safai B., Good R. A. (1981). Kaposi's sarcoma: a review and recent developments. CA **31**: 1–10.

Wright B. A., Jackson D. (1980). Neural tumours of the oral cavity. *Oral Surg.*, **49**: 509–522.

Chapter
22 *Miscellaneous oral disorders*

HALITOSIS

Oral sepsis can cause or modify breath odours. A few systemic diseases such as diabetic ketosis can also give a characteristic odour to the breath (Table 22.1) and, with halitosis from any cause, the patient may also complain of a bad taste in the mouth (Table 22.2; Chapter 29). The treatment is that of the underlying cause.

Potent causes of halitosis and bad taste include, smoking, eating various food and the following.

Table 22.1
Differential diagnosis of halitosis

Foods	Garlic
	Others
Smoking	
Oral infections	Chronic periodontitis
	Pericoronitis
	Acute ulcerative gingivitis
	Dry socket
	Oral abscesses
	Others
Starvation	
Drugs	Dimethyl sulphoxide and others
Organic diseases	Respiratory tract infections
	Nasal foreign bodies
	Oro-antral fistulae
	Cirrhosis
	Renal failure
	Diabetic ketosis
	Gastrointestinal disease
	Xerostomia
Psychogenic	

Periodontal sepsis

In the middle aged or elderly this is most usually the result of advanced periodontitis (pyorrhoea). In a young adult, halitosis may be caused by acute ulcerative gingivitis or pericoronitis, anaerobic infections which are particularly liable to be foul smelling.

Table 22.2
Causes of unpleasant taste

Local causes
Dental infections
   Chronic periodontitis
   Acute ulcerative gingivitis
   Chronic dental abscess
   Dry socket
   Others
Nasal disease
   Chronic sinusitis
   Oro-antral fistula
   Foreign bodies

Systemic causes
Salivary gland disorders causing xerostomia
   Sjögren's syndrome
   Irradiation damage
   Sialadenitis

Psychogenic causes
   Depression
   Anxiety states
   Psychoses
   Hypochondriasis
Drugs
   Drugs causing dry mouth (see Table 25.1)
   Metronidazole, lithium, gold etc.

Gastric regurgitation

Other types of oral sepsis

Infected extraction sockets are also likely to contain anaerobic infections and give rise to halitosis. Debris under a neglected or poorly designed dental bridge is another cause.

Dry mouth

Any patient with a dry mouth can have unpleasantly smelling breath. This may be made worse by supervening infections, particularly periodontal disease or acute ascending parotitis.

In acute gastrointestinal disease, especially acute appendicitis, the smell of the breath may be due to dryness of the mouth as much as to the gut lesion.

Starvation

Drugs

Smoking and alcohol are common causes of halitosis but some drugs are particularly noxious—perhaps the worst is dimethylsulphoxide.

Systemic disease

A range of systemic diseases can cause halitosis, particularly advanced cirrhosis and terminal renal failure. In diabetic ketosis the breath may smell of acetone.

Nasal sepsis or foreign bodies, or infection of the paranasal sinuses may also result in halitosis.

Psychogenic factors

The complaint of halitosis may be made by patients who do not have it but imagine it because of psychogenic disorders.

BLISTERS

Blistering, or vesiculobullous disorders, are discussed in detail elsewhere (especially in Chapter 16) since most are related to infection such as herpetic stomatitis, or to mucocutaneous diseases such as pemphigus and pemphigoid.

Blisters may also prove to be mucoceles or occasionally other cystic lesions (Chapter 5). Blood blisters may be caused by trauma, chemical or thermal burns, localized oral purpura (angina bullosa haemorrhagica: Chapter 16), platelet defects such as thrombocytopenia, or, rarely, amyloid disease (Table 22.3).

Table 22.3
Causes of oral blisters

Infections
Herpetic stomatitis
Chickenpox
Shingles

Mucocutaneous disorders
Pemphigus
Pemphigoid
Dermatitis herpetiformis and linear IgA disease
Erythema multiforme
Lichen planus (rarely)
Epidermolysis bullosa
Localized oral purpura (angina bullosa haemorrhagica)

Others
Purpura
Burns
Cysts
Amyloidosis
Mucocele

LOSS OF ELASTICITY OF ORAL TISSUES

Fibrosis of oral tissues can follow burns or irradiation (Volume 1; Chapter 15); may be associated with habits such as the chewing of betel-nut (areca), which predisposes to oral submucous fibrosis; may be caused by a connective tissue disorder (scleroderma) or, rarely, is occupational (polyvinylchloride workers). Epidermolysis bullosa and pemphigoid may cause scarring (Chapter 16).

Oral submucous fibrosis

Oral submucous fibrosis appears to be caused by exposure to constituents of the areca nut and is found virtually exclusively in persons from the Indian subcontinent.

It causes symmetrical fibrosis of the cheeks, lips or palate. In the early stages this may be symptomless and noted only by the dentist—as bands running through the mucosa. Fibrosis can, however, be so severe that the affected site becomes white and firm, and there may be severe restriction of opening of the mouth (Fig. 22.1). Oral submucous fibrosis appears to be restricted to the mouth, though many patients are also anaemic. There is evidence that it predisposes to the development of oral carcinoma.

Management is difficult: intralesional corticosteroids

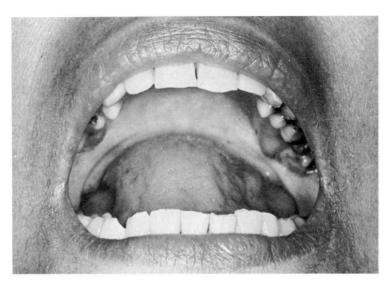

Fig. 22.1 *Oral submucous fibrosis, showing restricted oral opening and palatal fibrosis.*

and exercises may be useful, but surgery may be needed to relieve the fibrosis.

Systemic sclerosis (scleroderma; progressive systemic sclerosis)

Systemic sclerosis is a connective tissue disorder mainly affecting middle-aged or elderly women. The aetiology is unknown but it is probably immunologically mediated.

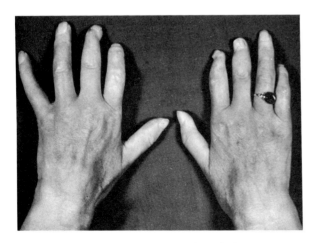

Fig. 22.2 *Scleroderma: atrophy of the digits.*

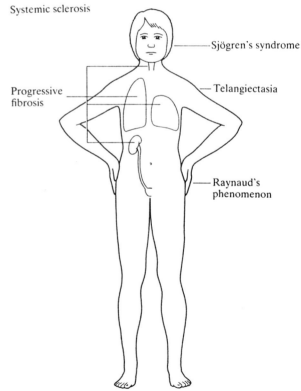

Fig. 22.3 *Features of systemic sclerosis.*

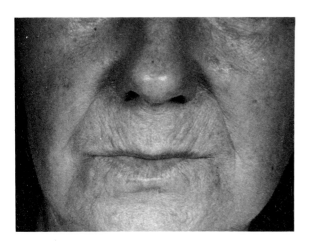

Fig. 22.4 *Systemic sclerosis: tightening and waxy appearance of skin.*

becomes stiff and thinned, has a waxy appearance and becomes pigmented and telangiectatic. Fibrosis also involves the lungs, heart, kidneys and gastrointestinal tract (Fig. 22.3).

The face and mouth are affected and oral opening may be restricted (Fig. 22.4) and the tongue stiffened. Sjögren's syndrome may be found in patients with systemic sclerosis. A minority of patients with systemic sclerosis have oral telangiectasia or widening of the periodontal space on radiography, though there is no increase in tooth mobility.

Management

The diagnosis is made primarily on clinical grounds, though some patients have autoantibodies, especially against RNA. Penicillamine is the usual treatment.

Clinical features

The most obvious feature of scleroderma is progressive fibrosis and stiffening of the skin, and Raynaud's phenomenon—intense vasoconstriction of the vessels of the digits, precipitated by the cold (Fig. 22.2). The skin

RARE FUNGAL INFECTIONS

Fungal infections apart from candidosis are rare and usually seen in the immunocompromised or debilitated patient (Table 22.4).

Table 22.4
Rare fungal infections

Infection	Manifestations
Aspergillosis	Aspergilloma Rhinocerebral type causes palatal necrosis Disseminated in immunocompromised patients
Blastomycosis: North America	Skin or mucosal ulcers, or suppurating granulomas
South America	Mucosal ulcers
(paracoccidioidomycosis)	Lymphadenopathy: lung, liver and spleen abscesses
Coccidioidomycosis	Disseminated through lungs, bones and CVS Rarely oral
Cryptococcosis	Meningitis in immunocompromised patients Mouth ulcers
Histoplasmosis	Lungs, spleen and adrenal granulomas in immunocompromised patients Lumps or ulcers in mouth
Phycomycosis (mucormycosis, zygomycosis)	Antral involvement with palatal ulceration in immunocompromised patients—especially diabetics
Sporotrichosis	Granulomas affecting mainly the limbs Oral lesions rare

FURTHER READING

Canniff J. P., Harvey W. (1981). The aetiology of oral submucous fibrosis: the stimulation of collagen synthesis by
  extracts of areca nut. *Int. J. Oral Surg.*, **10**: 163–167.
Pindborg J. J., Bhousle R. B., Murti P. R. *et al.* (1980). Incidence
  and early forms of oral submucous fibrosis. *Oral Surg.*, **50**:
  40–44.
Scully C., Cawson R. A. (1987). *Medical problems in dentistry*,
  2nd edn. Bristol: Wright.
Yen D. J. (1982). Surgical treatment of submucous fibrosis. *Oral
  Surg.*, **54**: 269–272.

Section III
Salivary Glands

Salivary gland development, anatomy and physiology

The salivary glands arise from invaginations of oral epithelium early in embryonic life: the parotid glands develop at around 4 weeks intrauterine life (i.u.l.), the submandibular glands around 6 weeks i.u.l., the sublingual glands around 8 weeks i.u.l., and the labial minor salivary glands around 12 weeks i.u.l. Although it is still somewhat controversial, the sublingual glands are thought to bud off the original invagination of oral mucosa which gives rise to the submandibular gland, and so frequently both the sublingual and submandibular glands have a common duct outlet.

Developmental disorders of the salivary glands are rare, as is aplasia of the major salivary glands. Although aplasia can be inferred on clinical grounds, functional studies such as radioisotope studies (scintiscanning) or sialography are required to confirm the diagnosis, and computerized tomography (CT) may be helpful (Volume 1). Even if major gland aplasia is demonstrated, xerostomia is only a problem if both parotid and both submandibular glands are absent.

Salivary gland tissue has, rarely, been reported at ectopic sites, including the middle ear, neck and vulva.

ANATOMY AND PHYSIOLOGY

Structure

Salivary tissue consists of acinar, ductal and other specialized cell types. The acinar tissue contains serous or mucous cells or a combination of the two. Under routine haematoxylin and eosin stain, mucous cells are darker than serous cells (Fig. 23.1).

With the exception of the minor salivary glands of Von Ebner, situated around the circumvallate papillae, all minor salivary glands are mucous in type. The sublingual

glands are also mucous; the submandibular glands are largely mucous, but the parotid glands are principally serous, though the number of mucous cells increases with

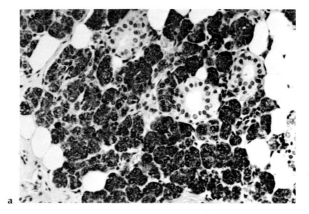
a

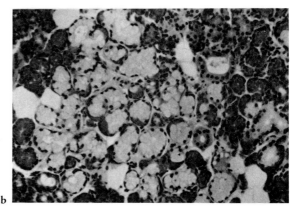
b

Fig. 23.1 *Comparative staining properties and histological appearance of (a) parotid serous cells and (b) submandibular mucous cells.*

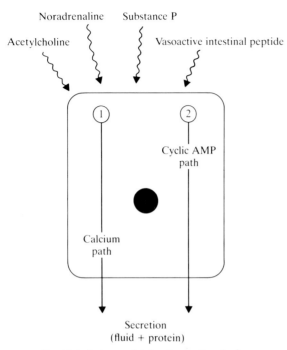

Fig. 23.2 *Factors modulating the secretion of saliva.*

ent on several modulatory influences which act via either a cyclic AMP or calcium-dependent pathway (Fig. 23.2).

The duct cells of salivary glands are specialized both in function and in structure (Fig. 23.3). In minor labial salivary glands, the cells closest to the acini are the intercalated duct cells which join adjacent lobules of acinar tissue and lead finally into an excretory duct. In major salivary glands other specialized duct cells are present between the intercalated ducts and the excretory ducts. One such cell is the striated duct cell, which selectively reabsorbs certain electrolytes, and contains numerous peptides such as epidermal growth factor and nerve growth factor, which may have biological significance (see below). Increased mitochondria in the intercalated duct cells, a normal age change, produce darkly-staining oncocytes. Other duct cells (such as the duct cell of Pfluger) are of unknown significance. As can be seen from Figures 23.4–23.6, ductal cell types have a specific histological appearance.

Myoepithelial cells, though not obvious in normal tissue on routine histological staining (Fig. 23.7), can be seen ultrastructurally around acini and extending down ducts. Intracellular myofilaments can be demonstrated. Myoepithelial cells probably originate from epithelium, have contractile properties, and help acinar cells to express saliva.

Physiology, innervation and applied anatomy

Control of salivary gland secretion is mainly neural, under the influence of the autonomic nervous system (Fig. 23.8), although various hormones and bradykinin may also modulate salivary composition. *In general, para-*

age. Mucous cells secrete mucins that give saliva from certain glands (such as the submandibular) a more viscous, sticky nature compared with the 'watery' secretion of serous glands (parotid). Acinar tissue produces the initial secretion of fluid, with an electrolyte composition similar to plasma possibly via a $Na^+/K^+/Cl^-$ co-transporter mechanism. Secretion appears to be depend-

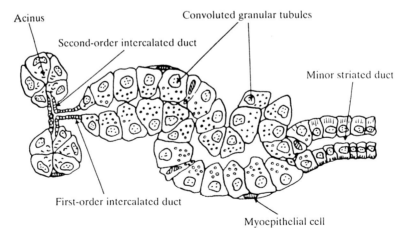

Fig. 23.3 *Diagrammatic representation of a major salivary gland.*

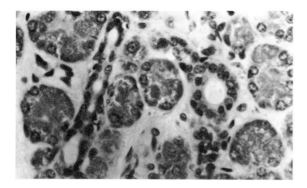

Fig. 23.4 *Intercalated duct cell which is cuboidal in shape.*

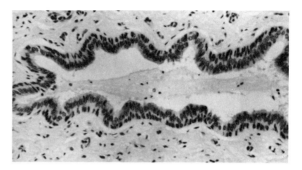

Fig. 23.6 *Excretory duct, which can have a pseudostratified appearance.*

sympathetic stimulation increases salivation; sympathetic stimulation depresses salivation.

Parasympathetic innervation to the parotid gland is via the inferior salivatory nucleus, through the glossopharyngeal nerve (tympanic branch) and the lesser petrosal nerves (Fig. 23.8). Synapse of preganglionic parasympathetic fibres occurs in the otic ganglion, with postganglionic fibres then reaching the parotid gland via the auriculotemporal nerve. The parotid gland itself receives *sensory* input via the auriculotemporal nerve, but the parotid fascia is innervated by the greater auricular nerve.

The lingual nerve carries the parasympathetic secretomotor supply to the submandibular and sublingual glands, the fibres originating in the superior salivatory nucleus and passing with the facial nerve and chorda tympani (Fig. 23.8). The lingual nerve also gives a sensory supply, both to the submandibular and sublingual glands.

Sympathetic supply to all glands is from the superior cervical ganglion and passes along the course of branches of the external carotid artery.

The major salivary glands have lymph nodes both on the surface and within the substance. Immediately superficial to the parotid fascia are the preauricular lymph nodes which drain to the jugulodigastric and other deep cervical lymph nodes. The submandibular gland drains lymph both to the jugulo-omohyoid and jugulodigastric nodes. Lymph from the sublingual glands drains to the submandibular and submental nodes and thence to the anterior deep cervical lymph nodes.

FUNCTIONS OF SALIVA

The most obvious function of saliva is to lubricate food and mucosa—dry mouth (xerostomia) causes great diffi-

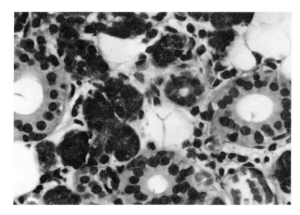

Fig. 23.5 *Striated duct cell which is columnar in shape and has many mitochondria.*

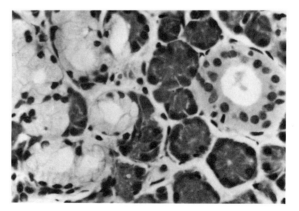

Fig. 23.7 *Myoepithelial cells surrounding salivary acini. These cells have intracellular myofilaments.*

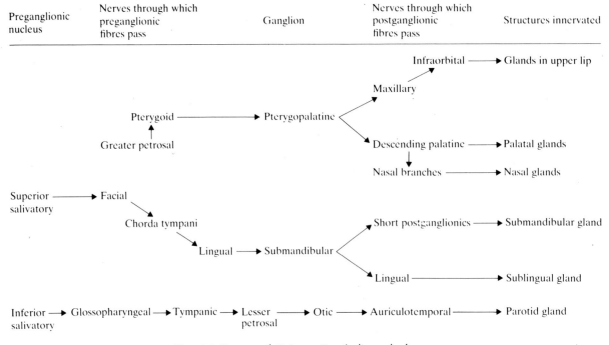

Preganglionic nucleus	Nerves through which preganglionic fibres pass	Ganglion	Nerves through which postganglionic fibres pass	Structures innervated
			Infraorbital → Glands in upper lip	
	Pterygoid → Pterygopalatine	Maxillary		
	Greater petrosal		Descending palatine → Palatal glands	
			Nasal branches → Nasal glands	
Superior salivatory → Facial	Chorda tympani		Short postganglionics → Submandibular gland	
	Lingual → Submandibular		Lingual → Sublingual gland	
Inferior salivatory → Glossopharyngeal → Tympanic → Lesser petrosal → Otic → Auriculotemporal → Parotid gland				

Fig. 23.8 *Parasympathetic innervation of salivary glands.*

culty in swallowing and speech—but there are a number of other functions.

Digestive

Salivary amylase probably has a very minor role in humans in the conversion of starch to maltose. Salivary lipase may assist the initiation of fat digestion.

However, the water, mucins and proline-rich glycoproteins do lubricate food and help swallowing. Saliva is now known not to be essential for normal taste perception.

Excretory

Some drugs are excreted in saliva, but this is important only in the context of the usefulness of saliva for monitoring blood levels of some drugs, e.g. anticonvulsants.

Maintenance of tooth integrity

Enamel maturation and remineralization are saliva dependent (Volume 3). The buffering capacity of saliva is also important in maintaining tooth integrity (Volume 3).

Hormonal

A polypeptide hormone—epidermal growth factor (EGF; urogastrone)—from the submandibular gland is, at least in animals, protective against gastric ulceration by inhibiting gastric acid secretion. Its role in humans is unclear, but it may be involved in wound healing. Homeostatic proteases such as kallikrein, renin and tonin may exert control on local vascularity and on water/electrolyte transport.

Protective

There is an obvious lubricative and mechanical washing effect of saliva, as well as its non-specific and immune protective mechanisms. Saliva is inhibitory to various microbial agents, including, for example, HIV. The mechanisms include the following.

Mucins

Salivary mucins aid lubrication, aggregate bacteria, are

antiviral and restrict mucosal permeability to various toxins.

Inhibitors of proteolytic enzymes

Cysteine-containing phosphoproteins in high concentrations in submandibular saliva, and antileukoprotease in submandibular and parotid saliva are, with mucins, protective against proteolytic enzymes from bacteria and leucocytes.

Bacterial aggregators

Salivary mucins, some salivary glycoproteins, and lysozyme can aggregate bacteria and prevent their attachment to oral surfaces.

Direct non-immune antimicrobial mechanisms

Lysozyme interacts with anions such as thiocyanate to disrupt bacterial cell membranes and lyse Gram-positive bacteria.

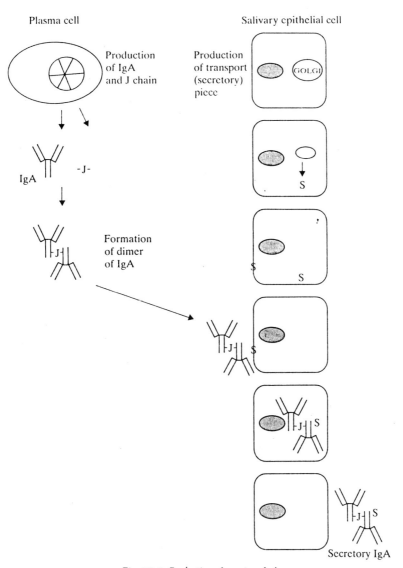

Fig. 23.9 *Production of secretory IgA.*

Histidine-rich peptides in parotid saliva also suppress oral bacteria and fungi.

Lactoferrin chelates iron and deprives bacteria of this essential factor.

Lactoperoxidase, with thiocyanate and hydrogen peroxide, disrupts bacterial metabolism. This system acts against some Gram-positive and Gram-negative bacteria, and yeasts.

Amylase may modulate bacterial growth; for example, it protects against *Neisseria gonorrhoeae.*

Immune protection (Chapter 13)

Secretory IgA is the main class of antibody in saliva and, overall, one-third is secreted by the minor salivary glands, two-thirds by the major glands. Salivary secretory IgA (sIgA) is produced locally by plasma cells in the salivary glands; the secretory piece is synthesized by the gland epithelium and facilitates transport of the sIgA into the gland lumen (Fig. 23.9).

Salivary tissue may form part of a common mucosal immune system, reacting not only to local antigenic stimuli but also in concert with gut-associated lymphoid tissue (GALT) and bronchial-associated lymphoid tissue (BALT). The overall system may be called the mucosal-associated lymphoid tissue (MALT).

Certainly, stimulation of one mucosal site (A) can cause a specific antibody response in a remote glandular site (B), presumably because immune-competent lymphocytes produced at A are seeded and migrate in lymph through the thoracic duct to the cardiovascular system and reach site B, and other sites. For example, sIgA antibodies against *Streptococcus mutans* can appear in saliva when the *Strep. mutans* is given by a gastric tube to animals. This is the basis of one proposed caries vaccine.

Local antigenic stimulation may involve a further possible immune mechanism, in the lymphoid tissue associated with salivary glands. For example, the instillation of *Strep. mutans* into the parotid duct of animals elicits a specific sIgA response in that gland. The minor salivary glands may also play a significant role since they have duct-associated lymphoid tissue (DALT), especially in relation to the interlobular and secretory ducts. Oral antigens may pass retrogradely into the salivary glands and initiate an immune response in periductal lymphocytes.

FURTHER READING

Carter B. L. *et al.* (1981). Computed tomography and sialography. 1. Normal anatomy. *J. Comput. Assist. Tomogr.,* **5**: 42–45.

Dardick I., Van Nostrand A. W. P. (1985). Myoepithelial cells in salivary glands revisited. *Head and Neck Surg.,* **7**: 395–408.

Garrett J. R. (1975). Recent advances in physiology of salivary glands. *Br. med. Bull.,* **31**: 152–155.

Weiffenbach J. M., Fox P. C., Baum B. J. (1986). Taste and salivary function. *Proc. Natl. Acad. Sci. USA,* **83**: 6103–6106.

Young J. A. (1982). Is Na^+/Cl^- cotransport the basis of transport in absorptive and secretory epithelia? In Case R. M., Garner A., Turnberg L. A., Young J. A. Electrolyte and Water Transport across Epithelia. Raven Press. New York. pp. 181–198.

Chapter
24 *Salivary gland swelling*

The causes of swelling of the salivary glands are summarized in Table 24.1 and Figure 24.1.

INFLAMMATORY CAUSES OF SALIVARY GLAND SWELLING

By far the commonest cause of salivary gland swelling is infection—usually mumps.

Table 24.1
Causes of salivary gland swelling

Local causes
Inflammatory
  Ascending sialadenitis
Neoplasms
Others
  Duct obstruction (e.g. calculus)

Systemic causes
Inflammatory
  Mumps
  Sjögren's syndrome
  Sarcoidosis
  Actinomycosis
  HIV parotitis

Others
  Sialosis
  Mikulicz disease (lymphoepithelial lesion) and syndrome
  Drug-associated (uncommon)
    Chlorhexidine
    Phenylbutazone
    Iodine compounds
    Thiouracil
    Catecholamines
    Sulphonamides
    Phenothiazines
    Methyldopa

Mumps (acute viral sialadenitis; epidemic parotitis)

This is an acute infectious disease which principally affects the parotid salivary glands of children, both sexes being affected equally. Mumps is caused by an RNA paramyxovirus and is endemic worldwide, with a seasonal increase in winter and spring. One infection confers immunity to further attacks.

Other viruses, including parainfluenza, Coxsackie A, echoviruses, Epstein–Barr virus and human immunodeficiency viruses can also, *rarely*, produce parotitis.

Transmission of mumps is by direct contact or by droplet spread from saliva. An incubation period of 2–3 weeks elapses before clinical features appear but many infections are sub-clinical.

Clinical features

Typically the patient suffers an acute onset of painful

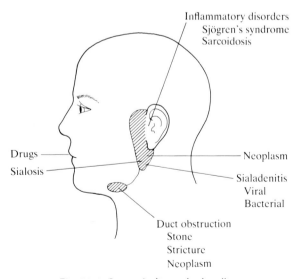

Fig. 24.1 *Causes of salivary gland swelling.*

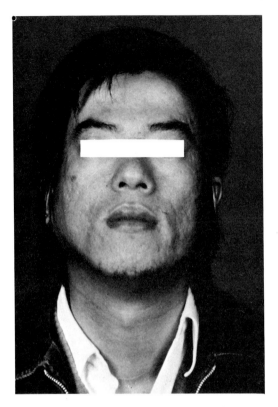

Fig. 24.2 *Clinical appearance of a patient with mumps involving one parotid gland only.*

parotitis, usually bilaterally, although in the early stages only one parotid gland may appear to be involved (Fig. 24.2). In approximately 10% of cases the submandibular glands are also affected; rarely, these may be the only glands involved. The salivary swelling may be accompanied by pain, trismus, fever and malaise, but there is no significant xerostomia. Generally, the salivary swelling persists for about 7 days and then gradually subsides.

Mumps less commonly involves organs other than the salivary glands. These extrasalivary manifestations include especially inflammation of the testes (orchitis), pancreatitis, and meningitis. Ensuing infertility from orchitis is *rare*.

Management

The diagnosis is on clinical grounds but confirmation, if needed, is by demonstrating a fourfold rise in serum antibody titres to mumps S and V antigens between acute serum and convalescent serum taken 3 weeks later.

Treatment is symptomatic, involving analgesics, ensuring adequate hydration and reducing the fever. No specific antiviral agents are available. Patient isolation for 6–10 days may be advised since the virus can be detected in saliva during this time.

Bacterial salivary gland infection (bacterial ascending sialadenitis)

The parotid glands are more commonly affected by

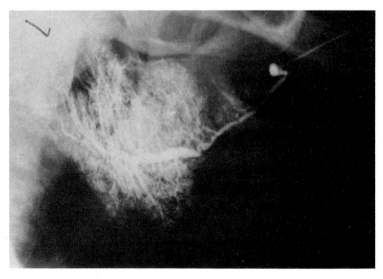

Fig. 24.3 *Sialographic appearance of a parotid gland in a patient previously presenting with acute parotitis. A benign stricture is present.*

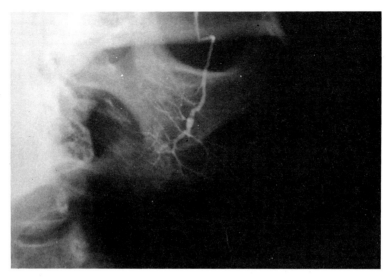

Fig. 24.4 *Sialographic appearance of a parotid gland in a patient previously presenting with acute parotitis. A mucus plug is present.*

ascending sialadenitis than are the submandibular salivary glands.

Parotitis

Acute bacterial parotitis was previously not uncommon in hospital in-patients, particularly following gastrointestinal surgery, because of dehydration. Infection subsequently ascended from the mouth. With better understanding of fluid balance and more widespread use of prophylactic antibiotics, acute parotitis is now uncommon in hospital in-patients, though it occasionally develops in patients receiving radiotherapy for parotid tumours. Infection in otherwise healthy patients is usually

due to abnormalities such as calculi, mucus plugs and benign duct strictures (Figs. 24.3 and 24.4). Reduced salivary flow also allows retrograde access of bacteria from the oral cavity. The organisms most commonly isolated are *Streptococcus viridans* and *Staphylococcus aureus*, the latter frequently being penicillin-resistant (Table 24.2).

Clinical features

Acute parotitis presents as painful parotid enlargement (Fig. 24.5). The affected gland is tender to palpation, and trismus and cervical lymphadenopathy may be present. One parotid gland is usually involved and patients are pyrexial, rarely toxaemic. The overlying skin may be reddened and, intra-orally, pus is seen exuding from the parotid duct orifice. If the infection localizes as a parotid abscess, it may point externally through the overlying skin (Fig. 24.6) or, rarely, into the external acoustic meatus.

Management

Pus should be sent for culture and sensitivity testing. Prompt antimicrobial therapy with flucloxacillin usually and, where fluctuation is present, surgical drainage are needed (Table 24.3; Volume 1) as there may be extensive glandular damage (Fig. 24.7)

Table 24.2
Organisms commonly isolated in cases of acute suppurative parotitis

α-Haemolytic streptococci	*Veillonella* species
Non-haemolytic streptococci	*Haemophilus* species
Anaerobic streptococci	*Bacteroides* species
Staphylococcus aureus	*Micrococcus* species
Elkenella corrodens	*Neisseria* species
Actinomyces odontolyticus/naeslundii	

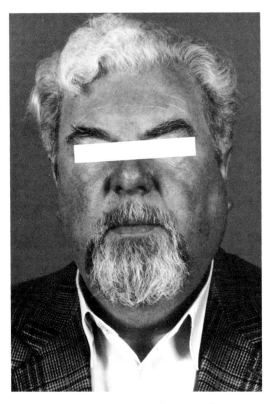

Fig. 24.5 Acute parotitis showing swelling.

Table 24.3
Management of acute bacterial sialadenitis

Collect pus for a stained smear, microbiological culture (aerobic and anaerobic) and antibiotic sensitivity testing

Axillary temperature should be noted and evidence of cervical lymphadenopathy sought

A history of allergy to antibiotics should be excluded

Antibiotic therapy should be commenced orally unless the patient requires hospital admission; the antibiotic of choice is flucloxacillin or amoxycillin, with erythromycin as an alternative if the patient is penicillin allergic

Choice of the antibiotic prescribed may be guided by the results of sensitivity tests

Supportive therapy, such as ensuring an adequate fluid intake, analgesics and attention to good oral hygiene are important

Once the acute condition has resolved, sialography should be undertaken to identify correctable factors such as mucus plugs, benign strictures or calculi

Submandibular sialadenitis

Acute bacterial infections of the submandibular salivary gland are rare and usually result from a predisposing cause such as a calculus (sialolith: Fig. 24.8). Salivary calculi are much commoner in the submandibular than in the

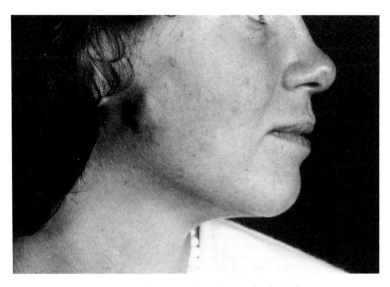

Fig. 24.6 *Pus has tracked subcutaneously producing a localized abscess in a case of acute suppurative parotitis.*

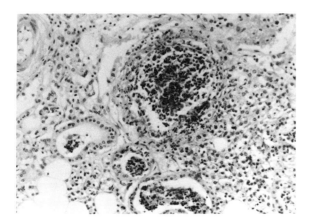

Fig. 24.7 *Acute parotitis showing acute inflammation and suppuration.*

parotid gland, are usually intraductal, but many also form within the gland itself and can reach a large size before producing symptoms (see below).

Chronic bacterial sialadenitis

Chronic bacterial sialadenitis may develop after acute sialadenitis, particularly if inappropriate antibiotics are used or predisposing factors are not eliminated. Unfortunately, serous acini may atrophy when salivary outflow is chronically obstructed and this further reduces function.

Recurrent parotitis of childhood

Chronic recurrent parotitis of childhood is an uncommon condition, characterized by repeated unilateral parotitis. Sialectasis is seen on sialography (Fig. 24.9). These cases often improve spontaneously around the time of puberty. The children are otherwise well, but the condition may be due to Epstein–Barr virus infection.

Sjögren's syndrome (see Chapter 25)

Sarcoidosis (see Chapters 26 and 31)

SALIVARY DUCT OBSTRUCTION

Salivary duct obstruction is not uncommon and is usually caused by a calculus in the submandibular duct. Strictures, mucus plugs or neoplasms are occasional causes.

Major ducts may be obstructed intraductally (material in the lumen), ductally (stenosis) or extraductally (pressure from without). The commonest causes of intraductal obstruction are mucus plugs and salivary calculi. Ductal causes of duct obstruction are benign stricture or duct wall fibrosis following trauma, radiation or chronic irritation by a calculus. Rarely, patients present with 'physiological' duct obstruction due either to duct spasm or an abnormal passage of the parotid duct through the buccin-

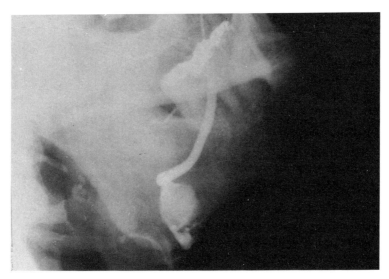

Fig. 24.8 *A large intraductal submandibular calculus producing almost complete duct outlet obstruction and predisposing to bacterial infection.*

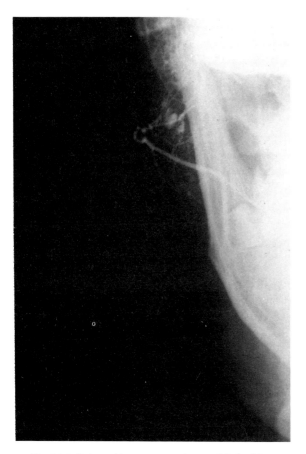

Fig. 24.9 *Sialographic appearance of a parotid gland in a child suffering from chronic recurrent parotitis of childhood. Multiple areas of dye pooling (sialectasis) are evident.*

ator or in relation to the masseter muscles. Extraductal causes of outlet obstruction, which are uncommon, include non-salivary tumours.

Prolonged duct obstruction produces atrophy, particularly of serous acini such as in the parotid gland. Even considerable degrees of submandibular gland obstruction may not, however, following resolution of the obstruction, leave a permanent acinar deficit.

Clinical features

A history of painful salivary gland swelling just before, or at, mealtimes is a classical feature of obstruction but, in older patients, this history is not always obtained. There may be dull pain over the affected gland, referred else-

where. Obstruction may occasionally mimic temporomandibular joint dysfunction (Chapter 9).

Management

It is rarely possible clinically to determine the cause of major duct obstruction except when a calculus is palpable. Plain radiographs may reveal a calculus if it is radiopaque (Fig. 24.10a). Sialography should help differentiate the various causes of major duct obstruction: intraductal or ductal causes are usually readily seen, but 'physiological' obstructions require pressure-monitored sialographic techniques for detection. Extraductal causes of obstruction may be clinically obvious or apparent only on sialography or combined (CT) sialography (Volume 1).

Intraductal and ductal causes of duct obstruction are usually correctable by the removal of the cause (e.g. mucus plug or calculi) or repeated duct dilatation in a benign stricture. To remove a stone the duct should be ligated temporarily between the stone and the gland to prevent the calculus being pushed distally. The duct is then incised longitudinally and the stone removed (Fig. 24.10b–e). The wound can often be left open. Extraductal causes of duct obstruction also require surgery.

Obstruction of minor salivary glands

Minor gland outlet obstruction is most commonly encountered when a mucocele is present (Fig. 24.11), although smoking and its accompanying nicotinic stomatitis produce transient palatal minor gland outlet obstruction also (Fig. 24.12).

Mucoceles are common. Most are caused by trauma to the duct of a minor salivary gland leading to extravasation of mucus and the appearance of a cystic lesion. It is not, however, lined by epithelium, and therefore is not a true cyst (Fig. 24.13). Occasional mucoceles are caused by saliva retention. Most mucoceles appear in the lower labial mucosa, buccal mucosa or ventrum of the tongue. They are fluctuant, bluish lesions and either resolve spontaneously or can be excised, or treated with cryosurgery.

NEOPLASMS

Although a wide range of different neoplasms can affect the salivary glands, most present as unilateral swelling of the parotid and are benign. The 'rule of nines' is an approximation that states that 9 out of 10 tumours affect the parotid, 9 out of 10 are benign, and 9 out of 10 are pleomorphic adenomas.

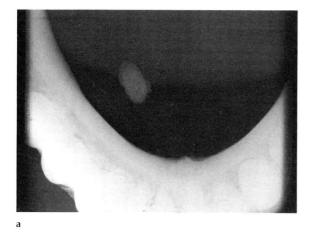

a

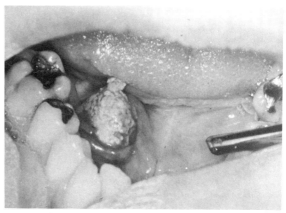

d

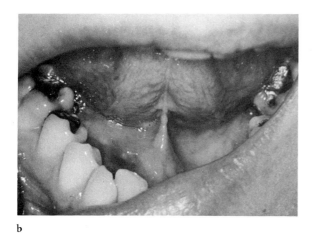

b

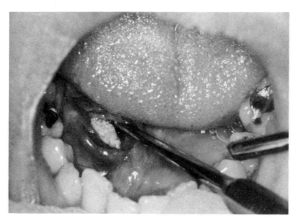

c

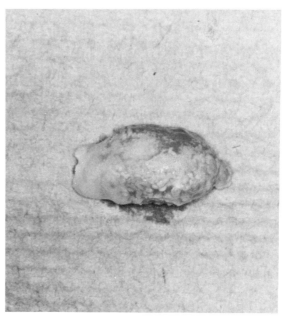

e

Fig. 24.10 (a) *Radiograph of submandibular calculus.* (b) *Clinical appearance of calculus.* (c) *Incision over the duct reveals calculus.* (d) *Calculus shelled out.* (e) *Calculus.*

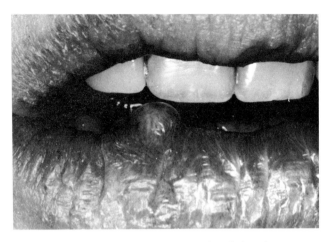

Fig. 24.11 *Clinical appearance of a mucocele of the lip. This patient has further traumatized the lesion by lip biting.*

In the major salivary glands the commonest tumour is the pleomorphic salivary adenoma, the next most common being carcinoma which, in some cases, arises in a longstanding pleomorphic salivary adenoma. For this reason, suspected pleomorphic salivary adenomas require early removal.

Submandibular gland tumours are also usually pleomorphic salivary adenomas but malignant neoplasms constitute up to one-third of all submandibular tumours.

Sublingual gland tumours are exceedingly rare, but virtually all are malignant.

Apart from these tumours, other neoplasms of the major salivary glands are usually monomorphic adenomas (such as adenolymphomas), mucoepidermoid tumours or acinic cell tumours.

Minor salivary gland tumours most commonly arise in the palate but may be seen in the buccal mucosa or upper lip; those of the tongue or lower lip are extremely rare.

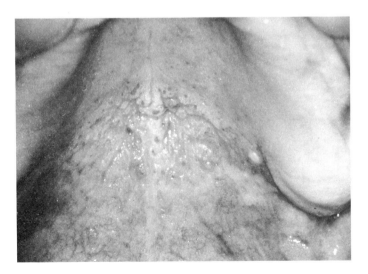

Fig. 24.12 *Minor palatal salivary duct obstruction due to smoking.*

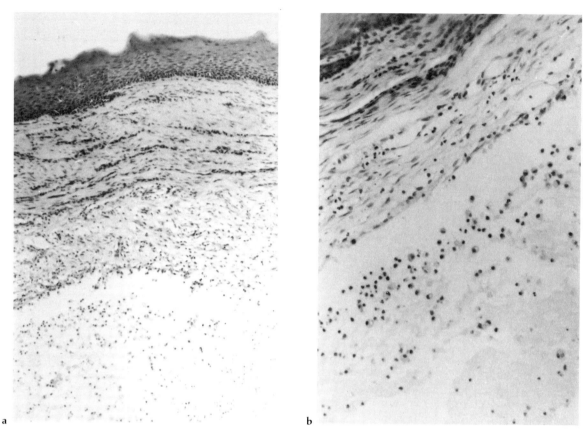

a   b

Fig. 24.13 *Mucocele: (a) collection of mucus beneath mucosa; (b) high power.*

Although pleomorphic adenomas are also common in minor salivary glands, malignant tumours such as carcinomas and adenoid cystic carcinomas are relatively more common—accounting for about 50% of all neoplasms in minor salivary glands.

Bilateral salivary neoplasms are rare, except in the case of adenolymphoma which is exclusively a tumour of the parotid glands, usually in elderly males.

Apart from the above epithelial neoplasms, lymphomas are the next most common neoplasms found in salivary glands. Sjögren's syndrome is recognized as predisposing to lymphomas, which have arisen in up to 6% of patients over 10 years in some studies. An intermediate stage between the salivary gland swelling in Sjögren's syndrome and lymphomas is termed the benign lymphoepithelial lesion, a histological rather than a clinical condition. It has recently been suggested that the lymphoepithelial lesion represents a *localized* lymphomatous process.

Aetiology of salivary gland neoplasm

The aetiology is unknown but the following facts can be stated.

1. Salivary gland tumours have increased in incidence in survivors of the atomic explosions in Japan.

2. Rarely, the use of 131-iodine in the treatment of thyroid malignancy appears to predispose to salivary gland neoplasia.

3. Salivary gland tumours occasionally follow radiotherapy to the head and neck.

4. Salivary gland tumours are more common in certain geographical locations. Eskimos, for example, have an increased prevalence and this has been suggested to be related to Epstein–Barr virus infection.

5. In mice, certain viruses such as polyomavirus may produce salivary gland tumours.

6. There is a correlation between salivary gland and breast cancer.

Table 24.4
Classification of salivary gland tumours (after WHO)

Epithelial tumours	Non-epithelial tumours	Unclassified tumours	Allied conditions
Adenomas	see text	see text	
Pleomorphic			Benign lympho
Monomorphic			epithelial lesion
Adenolymphoma			Sialosis
Oxyphilic			
Others			Oncocytosis
Mucoepidermoid			
Acinic cell tumours			
Carcinomas			
Adenoid cystic			
Adenocarcinoma			
Epidermoid			
Undifferentiated			
Carcinoma in pleomorphic adenoma			

Classification

The World Health Organization classification is the most widely used (Table 24.4), and the epithelial tumours, which are the most important, can be memorized by the mnemonic: *A Most Acceptable Classification*:

Adenomas	benign
Mucoepidermoid tumour	intermediate (see below)
Acinic cell tumour	intermediate (see below)
Carcinomas	malignant.

The subdivisions of this classification are shown in Table 24.4.

Adenomas

Pleomorphic adenoma (mixed salivary gland tumour)

The pleomorphic salivary adenoma (PSA) is the most common salivary gland neoplasm, and is usually slow growing and benign (Fig. 24.14). However, it can recur if excision is inadequate. The tumour is poorly encapsulated and parotid adenomas are in intimate relationship with the facial nerve—both facts making complete excision difficult to achieve.

Most pleomorphic adenomas are lobulated, rubbery swellings with normal overlying skin or mucosa but a bluish appearance if intra-oral (Fig. 24.15). They are not fixed to deeper tissues.

Malignant change is uncommon but is suggested clinically by:

(a) rapid growth,
(b) pain,
(c) fixation to deep tissues,
(d) facial palsy.

Histopathology

Pleomorphic adenoma appears to originate from ductal epithelium and myoepithelial cells which proliferate to contribute many duct-like spaces, sheets of epithelial cells and sometimes areas of squamous metaplasia (Fig. 24.16). There are also areas reminiscent of connective tissue such as cartilage (Fig. 24.17). The admixture of epithelial elements with what resembles fibrous, myxoid or cartilage tissue, leads to the name mixed tumour. These lesions usually have a thin fibrous capsule but this is not complete, and neoplastic cells may be seen in or outside the capsule (Fig. 24.18).

Malignant change is shown by obvious malignant features within the benign cellular picture.

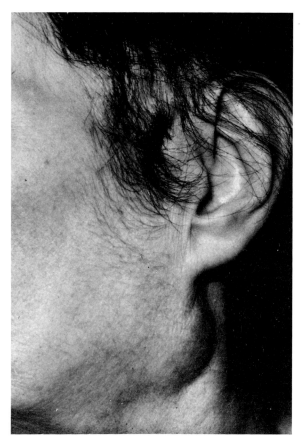

Fig. 24.14 *Pleomorphic salivary adenoma in the parotid gland.*

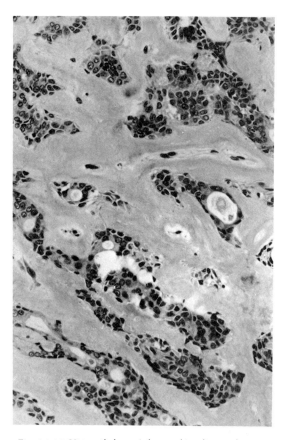

Fig. 24.16 *Histopathology of pleomorphic salivary adenoma.*

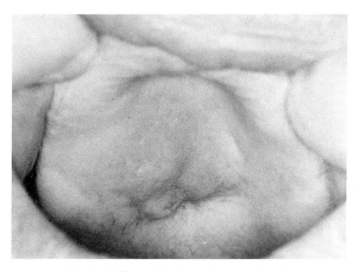

Fig. 24.15 *Pleomorphic salivary adenoma in the palate.*

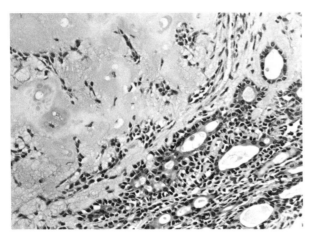

Fig. 24.17 *Cartilaginous areas in pleomorphic adenoma.*

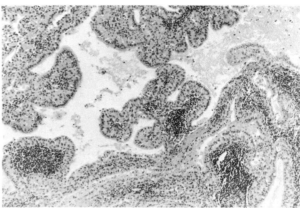

Fig. 24.19 *Adenolymphoma: cystic spaces and papillary epithelial-lined infoldings.*

Monomorphic adenomas

Unlike the *pleo*morphic adenoma, these tumours have a uniform cellular structure of epithelial elements (*monomorphic*).

1. *Adenolymphoma* (papillary cystadenoma lymphomatosum or Warthin's tumour). This neoplasm is found only in the parotid where it accounts for about 1 in 20 tumours. It is benign. Histopathologically, it consists of columnar cells surrounding lymphocytes in a folded (papillary) lining to cystic spaces (Figs. 24.19 and 24.20).

2. *Oxyphil adenoma.* This neoplasm is found virtually only in the parotid. It is extremely rare and affects mainly the elderly. It is benign. Histopathologically, the characteristic of this tumour is that it consists of cords of large eosinophilic cells with small nuclei (oncocytes).

Mucoepidermoid tumour

This tumour accounts for up to 10% of salivary gland tumours and is usually a slow-growing tumour of low grade malignancy or is benign.

The mucoepidermoid tumour consists of large pale mucus-secreting cells (hence 'muco'), surrounded by squamous epithelial cells (hence 'epidermoid') (Figs. 24.21 and 24.22).

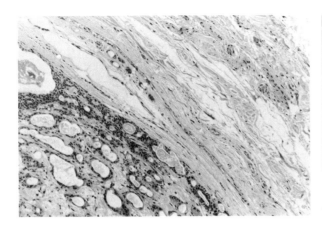

Fig. 24.18 *Photomicrograph showing tumour cells in capsule wall of pleomorphic salivary adenoma.*

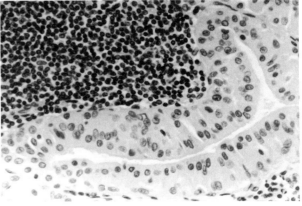

Fig. 24.20 *High power photomicrograph of adenolymphoma.*

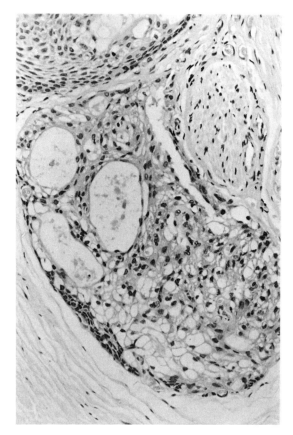

Fig. 24.21 *Mucoepidermoid tumour: mucous and epidermoid cells.*

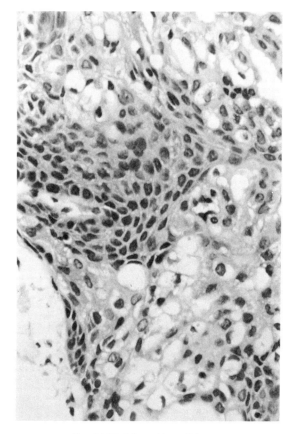

Fig. 24.22 *Mucoepidermoid tumour.*

Acinic cell tumours

Acinic cell tumours are very rare tumours that are usually benign, though all grades of malignancy have been reported. They are composed of large cells with a granular basophilic cytoplasm with spaces between some cells. The cells resemble serous cells of normal salivary glands (Figs. 24.23 and 24.24).

Carcinomas

Salivary carcinomas are uncommon and usually adenoid cystic or adenocarcinomas.

Adenoid cystic carcinoma (cylindroma)

This is a slow-growing malignant tumour (Fig. 24.25)

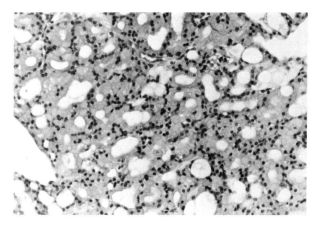

Fig. 24.23 *Acinic cell tumour showing uniform pattern of serous-type cells.*

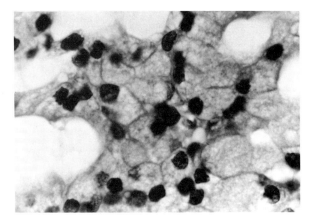

Fig. 24.24 *Acinic cell tumour showing granular cytoplasm of serous-type cells.*

which has a tendency to infiltrate, spread perineurally, and metastasize.

Histopathologically, rounded islands of small darkly staining cells surrounding multiple clear areas of varying size (Swiss-cheese appearance) are characteristic of adenoid cystic carcinoma (Figs. 24.26 and 24.27).

Adenocarcinoma

These are rapidly growing tumours of more malignant behaviour than adenoid cystic carcinomas. Their histopathological appearances can resemble mucoepidermoid, acinic cell or other tumours.

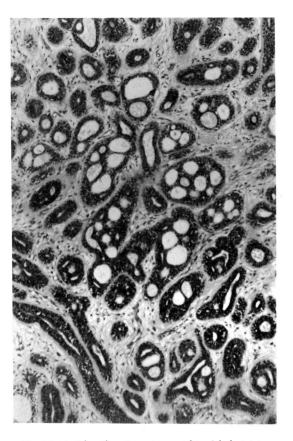

Fig. 24.26 *Adenoid cystic carcinoma: islets of dark-staining epithelial cells and 'Swiss-cheese' appearance.*

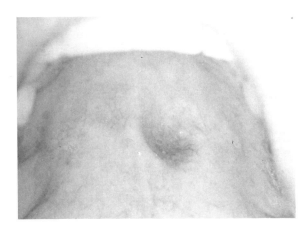

Fig. 24.25 *Adenoid cystic carcinoma in the palate.*

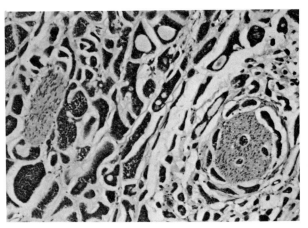

Fig. 24.27 *Adenoid cystic carcinoma: tumour cells have very little cytoplasm.*

Epidermoid carcinoma

These are often undifferentiated, highly malignant tumours.

Other salivary tumours

These are referred to elsewhere in the text but include:

   non-epithelial tumours (lymphomas, juvenile haemangioma),
   unclassified tumours,
   allied conditions (benign lymphoepithelial lesion, sialosis, oncocytosis).

Diagnosis of salivary gland neoplasms

A swelling of a salivary gland, especially if localized, firm and persistent, may be a neoplasm. Features suggestive of malignancy are noted above.

A detailed history is essential: a long history of gradual gland enlargement suggests a benign process, while pain or facial nerve palsy is ominous and suggests carcinoma (see above and Table 24.5). Some tumours may be small and the presentation may be of pain only. However, clinical examination may reveal an obvious swelling—in the case of the parotid, outlining the gland anteriorly to the ear, and causing eversion of the ear lobe. Sialography may reveal an obvious filling defect or displacement of the gland but is a relatively imprecise means of tumour detection. Computerized tomography alone, or in conjunction with sialography, is a more sensitive means of tumour detection. Radionuclides such as technetium, selenomethionine or gallium have been reported to be selectively taken up by some or excluded by other tumours, but in fact both false positive and negative results make the current techniques unsatisfactory. Pre-operative needle biopsy, sometimes CT guided, has a high tumour detection rate, but only in experienced hands. Ultrasonography has a limited application, being more suited for detecting cysts. The diagnosis can often best be firmly established by open biopsy.

Management of salivary gland neoplasms

Early detection carries a good prognosis, since most tumours metastasize late. Some tumours, such as adenoid cystic carcinoma, invade bone and neural tissues preferentially.

The treatment of choice for salivary gland tumours of major or minor gland origin is surgical excision, since the tumours are relatively radioresistant. However, radiotherapy is sometimes used as an adjunct.

Chemotherapy is used on a very limited basis only for some salivary gland tumours such as adenocarcinoma or adenoid cyst carcinoma, and then is used with surgery and/or radiotherapy.

SIALOSIS (SIALADENOSIS)

Sialosis is a benign, non-inflammatory, non-neoplastic, bilaterally symmetrical and painless recurrent enlargement of salivary glands, which usually affects the parotids. Salivary secretion is not impaired and sialographic examination reveals enlarged but otherwise normal glands.

Aetiology

A variety of causes of sialosis are recognized (Table 24.6), including alcohol abuse with or without accompanying liver cirrhosis; diabetes mellitus; and sympathomimetic drugs such as isoprenaline. In children, sialosis has been reported both in cystic fibrosis and in malnutrition. In

Table 24.5
Diagnostic significance of facial nerve palsy in patients with salivary gland tumours

	Incidence of palsy (%)
Poorly differentiated carcinoma	24
Adenoid cystic carcinoma	24
Carcinoma in pleomorphic salivary adenoma	11
Adenocarcinoma	10
Mucoepidermoid	8

Table 24.6
Causes of sialosis

Liver dysfunction and/or alcohol abuse
Uraemia
Diabetes mellitus
Acromegaly
Pregnancy
Starvation, e.g. anorexia nervosa
Pancreatitis
Cystic fibrosis
Drugs, e.g. phenylbutazone, isoprenaline and phenothiazines

adults, it may also be seen in hormonal disorders other than diabetes, such as acromegaly, or following oophorectomy. Anorexia nervosa or bulimia with malnutrition are rare causes of sialosis. Dysregulation of the autonomic innervation of the salivary glands is the unifying factor in all forms of sialosis.

Clinical features

Clinically there is soft, painless general enlargement of the involved glands. A useful guide to whether the patient is simply obese or has parotid enlargement is to observe the outward deflection of the ear lobe which is seen in true parotid swelling (Fig. 24.28).

Diagnosis

The diagnosis of sialosis is one of exclusion, based mainly on history and clinical examination. Appropriate blood examination for raised glucose levels or abnormal liver function may point to an underlying cause. Salivary gland function is normal but sialography is likely to show enlarged normal glands. Rarely, a bilateral space-occupying lesion such as a salivary neoplasm, cyst or lymphoid neoplasm may present difficulties in differentiation from sialosis, but biopsy is not usually needed. The affected gland in sialosis shows acinar hypertrophy and parotid sialochemistry may show raised potassium and calcium levels which would not be present in parotid enlargement due to other causes.

Management

No treatment is available. If the parotid swelling is only of salivary tissue and investigations have revealed a likely cause, such as alcoholism or diabetes, then the sialosis may resolve when alcohol intake is reduced or glucose control is instituted.

MIKULICZ SYNDROME

Leukaemic infiltration of the parotids and lacrimal glands is sometimes termed Mikulicz syndrome.

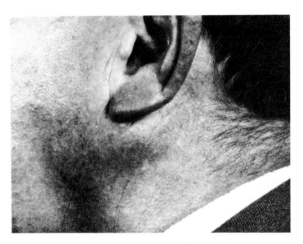

Fig. 24.28 *Sialosis: the ear lobe is everted.*

DRUGS

Drugs are a rare cause of salivary gland swelling, but chlorhexidine and methyldopa are occasionally implicated.

FURTHER READING

Batsakis J. G. (1988). Sialadenosis. *Ann. Otol. Rhinol. Laryngol.* **97**: 94–95.

Eveson J. W., Cawson R. A. (1985). Tumours of the minor (oropharyngeal) salivary glands: a demographic study of 336 cases. *J. oral Pathol.*, **14**: 500–509.

Eveson J. W., Cawson R. A. (1985). Salivary gland tumours: a review of 2410 cases with particular reference to histological types, site, age and sex distribution. *J. Path.*, **146**: 51–58.

Ferguson M. M., MacDonald D. G. (1978). Persistent sialadenitis in an accessory parotid gland. *Oral Surg., oral Med., oral Path.*, **45**: 696–700.

Gates G. A. (1982). Malignant neoplasms of the minor salivary glands. *N. Engl. J. Med.*, **306**: 718–722.

Gorlin R. J., Goldman H. M. (1970). *Thoma's oral pathology*, Vol. 1, 6th edn. St Louis, Miss.: C. V. Mosby.

Owens O. T., Calcaterra T. C. (1982). Salivary gland tumours of the lip. *Arch. Otolaryngol.*, **108**: 45–47.

Chapter
25   *Dry mouth (xerostomia)*

The complaint of a dry mouth is not uncommon but cannot always be objectively confirmed. There is a range of causes of a reduction in salivary flow (Fig. 25.1) but there is no doubt that *drugs are a common cause* (Table 25.1).

DRUGS

The drugs commonly implicated in causing a dry mouth are those with sympathomimetic or anticholinergic activity, especially tricyclic antidepressants and antihypertensive agents (Table 25.1). There is usually a fairly close temporal relationship between starting treatment with certain drugs and experiencing a dry mouth. Some patients report a dry mouth following an increase in dose

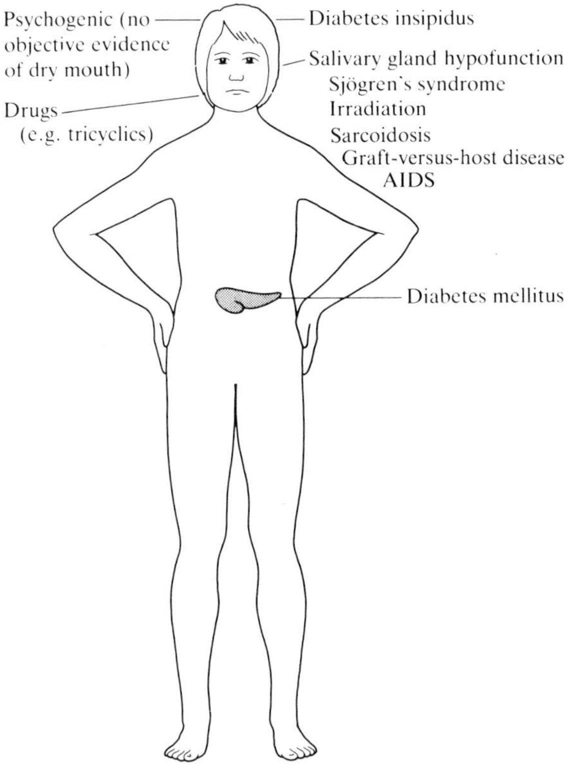

Psychogenic (no objective evidence of dry mouth)

Drugs (e.g. tricyclics)

Diabetes insipidus

Salivary gland hypofunction
Sjögren's syndrome
Irradiation
Sarcoidosis
Graft-versus-host disease
AIDS

Diabetes mellitus

Fig. 25.1 *Causes of a dry mouth.*

Table 25.1
Causes of dry mouth

Drugs with anticholinergic effects
  Atropine and analogues
  Tricyclic antidepressants
  Antihistamines
  Antiemetics
  Major tranquillizers
  Some antihypertensives
  Lithium

Drugs with sympathomimetic actions
  Ephedrine
  Decongestants
  Bronchodilators
  Amphetamines and other appetite suppressants

Dehydration
  Diabetes mellitus
  Diarrhoea and vomiting
  Severe haemorrhage

Psychogenic
  Anxiety states
  Depression
  Hypochondriasis

Organic disease of glands
  Sjögren's syndrome
  Irradiation damage or Cytotoxic drugs
  Mumps and other infections (temporary)
  Sarcoidosis
  Graft-versus-host disease
  AIDS

of a drug they have been taking for some time. However, the cause for which the drug is being taken may also be important. For example, patients with anxiety states or depressive conditions may complain of a dry mouth even in the absence of drug therapy or evidence of reduced salivary secretion.

IRRADIATION

Patients who have received head and neck irradiation for neoplastic conditions often develop a dry mouth (see Chapter 15). Fortunately, the more recent cone techniques of radiotherapy restrict unwanted irradiation of salivary tissue to one side alone and this preserves contralateral salivary function.

Patients who have received radiotherapy to the salivary glands and mouth have a dry oral mucosa and show signs of prolonged reduced salivary flow such as mucosal atrophy. Mucositis is also an early feature (Chapter 15, and Volume 1).

SJÖGREN'S SYNDROME

Sjögren's syndrome is a chronic multi-system inflammatory disease which appears to be the result of lymphocyte-mediated destruction of salivary, lacrimal and other exocrine glands (Fig. 25.2). The most common type of Sjögren's syndrome comprises dry eyes and dry mouth and a connective tissue or autoimmune disease, usually rheumatoid arthritis or primary biliary cirrhosis. The same clinical features in the absence of a systemic disease are frequently termed sicca syndrome (Fig. 25.3). Sicca syndrome is often now referred to as primary Sjögren's syndrome (SS–1), while if a connective tissue or other autoimmune disease is present, the term secondary Sjögren's syndrome (SS–2) is used. The general term of Sjögren's syndrome is often used to encompass both types, but the secondary type is by far the most common.

The two subgroups, though they have much in common, have several clinical, genetic and immunological differences (Table 25.2), but the important differences are that sicca (primary Sjögren's) syndrome is characterized by more severe ocular and oral manifestations and is more likely to be complicated by lymphoproliferative disease.

The term Sjögren's syndrome is used for both subtypes in the discussion below.

Sjögren's syndrome predominantly affects middle-aged and elderly women. Rheumatoid arthritis is by far the most common connective tissue disease associated

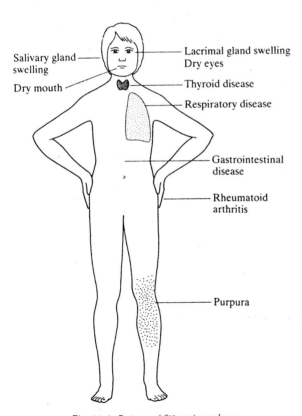

Fig. 25.2 *Features of Sjögren's syndrome.*

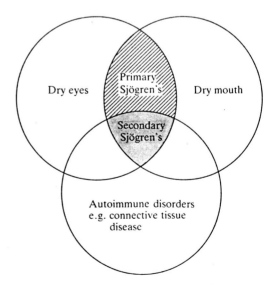

Fig. 25.3 *Components of Sjögren's syndrome.*

Table 25.2
Sjögren's syndrome: comparison of subtypes

Feature	Primary	Secondary
Connective tissue disease	−	+
Oral involvement	More severe	Less common
Recurrent sialadenitis	More common	Less common
Eye involvement	More common	Less common
Lymphoma	More common	Less common

Table 25.3
Sjögren's syndrome: some associated disorders

Rheumatoid arthritis
Systemic lupus erythematosus
Systemic sclerosis
Mixed connective tissue disease
Primary biliary cirrhosis

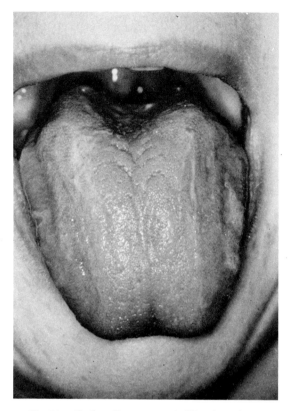

Fig. 25.4 *Frothy saliva on tongue in Sjögren's syndrome.*

with it, but many other autoimmune diseases may be associated (Table 25.3) and primary biliary cirrhosis is the most common in some studies.

Clinical features

Oral complaints are frequently the presenting features of Sjögren's syndrome and include:

(a) xerostomia;
(b) unpleasant taste or loss of sense of taste (Chapter 29);
(c) difficulty eating dry foods such as biscuits (the 'cracker sign');
(d) soreness of the mouth;
(e) difficulties in controlling dentures;
(f) the salivary glands may swell at some time in up to 30% of patients;
(g) difficulties in speech and swallowing.

Oddly, some patients with apparent total absence of saliva may not complain of any discomfort at all.

Clinically, the mouth may appear dry and, on examination, there may be lack of the usual pooling of saliva in the floor of the mouth, and thin lines of frothy saliva may form along lines of contact of the oral soft tissues (Fig. 25.4). In advanced cases, the mucosa is obviously dry and glazed.

The dryness of the mouth may be recognized by the 'clicking' quality of the speech as the tongue tends to stick to the palate. The mucosa also tends to stick to a dental mirror.

The tongue typically also develops a characteristic lobulated, usually red, surface with partial or complete depapillation (Fig. 25.5).

Soreness and redness of the oral mucosa are usually the result of candidosis, which is commonly associated with angular stomatitis and often with denture-induced stomatitis.

In dentate patients, dental caries (Fig. 25.6) tends to be severe and difficult to control.

Ascending (suppurative) sialadenitis is a hazard: Sjögren's syndrome is now the most common underlying cause in ambulant patients with acute bacterial sialadenitis (Chapters 24 and 26). However, the major salivary glands often swell in Sjögren's syndrome in the absence of bacterial infection (Fig. 25.7).

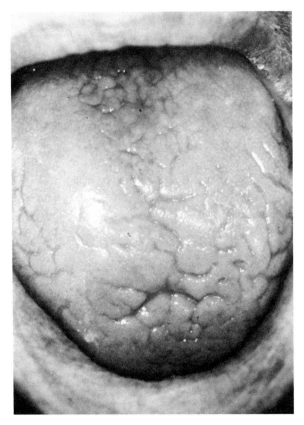

Fig. 25.5 *Dryness, depapillation and lobulation of tongue in Sjögren's syndrome.*

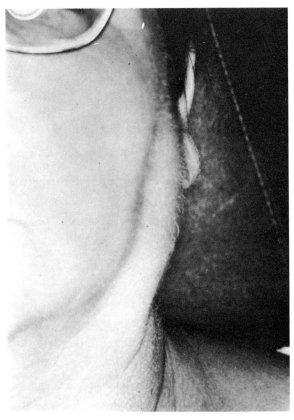

Fig. 25.7 *Swollen parotid salivary gland in Sjögren's syndrome.*

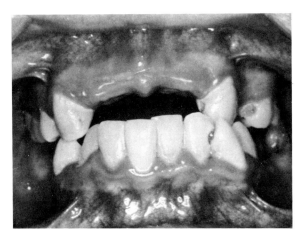

Fig. 25.6 *Caries and loss of teeth as a consequence in Sjögren's syndrome.*

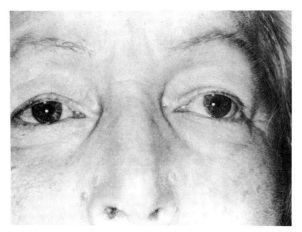

Fig. 25.8 *Dry, red eyes in Sjögren's syndrome.*

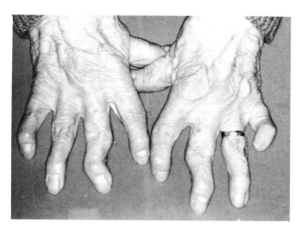

Fig. 25.9 *Rheumatoid arthritis in Sjögren's syndrome.*

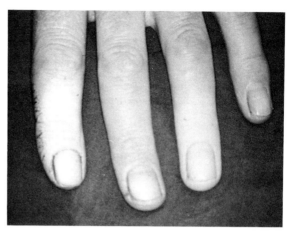

Fig. 25.11 *Raynaud's phenomenon: blanching of the digits due to intense vasoconstriction precipitated by the cold. This is a feature of several disorders, including connective tissue diseases.*

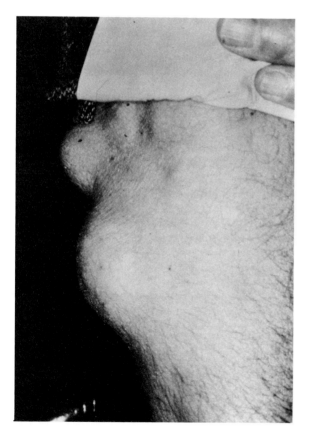

Fig. 25.10 *Rheumatoid nodules at the elbow in Sjögren's syndrome.*

Ocular complaints include sensations of grittiness, soreness or dryness of the eyes. The eyes may be red, with infection of the conjunctivae and soft crusts at the canthi (keratoconjunctivitis sicca: Fig. 25.8). Ophthalmological examination is essential.

In those with secondary Sjögren's syndrome, rheumatoid arthritis or other connective tissue disease is typically longstanding and should be clinically obvious (Figs. 25.9, 25.10). Rheumatoid arthritis may present with small-joint polyarthralgia and typical ulnar deviation and deformities of the fingers. Raynaud's phenomenon is common (Fig. 25.11; see also Chapter 22).

The connective tissue disease in secondary Sjögren's syndrome usually precedes the onset of dry eyes and dry mouth and, therefore, patients presenting with dry eyes and dry mouth alone probably have primary Sjögren's syndrome, unless a connective tissue disease manifests within about 1 year.

Sjögren's syndrome is a generalized disorder that may involve many exocrine and non-exocrine tissues (see Fig. 25.2).

Aetiology and pathogenesis

The lesion in Sjögren's syndrome is an immunologically mediated inflammatory exocrinopathy which starts with periductal infiltration of the salivary tissue by lymphocytes and plasma cells (Fig. 25.12). The infiltrate is initially mainly of B but later mainly of T lymphocytes.

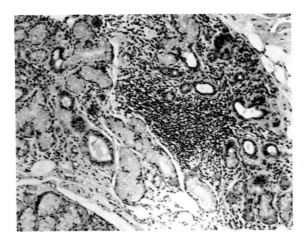

Fig. 25.12 *Glandular acinar atrophy and focal lymphocytic infiltrate in Sjögren's syndrome.*

One theory is that Sjögren's syndrome is caused by a deficiency of suppressor T lymphocytes and subsequent overactivity of B lymphocytes and the production of autoantibodies.

The glandular acini atrophy and progressively disappear, and are ultimately replaced by a dense infiltrate of lymphocytes. The salivary ductal epithelium, however, tends to persist and proliferates sometimes to the extent that the duct lumens may become obliterated, producing islets of epithelium known as epimyoepithelial islands. The fully developed lesion of Sjögren's syndrome in major glands therefore appears as a dense mass of lymphocytes interspersed with islands of epithelium, a pattern termed the benign lymphoepithelial lesion. Occasionally the benign lymphoepithelial lesion is present in the absence of serological and other features of Sjögren's syndrome.

Sjögren's syndrome is characterized also by various serological features, especially several autoantibodies—particularly antinuclear factor and rheumatoid factor and, consequently, a polyclonal hyperglobulinaemia. Antinuclear antibodies known as the SS-A (Ro) and SS-B (La) antibodies are found especially in primary Sjögren's syndrome, may have diagnostic value in patients with unexplained parotid swelling, and may antedate clinical evidence of Sjögren's syndrome by months or years.

Salivary duct autoantibodies are another characteristic finding, but in sicca syndrome (where oral symptoms are typically more severe) salivary duct autoantibodies are less frequently found than in secondary Sjögren's syndrome, suggesting that these antibodies may be unrelated to the duct damage.

Lymphoproliferative malignancy in Sjögren's syndrome

Although mild enlargement of salivary glands is not uncommon in Sjögren's syndrome, it is occasionally massive and associated with enlargement of the regional lymph nodes, a condition called pseudolymphoma. The B cell lymphoproliferation may actually be malignant, with a true lymphoma in up to 6% of cases in some series, though experience in the UK suggests a lower rate.

Diagnosis of Sjögren's syndrome

The diagnosis of Sjögren's syndrome is mainly on the history and clinical examination.

Examination of the eyes is most important and a routine autoantibody profile (rheumatoid and antinuclear factors, and anti-SS-A and anti-SS-B antibodies); haematological investigation to exclude anaemia; and erythrocyte sedimentation rate (ESR) or plasma viscosity (usually raised) are indicated. Biopsy and salivary studies may be indicated (see below).

A rinse or swab from the oral mucosa should be taken to confirm the presence of candidosis if there is soreness and signs of inflammation. Examination of any pus is also, of course, essential as a guide to antimicrobial treatment if ascending sialadenitis develops (Chapters 24 and 26).

OTHER CAUSES OF XEROSTOMIA

The importance of other causes of xerostomia has in the past been overemphasized. Dehydration with a reduction in extracellular volume will lead to xerostomia, but only if severe, and such patients require hospitalization or are already hospitalized. Systemic conditions which have polyuria as a feature, such as diabetes mellitus, may produce xerostomia, especially in poorly controlled diabetics. Sarcoidosis is discussed in Chapter 26. Graft-versus-host disease and AIDS may also produce xerostomia (Volume 1). *Obstruction or removal of a major salivary gland does **not** cause xerostomia.*

DIAGNOSIS OF XEROSTOMIA

Salivary function studies (Table 25.4, and Volume 1).

Salivary flow rates (sialometry)

When there is no gross xerostomia, salivary flow rate estimation is a sensitive indicator of salivary gland function. It is most satisfactorily carried out using a Lashley or

Table 25.4
Sjögren's syndrome: salivary studies

Investigation	Comments	Findings typical of Sjögren's syndrome
Salivary flow rate (sialometry)	Non-invasive, simple and cheap; sensitive but non-specific	Reduced
Labial salivary gland biopsy	Relatively simple; specific	Focal lymphocytic infiltrate
Scintiscanning (scintigraphy)	Non-invasive but expensive; exposure to radionuclide; little advantage over the above investigations	Reduced uptake of $^{99}Tc^m$ (technetium)
Sialography	Relatively simple and non-invasive but non-specific and may cause glandular damage or infection occasionally	Sialectasis
Sialochemistry	Results thus far offer little, if any, practical advantage over other investigations	β_2 microglobulin increased

Carlsson–Crittenden suction cup (Fig. 25.13) to obtain parotid saliva after stimulation with a few drops of lemon juice or 1 ml of 10% citric acid on the tongue. The reason for measuring parotid flow is that the parotids make the major contribution to the total salivary flow, are responsible for stimulated flow, and are the most consistently affected glands in Sjögren's syndrome. Moreover, there is no simple and reliable method of measuring mixed (total) salivary flow rates. Stimulated parotid flow rates in symptomatic primary and secondary Sjögren's syndrome are usually below 0.5–1.0 ml/min (normal 1–2 ml/min).

Sialometry has the advantage of simplicity and of being non-invasive but is relatively crude and does not distinguish between various causes of xerostomia.

Sialochemistry

In practical terms, sialochemistry (studies of constituents of saliva) is currently of very limited value in diagnosis or management, mainly because of its lack of specificity.

Sialography

If the salivary flow rate is equivocal, sialography can be used to detect duct damage. Normal sialograms are described and shown in Volume 1. Radiopaque dye is introduced into the salivary duct. The most consistent

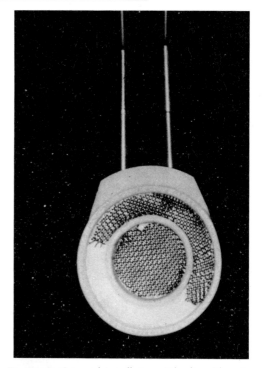

Fig. 25.13 *Cup used to collect parotid saliva. The outer chamber is a suction ring to hold the cup to the mucosa around Stensen's duct. Saliva is collected from the inner cup—which overlies the duct.*

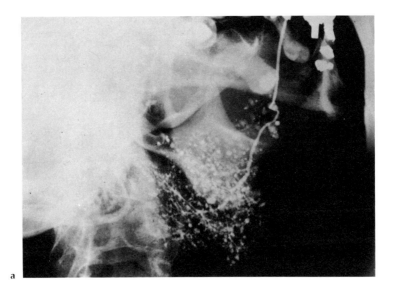

a

b

Fig. 25.14 Sialograms in Sjögren's syndrome showing sialectasis.

finding in Sjögren's syndrome is that of dye extravasation (sialectasis), which typically produces a snowstorm appearance as a result of leakage of contrast medium through the damaged ducts (Fig. 25.14). Sialectasis is described as punctate, globular or cavitary and is non-specific.

Atrophy (reduction in the size of the ductal tree) may also be seen.

Salivary scintiscanning

Salivary scintiscanning with technetium pertechnetate correlates both with salivary flow rate and labial gland changes (see below) and offers the additional advantage that all major salivary glands are examined non-invasively, simultaneously and, if necessary, continously (Fig. 25.15). However, it is expensive and there is a small radiation hazard from the use of radionuclides.

Salivary biopsy

Biopsy of a parotid gland has attendant hazards of damage to the facial nerve, the production of a salivary fistula, and facial scarring. For these reasons, biopsy of minor salivary glands is usually chosen since this is a relatively simple technique with few complications (Volume 1). The glands selected are the labial glands in the lower labial mucosa since they are easily biopsied through a simple incision (Fig. 25.16) and the changes effect those in the major glands.

Typical findings include (see Fig. 25.12):

(a) focal lymphocytic infiltrate—the most significant;
(b) acinar loss;
(c) duct dilatation;
(d) periductal fibrosis.

The advantages and disadvantages of, and typical results of, salivary studies in Sjögren's syndrome are summarized in Table 25.4.

MANAGEMENT OF PATIENTS WITH SEVERE XEROSTOMIA

Control of infections

Candidosis

Oral candidosis is almost invariable in severe xerostomia, and antifungals are indicated. Angular stomatitis is common and, since it is often associated with staphylococci and streptococci as well as *Candida albicans*, miconazole is the preferred treatment. The dentures should be left out of the mouth at night and stored in sodium hypochlorite solution or chlorhexidine. An antifungal such as miconazole gel or amphotericin or nystatin ointment should be spread on the denture before re-insertion and a topical antifungal preparation such as nystatin or amphotericin suspension or lozenges used four times daily. Denture hygiene is crucial to success (Volume 3).

Oral hygiene should be improved and the use of an 0.2% aqueous chlorhexidine mouthwash helps control candidosis and periodontal disease.

Bacterial sialadenitis

Acute sialadenitis needs treating with a penicillinase-resistant antibiotic such as flucloxacillin (Chapters 24 and 26).

Dental caries

Oral hygiene measures alone are inadequate to prevent caries. Dietary control of sucrose intake, and the use of fluorides, are essential to control dental caries in patients with severe xerostomia. The daily use of 1% sodium

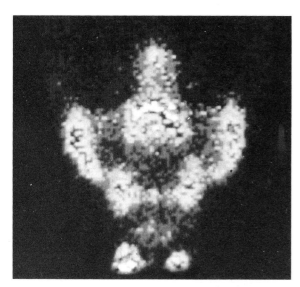

Fig. 25.15 *Salivary scan showing all major salivary glands, radionuclide centrally in the mouth and nose and both lobes of the thyroid.*

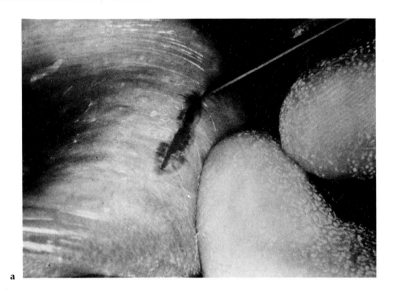

a

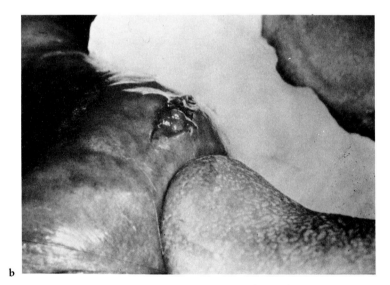

b

Fig. 25.16 *Labial gland biopsy. (a) Incision can be as shown, or at 90°.*
(b) Glands appear and at least 4 are excised. (c) Simple black silk suture closure.

fluoride gels or 0.4% stannous fluoride gels has been efficient in controlling xerostomia-associated caries (Volume
3).

Periodontal disease

Oral hygiene procedures and the use of 0.2% aqueous

chlorhexidine mouthwashes are essential to control periodontal disease (Volume 3).

Treatment of xerostomia

Items to avoid

Any drugs that may produce xerostomia (for example tri-

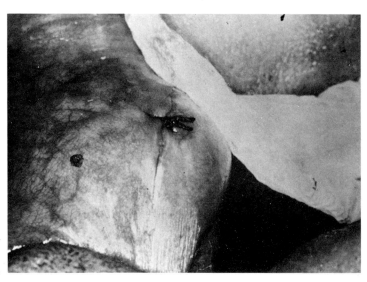

Fig. 25.16 c

cyclic antidepressants) clearly should not be prescribed for patients with a dry mouth. Alternative medication with less anticholinergic effect (such as trazolone) should be prescribed, if antidepressants are indicated.

Dry foods such as biscuits are best avoided, and alcohol and smoking should be reduced since they may worsen xerostomia.

Symptomatic treatment

Cholinergic drugs that stimulate salivation (sialogogues), such as pilocarpine, unfortunately may cause other cholinergic effects such as lacrimation and bradycardia. The anticholinesterase pyridostigmine is of greater benefit since it is longer acting and associated with fewer adverse effects. Salivation may be stimulated by using chewing gums (containing sorbitol, not sucrose) or sucking diabetic confectionery. Anetholetrithione increases cholinergic receptors in salivary glands and appears to produce clinical benefit.

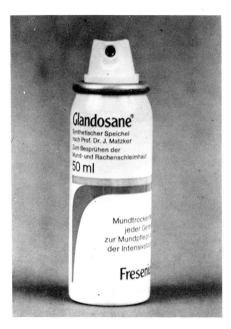

Fig. 25.17 One available saliva substitute.

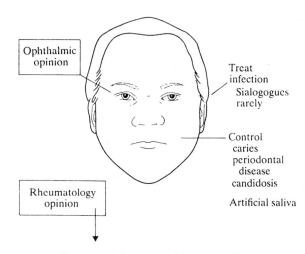

Fig. 25.18 Management of Sjögren's syndrome.

Some patients benefit from frequent small sips of water and this may be as useful as many of the other agents that have been evaluated. Salivary replacement using methylcellulose, mucin, polyethylene oxide or lemon and glycerin can be of significant help. Various sprays are available (Fig. 25.17).

Consultation with other disciplines (Fig. 25.18).

FURTHER READING

Glass B. J. *et al.* (1984). Xerostomia: diagnosis and treatment planning consideration. *Oral Surg.,* **58**: 248–252.

Manthorpe R. *et al.* (1981). Sjögren's syndrome: a review with emphasis on immunological features. *Allergy,* **36**: 139–153.

Navazesh M., Ship I. I. (1983). Xerostomia: diagnosis and treatment. *Am. J. Otolaryngol.,* **4**: 283–292.

NIH Conference (1980). Sjögren's syndrome (sicca syndrome): current issues. *Ann. int. Med.* (part 1), **92**: 212–226.

Scully C. (1986). Sjögren's syndrome: review of immunopathogenesis, clinical and laboratory features and management in relation to dentistry. *Oral Surg.,* **62**: 510–523.

Scully C. (1989). Oral parameters in the diagnosis of Sjögren's syndrome *Clin. Exp. Rheumatol.* (in press).

Strand V., Talal N. (1980). Advances in the diagnosis and concept of Sjögren's syndrome (autoimmune exocrinopathy). *Bull. Rheum. Dis.,* **30**: 1046–1052.

Miscellaneous salivary complaints

SALIVARY GLAND PAIN

Duct obstruction

Salivary gland pain due to obstruction of a duct of a major gland is usually a dull pain which can last hours (Chapter 24). Typically, pain is encountered at mealtimes but lesser degrees of obstruction produce pain during a meal. Some patients obtain relief from pain by massaging the affected gland or applying local heat.

Such a history should elicit a search for a local cause by examination, radiography and sialography. If, after removal of the cause, salivary flow from the affected gland does not return to normal, there is probably damage from longstanding disease (Fig. 26.1).

Sialadenitis

Sialadenitis is usually due to mumps or to bacterial infection, which have been described earlier (Chapter 24). Clear saliva is produced in mumps, whereas in bacterial

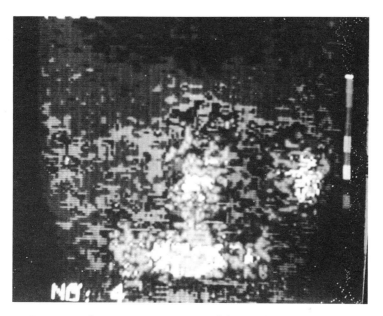

Fig. 26.1 *Technetium scan in a patient with longstanding parotitis showing complete loss of function in one parotid gland.*

infection frank pus is usually evident or there is no secretion. Pain is more constant than in duct obstruction and may be accompanied by obvious gland tenderness, fever and lymphadenopathy. Most viral sialadenitis is self-limiting, but bacterial sialadenitis may be chronic. Investigations such as sialography are contraindicated in acute viral or bacterial infections.

Neoplasms

Small neoplasms may produce unilateral pain. The pain of such lesions is constant and unrelated to mealtimes and, even with large salivary tumours, gland function can be remarkably well preserved. Neoplasms may be detected clinically or on sialography, CT-sialography or scinti-scanning (Chapter 24).

Drugs

Certain drugs, particularly chemotherapeutic agents such as vinca alkaloids, can occasionally produce salivary gland pain (Table 26.1).

Sarcoidosis (see also Chapter 31)

Sarcoidosis is a poorly understood disorder, characterized by widespread non-caseating granulomas (Fig. 26.2). Only a minority of patients with sarcoidosis have salivary gland involvement, but this is one of the few causes of unilateral or bilateral persistent salivary gland pain and may present with parotid swelling (Fig. 26.3) or xerostomia. If associated with fever and uveitis, the condition is termed uveoparotid fever, or Heerfordt's syndrome. Sublingual glands may also enlarge in sarcoidosis (Fig. 26.4).

The cause of the salivary gland pain in sarcoidosis is unclear, but it may be that granulomatous deposits in the duct wall produce a chronic obstruction. Granulomas within the gland themselves may also contribute to the pain. Salivary gland function in these patients is normal or reduced.

Granulomas may be present in minor salivary glands of patients with sarcoidosis, even when there are no

Table 26.1
Drugs which may produce salivary gland pain

Antihypertensives, e.g. methyldopa, guanethidine

Cytotoxic drugs, e.g. vincristine

Centrally acting antihypertensives, e.g. clonidine

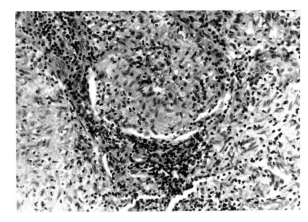

Fig. 26.2 *Sarcoidosis: non-caseating granuloma.*

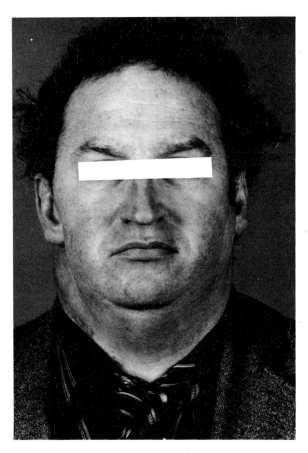

Fig. 26.3 *Bilateral painful parotid gland enlargement in a patient with sarcoidosis.*

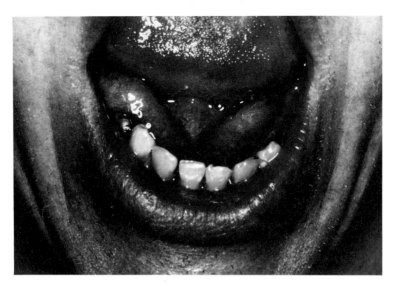

Fig. 26.4 *Bilateral sublingual gland enlargement in a patient with sarcoidosis.*

obvious oral clinical manifestations of sarcoidosis. Oral minor gland biopsy can, therefore, sometimes help diagnosis of sarcoidosis.

Psychogenic

Some patients may have a psychogenic basis for salivary pain. In some the pain has no physical basis, whilst in others it is self-induced. Deliberate cheek-biting may lead to oedema of the parotid duct and produce symptoms from duct obstruction (Fig. 26.5).

Even more bizarre are patients who have learnt to introduce air into their parotid glands in order, for example, to fail a medical examination such as enrolment into the

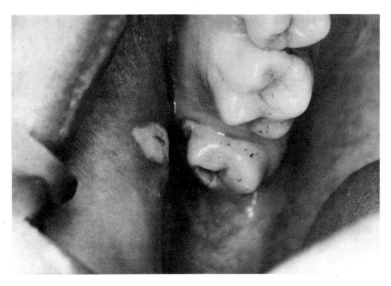

Fig. 26.5 *Chronic biting of the parotid papilla has produced oedema of the papilla and prevented the outflow of saliva.*

armed forces. Such a situation has only been described in the parotid and is known as pneumoparotid. This can also be an occupational hazard in glass-blowers.

SIALORRHOEA (PTYALISM)

The complaint of excess salivation is much less common than that of xerostomia (Fig. 26.6). In some cases it is not due to excess saliva production but to an inability to swallow saliva as a result of muscular inco-ordination, pharyngeal obstruction, or reduced swallowing rate. Typically, drooling is seen in these cases and the under-lying condition is often a neurological or muscular dis-order such as Parkinson's disease. myasthenia gravis, cerebral palsy, bulbar palsy, or mental retardation. Extremely rare causes are rabies and mercury poisoning.

Sialorrhoea is common in infants, especially when 'teething', and is common at any age where there are oral ulcers or when foreign bodies such as new dentures have been introduced into the mouth. Drugs such as anticholin-esterases, sympathomimetics, buprenorphine, meptazinol, and cocaine are rare causes.

In other patients the complaint of sialorrhoea seems to have no physical basis but reflects an underlying psycho-logical problem. Antidepressant therapy may help the underlying condition and perhaps also pharmacologically reduces salivary flow.

In other severe cases, atropinics, though theoretically useful, are of less practical value because of side-effects, and therefore surgical operations have been devised, for example to reroute the submandibular gland duct. How-ever, these do not have widespread application.

SALIVARY FISTULA

Salivary fistula is an abnormal communication between the gland or ducts and skin or mucous membrane. In-ternal fistulae are uncommon and asymptomatic. Trauma to the major glands may (rarely) cause a persistent fistula

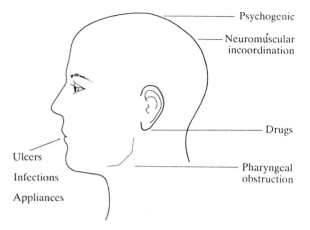

Fig. 26.6 *Causes of sialorrhoea.*

that is unpleasant and may lead to infection. Surgical re-pair is then indicated.

NECROTIZING SIALOMETAPLASIA

This is a benign inflammatory condition that affects pre-dominantly adult Caucasian males in the 4th–5th decade. It presents as a rapidly developing, large ulcer at the junc-tion of the hard and soft palate. This clinically and histo-logically resembles carcinoma but heals spontaneously.

FREY'S SYNDROME

This is discussed in Chapter 30.

FURTHER READING

Galili D., Marmary Y. (1986). Juvenile recurrent parotitis: clinicoradiologic follow-up study and the beneficial effect of saliva. *Oral Surg.*, **61**: 550–556.

Rabinov K., Weber A. L. (1985). *Radiology of the salivary glands.* Boston: G. K. Hall.

Section IV
Facial Pain and Neurological Disease with Orofacial Manifestations

Chapter
27   *Orofacial pain and headache*

The next four chapters discuss briefly the anatomy and disorders of the cranial nerves, with emphasis on those of particular concern to the dental surgeon, and relevant complaints such as pain, facial palsy and disturbances of taste sensation.

The dental surgeon should be able to recognize abnormalities involving particularly the trigeminal, facial, glossopharyngeal, vagal and hypoglossal nerves (Table 27.1). For example, patients with maxillofacial or head injuries may have brain damage with impaired eye movements or pupil reactions and loss of sense of smell (anosmia); and patients with orofacial pain often seek treatment from the dental surgeon. Knowledge of neurological disease, particularly in relation to the cranial nerves, therefore is essential to the dental surgeon.

Pain, paralysis, paraesthesia ('pins and needles' and other abnormal sensations—*not* sensory loss), and loss of sensation (hypaesthesia and anaesthesia) are the main manifestations of neurological disease. Loss of the special senses such as of smell, sight and taste are extremely handicapping.

OROFACIAL PAIN

Pain in the teeth, mouth or face is the main reason why many patients consult their dental surgeon. Mostly there is a local cause for the pain—usually the sequelae of dental caries (Fig. 27.1). However, a wide range of diseases apart from local disorders can cause orofacial pain, particularly neurological, vascular and psychogenic disorders (Fig. 27.2). Pain and pain control are discussed in Volume 1.

Nerve fibres concerned with perception of orofacial pain arise from pain receptors and pass in the trigeminal nerve via the brainstem sensory nuclear complex and via trigemino–reticulo–thalamic pathways to higher centres—especially the thalamus (Fig. 27.3; see also Volume 1).

Free nerve endings are found in most orofacial tissues. Three classes of nociceptive afferents are recognized.

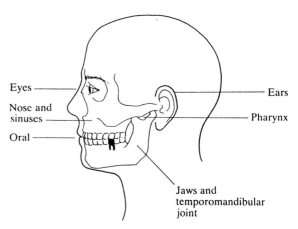

Fig. 27.1 *Local causes of orofacial pain.*

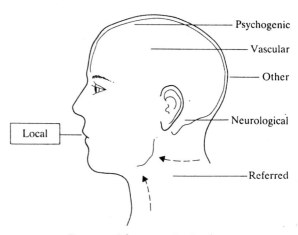

Fig. 27.2 *Other causes of orofacial pain.*

Table 27.1
Cranial nerve functions

Nerve	Modality carried
I. Olfactory	Sense of smell
II. Optic	Sense of sight
III. Oculomotor	(a) Motor nerve to extraocular muscles (except superior oblique and lateral rectus) and to levator palpebrae superioris (b) carries parasympathetic supply
IV. Trochlear	Motor nerve to superior oblique muscle
V. Trigeminal	(a) Motor nerve to muscles of mastication, tensor palati and tensor tympani (b) Sensory to oral cavity, face, orbital and nasal cavities and paranasal sinuses (c) Carries parasympathetic supply (d) Carries sense of taste
VI. Abducens	Motor nerve to lateral rectus
VII. Facial	(a) Motor nerve to muscles of facial expression, platysma, stylohyoid, stapedius and posterior belly of digastric (b) Sense of taste (anterior 2/3 tongue and palate) (c) Carries parasympathetic supply to lacrimal, nasal and palatal mucous, and submandibular and sublingual glands
VIII. Vestibulocochlear	Senses of hearing and balance
IX. Glossopharyngeal	(a) Motor nerve to stylopharyngeus (b) Sensory to back of tongue, tonsil, upper pharynx, middle ear mastoid air cells and Eustachian tube (c) Sense of taste (posterior 1/3 tongue) (d) Carries parasympathetic supply to parotid
X. Vagus	(a) Motor nerve to smooth muscle of respiratory system, gastrointestinal tract to colon, and to cardiac muscle (b) Sensory to tympanic membrane, lower pharynx and larynx (c) Carries parasympathetic supply to respiratory, cardiac and gastrointestinal systems
XI. Accessory	Motor nerve to sternomastoid, trapezius, muscles of soft palate including palatoglossus (except tensor palati), pharynx and larynx
XII. Hypoglossal	Motor nerve to muscles of tongue (except palatoglossus)

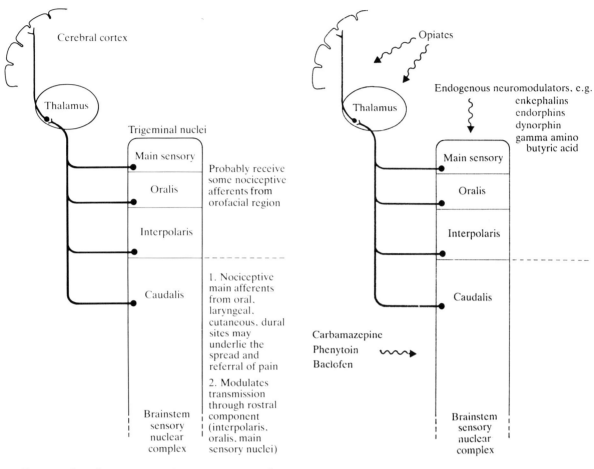

Fig. 27.3 *Central transmission of pain from orofacial region.*

Fig. 27.4 *Modulation of central transmission of orofacial pain.*

1. A-delta mechanothermal afferents (modulate mechanical and thermal stimuli).

2. C polymodal (modulate mechanical, thermal and chemical stimuli).

3. High-threshold mechanothermal afferents.

Impulses are relayed from the thalamus predominantly to: (a) the cerebral cortex, where the nature and site of the pain are perceived, memory is stored, and emotional responses are initiated; and (b) the hypothalamus, which is involved in the autonomic responses to pain.

Patients vary widely in their tolerance of, and response to, pain. Psychogenic and other factors, including drugs, modulate this response (Fig. 27.4; see also Volume 1).

TRIGEMINAL NERVE

The trigeminal nerve supplies sensation to most of the scalp, face and mouth (Fig. 27.5). The two roots of the trigeminal nerve emerge at the pons and enter Meckel's cave at the tip of the petrous temporal bone and the foramen lacerum, where the ganglion (Gasserian ganglion) of the sensory root lies. Motor fibres run only with the mandibular division.

Ophthalmic division

The ophthalmic division runs through the cavernous sinus close to the IIIrd, IVth and VIth cranial nerves and

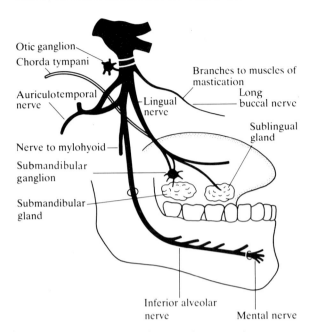

Otic ganglion
Chorda tympani
Auriculotemporal nerve
Branches to muscles of mastication
Lingual nerve
Long buccal nerve
Sublingual gland
Nerve to mylohyoid
Submandibular ganglion
Submandibular gland
Inferior alveolar nerve
Mental nerve

Fig. 27.5 *Mandibular division of the trigeminal nerve.*

the internal carotid artery. It then divides into the lacrimal, frontal and nasociliary branches which enter the orbital cavity through the superior ophthalmic (orbital) fissure between the lesser and greater wings of the sphenoid bone.

The lacrimal branch is joined by secretomotor parasympathetic fibres from the zygomatic branch of the maxillary division of the trigeminal and supplies the lacrimal gland and the skin and conjunctiva of the lateral sides of the eyelids. The frontal branch divides into a supraorbital and supratrochlear branch.The former leaves the orbital cavity through the supra-orbital notch or foramen, supplies the tissues of the forehead and scalp, and gives a branch to the frontal sinus. The supratrochlear branch leaves the orbital cavity at its medial angle to supply the upper eyelid and forehead above the root of the nose. The nasociliary branch supplies the mucous membrane of the sphenoidal and ethmoidal air sinuses. The larger anterior ethmoidal branch supplies the mucous membrane of the roof of the nasal cavity and small areas of the lateral and medial walls of the nasal cavity. A branch leaves the nasal cavity between the bony nasal margin and the alar cartilage to supply an area of skin over the lower half of the nose, and another supplies skin and conjunctiva at the medial angle of the eye, the lacrimal sac, the upper part of the nasolacrimal duct, and the skin over the upper half of the nose.

Maxillary division

The maxillary division of the trigeminal nerve runs for a short distance in the base of the cavernous sinus, giving off a meningeal branch to the dura mater of the middle cranial fossa. It leaves the middle cranial fossa through the foramen rotundum in the great wing of the sphenoid bone to enter the pterygopalatine fossa which it crosses to leave through the inferior opthalmic fissure as the infra-orbital nerve.

The branches of the maxillary division in the pterygopalatine fossa are as follows.

1. Posterior superior alveolar nerve (to the upper molars and part of the maxillary antrum).
2. Palatine nerves (to the palate).
3. Nasal nerves (sphenopalatine nerves).
4. Pharyngeal nerves (to the mucous membrane of the upper pharynx).
5. Zygomatic nerve, which enters the orbit by the inferior ophthalmic fissure and divides into a posterior (temporal) branch which enters the front of the temporal fossa behind the orbital cavity and then pierces the temporal fascia at the anterior margin of the temporal muscle to supply the skin between the eye and the ear. The other anterior (facial) branch appears through foramina on the facial surface of the zygomatic bone and supplies the overlying area of the skin. Parasympathetic fibres derived from the pterygopalatine ganglion run with the zygomatic nerve and join the lacrimal nerve as secretomotor fibres to the lacrimal gland.

The branches of the infra-orbital nerve are the middle and anterior superior dental nerves to the maxillary antrum, upper incisor, canine and premolar teeth and buccal gingiva, and three terminal branches, the labial, nasal and palpebral nerves, which supply the upper lip, cheek and lower eyelid.

Mandibular division (Fig. 27.5)

The mandibular division of the trigeminal nerve contains sensory and motor fibres. It leaves the middle cranial fossa through the foramen ovale in the greater wing of the sphenoid bone to give off branches to the tensor palati and tensor tympani muscles, the otic ganglion, the medial pterygoid muscle, and a recurrent sensory branch (nervus spinosus) which passes through the foramen spinosum to supply dura mater in the middle cranial fossa. The mandibular division lies on the outer surface of the tensor palati muscle with the otic ganglion between the nerve trunk and the muscle. Behind it lies the middle meningeal artery and laterally is the upper head of the lateral pterygoid muscle. The auditory (Eustachian) tube lies close to the nerve trunk as it emerges from the foramen ovale.

The mandibular nerve trunk then divides into a larger posterior division, giving off the auriculotemporal, inferior alveolar and lingual branches, and a smaller anterior division, which provides motor supply to the temporal, lateral pterygoid and masseter muscles and continues on as the sensory buccal nerve (long buccal nerve).

Taste fibres from the anterior two-thirds of the tongue, and secretomotor parasympathetic fibres to the submandibular and sublingual salivary glands, pass with the lingual nerve for part of its distal course (Fig. 27.5).

LOCAL CAUSES OF OROFACIAL PAIN
(Table 27.2)

The receptor mechanism(s) for dental pain appear to be within the dentine and pulp. Nerve fibres in the pulp include pain-associated fibres as well as fibres of uncertain function. Some nerve fibres appear to enter dentinal tubules where they are seen especially in the pulpal third and above the pulp horns. It is unclear whether these nerves subserve dentine sensitivity. Present evidence suggests that there are two classes of receptor—one sensitive to movement of the contents of dentinal tubules (which can be induced by, for example, touch and osmotic stimuli) and the other sensitive to heat changes (Fig. 27.6).

Table 27.2
Differential diagnosis of oral pain

Source of pain	Character	Exacerbating factors	Ability to locate	Associated signs	Pain provoked by	Radiography
Dental						
Dentinal	Evoked, does not outlast stimulus	Hot/cold, sweet, sour	Poor	Caries, defective restorations, exposed dentine	Hot/cold, probing dentine	May show interproximal caries, defective restorations
Pulpal	Severe, intermittent, throbbing	Hot/cold, sometimes biting	Poor	Deep caries, extensive restoration	Hot/cold, caries probing, sometimes percussion	May show deep caries or deep restoration
Periodontal						
Periapical	For hours at same intensity; deep, boring	Biting	Good	Periapical swelling and redness, tooth mobility	Percussion, palpation of periapical area	Periapical views may show periapical changes
Lateral	For hours at same level; boring	Biting	Good	Periodontal swelling, deep pockets with pus exuding, tooth mobility	Percussion, palpation of periodontal area	Useful when x-rayed with probe inserted into pocket
Gingival	Pressing, annoying	Food impaction, tooth-brushing	Good	Acute gingival inflammation	Touch, percussion	N.A.
Mucosal	Burning, sharp	Sour, sharp and hot food	Good	Erosive or ulcerative lesions, redness	Palpation	N.A.

N.A. = not applicable.

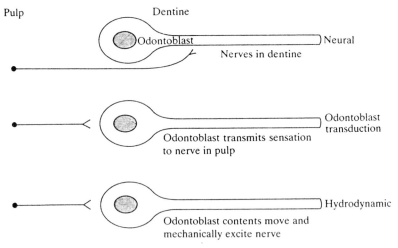

Fig. 27.6 *Hypotheses of dentine pain perception.*

Periodontal ligament nerves join the pulpal nerve fibres at the tooth apex, though some pass in the alveolar bone to join other nerves.

Dentinal pain

Pain originating in dentine is sharp and deep, usually evoked by an external stimulus and subsiding within a few seconds. Natural external stimuli are normally evoked by food and drinks which are hot, cold, sweet, sour and sometimes salty. Although extreme changes in temperature (e.g. hot soup followed by ice cream) may cause pain in intact, non-affected teeth, pain evoked by natural stimuli usually indicates a hyperalgesic state of the tooth. The pain may be poorly localized, often only to an approximate area within two to three teeth adjacent to the affected tooth. Frequently, the patient is unable to distinguish whether the pain originates from the lower or the upper jaw. Pain from affected posterior teeth is more difficult to localize than that from anterior teeth. However, patients rarely make localization errors across the midline.

Pulpal pain

Pain associated with pulp disease is spontaneous, strong, often throbbing and is exacerbated by temperature change and pressure on a carious lesion. When pulpal pain is evoked it outlasts the stimulus (unlike stimulus-induced dentinal pain) and can be excruciating for many minutes. Localization is poor, particularly when pain

becomes more intense, and the pain tends to radiate or refer to the ipsilateral ear, temple and cheek but does not cross the midline. Pain may be described by patients in different ways, and a continuous dull ache can periodically be exacerbated (by stimulation or spontaneously) for short (minutes) or long (hours) periods.

Pain may increase and throb when the patient lies down and in many instances wakes the patient from sleep. The pain of pulpitis is frequently discontinuous and abates spontaneously; the precise explanation for such abatement is not clear.

Periodontal pain

Pain originating in the periodontium is more readily localized than is pulpal pain; the affected teeth are often also tender to pressure.

Acute periapical periodontitis

Pain associated with acute periapical inflammation is spontaneous, and moderate to severe in intensity, for long periods of time (hours). Pain is exacerbated by biting on the tooth and, in more advanced cases, even by closing the mouth and bringing the affected tooth gently into contact with the opposing teeth. In these cases, the tooth feels 'high' (extruded) and is very sensitive to touch. Frequently there has been preceding pulpal pain. Periodontal pain, although of a more continuous nature, is usually better tolerated than the paroxysmal and excruciating pain of pulpitis; localization of periodontal pain is usually precise and the patient able to indicate the affected tooth. The improved ability to localize the source of pain may be attributed to the proprioceptive and mechanoreceptive sensibility of the periodontium that is lacking in the pulp. However, although localization of the affected tooth is often precise, in up to half the cases the pain is diffuse and radiates into the jaw on the affected side.

During examination the affected tooth is located readily by means of tooth percussion. The tooth is usually non-vital and the periapical buccal vestibular area often tender to palpation. In more severe cases there is swelling of the face, associated with cellulitis sometimes connected with fever and malaise. Usually, when the face swells, pain diminishes in intensity due to rupture of the pus through the periosteum of the bone around the affected tooth and the consequent decrease in pressure of the tooth apex (Volume 1).

Lateral periodontal abscess

The pain of a lateral periodontal abscess is similar to that of acute periapical periodontitis, well localized and with swelling and redness of the gingiva. However, the swelling is usually located more gingivally than in the case of the acute periapical lesion. The affected tooth is sensitive to percussion and is often mobile and slightly extruded, and there is a deep periodontal pocket. Probing the pocket may cause pus exudation and subsequent relief from pain. The tooth pulp is usually *vital* (Volume 3).

Food impaction

The patient complains of localized pain that develops between or in two adjacent teeth after meals, especially when food is fibrous (e.g. meat). The pain is associated with a feeling of pressure and discomfort, may gradually disappear until being evoked again at the next meal, or may be relieved immediately by removing the impacted food. Examination shows a faulty contact between two teeth and often food trapped between these teeth; the gingival papilla is tender to touch and bleeds easily. The adjacent teeth are usually sensitive to percussion. The cause of the faulty contact between the teeth is often caries or poor restorations.

Cracked tooth

Teeth can crack under trauma and can give rise to severe pain, which is worse on biting (Volume 3). The cause of pain is often difficult to ascertain.

Pericoronitis

Acute pericoronal infections are common, related to incompletely erupted teeth partially covered by flaps of gingival tissue (operculum), particularly lower third molars. Pain is spontaneous and may be exacerbated by closing the mouth. In more severe cases, pain is aggravated by swallowing, and there may be trismus.

Examination shows an operculum that is acutely inflamed, red and oedematous. Frequently, an opposing upper tooth indents or ulcerates the oedematous operculum. Occasionally, fever and malaise are associated. Pericoronitis is discussed in Volume 1.

Acute necrotizing gingivitis (Chapter 16)

Soreness and pain at the gingival margin are usually accompanied by profuse gingival bleeding in acute necrotizing gingivitis. In the early stages some patients may complain of a feeling of tightness around the teeth. Metallic taste is sometimes experienced and usually there is halitosis. Pain is fairly well localized to the affected areas. Fever and malaise are sometimes present. Examination shows necrosis and ulceration of the marginal gingiva with different degrees of gingival papillary destruction (see Volume 3, and Chapter 16).

Mucosal pain

Pain from the oral mucosa can be either localized or diffuse. Localized pain is usually associated with an erosion or ulcer. Diffuse pain may be associated with a widespread infection, mucosal atrophy or erosion, a systemic underlying deficiency disease or other factors, and is usually described as 'soreness' or sometimes 'burning' (see Chapter 14–17).

Mucosal pain may be aggravated mechanically or by sour, spicy, salty or hot foods.

Other local causes of orofacial pain

Jaws

Pain from the jaws can be caused by acute infection, malignancies and direct trauma. Lesions such as cysts, retained roots and impacted teeth are usually painless unless associated with infection or fracture of the jaw. Odontogenic and other benign tumours of the bone do not normally produce pain, but malignant tumours usually produce deep, boring pain, sometimes associated with paraesthesia or anaesthesia.

Radiation therapy may result in severe pain due to

infection and osteomyelitis associated with osteoradio-necrosis.

Temporomandibular joint (Chapter 9)

Pain from the temporomandibular joint is usually intensi-fied by movement of the mandible; the joint may be ten-der to palpation via the external auditory meatus. Pain may result from dysfunction, acute inflammation, trauma, primary or secondary malignant tumours. When acutely inflamed, the joint may also be swollen and warm to touch. A splinting protective mechanism by the mastica-tory muscles may result in muscle spasm, producing secondary pain and trismus (Chapter 9).

Salivary glands (Chapters 24 and 26)

Pain from salivary glands is localized to the affected gland, may be quite severe, and may be intensified by in-creased saliva production such as before and with meals. The salivary gland is swollen and sensitive to palpation. In acute parotitis, mouth-opening causes severe pain, and thus there is a degree of trismus. Salivary flow from the affected gland is usually reduced. Pain may be associated with fever and malaise. In children, the most common cause is mumps. In adults, pain from salivary glands re-sults usually from blockage of a salivary duct by calculus or mucus plug.

Sinuses and pharynx (Chapter 10)

Disease of the paranasal sinuses and nasopharynx can cause oral and/or facial pain. In acute sinusitis there has usually been a preceding cold followed by local pain and tenderness (but not swelling) and radio-opacity of the affected sinuses, sometimes with an obvious fluid level. With maxillary sinusitis, pain may be felt in related upper molars, which may be tender to percussion. The pain of ethmoidal or sphenoidal sinusitis is deep in the nose; that of frontal sinusitis causes an anterior headache with tenderness at the root of the nose. Pain in any type of acute sinusitis may be aggravated by change of position of the head.

Tumours of the sinuses or nasopharynx can also cause facial pain. These tumours are often carcinomas which infiltrate various branches of the trigeminal nerve and can remain undetected until too late. Nasopharyngeal carcin-oma often presents late, with facial pain, paraesthesia, ipsilateral deafness and/or cervical lymph node enlarge-ment (Trotter's syndrome: Chapter 15).

Pressure on mental nerve

Rarely, pain is caused by constriction of the mental fora-men in, for example, Paget's disease of bone. More common is pressure from a denture on the nerve which comes to lie on the crest of the ridge as the alveolar bone is resorbed in the edentulous mandible. Either the denture should be relieved from the area or, occasionally, it is necessary to resite the nerve surgically.

Styloid process (stylalgia)

Eagle's syndrome, a rare disorder due to an elongated styloid process, may cause pain on chewing, swallowing or turning the head.

Eyes

Pain from the eyes can arise from disorders of refraction, retrobulbar neuritis (for example in multiple sclerosis), or glaucoma (raised intra-ocular pressure), and can radiate to the orbit or frontal region.

Ears

Middle ear disease may cause headaches, Conversely, oral disease may cause pain referred to the ear, particu-larly from lesions of the posterior tongue.

Neck

Neck pain, usually from cervical vertebral disease, especially cervical spondylosis, very occasionally causes pain referred to the face.

NEUROLOGICAL CAUSES OF FACIAL PAIN

Sensory innervation of the mouth, face and scalp depends on the trigeminal nerve, so that involvement of this nerve can cause orofacial pain or indeed sensory loss—sometimes with serious implications.

Facial neuralgia caused by intracranial tumours or other lesions

Lesions affecting the trigeminal nerve from the trigeminal nuclei anywhere from the pons, through the posterior and middle cranial fossa, to the foramen ovale and rotun-dum, and to the superior orbital fissure can cause facial pain. The clinical features vary with the site and extent of the lesion. Commonly, there is facial pain associated with a facial sensory deficit and impaired corneal reflex on the affected side (the cornea is supplied by the trigeminal nerve). Anatomically closely related cranial nerves such as III, IV, VI and VII are frequently involved.

Severe facial pain suggestive of trigeminal neuralgia but with physical signs such as facial sensory or motor impairment can result from brainstem ischaemia or infarction in cerebrovascular disease, demyelinating disorders such as multiple sclerosis, infections such as AIDS, or neoplasms.

Lesions in the posterior cranial fossa, such as cerebello-pontine angle tumours (acoustic neuroma or meningioma), can cause facial pain associated with an absent corneal reflex (Vth nerve); deafness, tinnitus and vertigo (from involvement of the VIIIth nerve); facial palsy (VIIth nerve); ataxia, intention tremor and nystagmus (due to cerebellar involvement); and spasticity of the leg (pyramidal tract involvement).

Middle cranial fossa lesions can involve the Vth with the VIth nerves (when there is also a lateral rectus palsy). Carotid aneurysms, especially those in the cavernous sinus, or cavernous sinus thrombosis, may cause facial pain with lesions of the IIIrd, IVth and VIth nerves.

Facial neuralgia caused by extracranial tumours or other lesions

Any lesion affecting the trigeminal nerve, whether it be traumatic, inflammatory or neoplastic (for example a nasopharyngeal or antral carcinoma), may cause pain. These are discussed in Chapters 10 and 15.

Idiopathic trigeminal neuralgia (benign paroxysmal trigeminal neuralgia; tic douloureux)

This is the most common neurological cause of facial pain, with the following characteristics.

1. Electric shock-like, brief, stabbing (lancinating) orofacial pains.
2. Pain-free intervals between attacks.
3. Unilateral pain.
4. Pain of abrupt onset and abrupt termination.
5. Pain restricted to the trigeminal nerve distribution.
6. Triggering of pain from the oral or perioral region on the ipsilateral side in some patients.
7. *No sensory loss in the trigeminal region nor other neurological abnormalities.*

Idiopathic trigeminal neuralgia is slightly more common in women (55% of patients); most are in the 50–70-year age group. The pain usually involves the mandibular and, rarely, the other divisions of the trigeminal nerve. Pain is unilateral, though, in a very small percentage (about 3%), pain may after some years move to the other side of the face.

The trigger site bears no necessary relation to the painful area and may not be in the area of distribution of the affected trigeminal nerve division, but is always ipsilateral to the pain. Patients do not necessarily recognize the trigger for what it is, and may find that pain is brought on by chewing, talking, swallowing, smiling or exposure to temperature change—usually cold air.

Tic douloureux is often an intermittent disease with apparent remissions for months or years. However, recurrence is common and very often the pain spreads to involve a wider area over time and the intervals between episodes tend to shorten. Some patients never have remissions. Emotional or physical stress usually increases the frequency and severity of attacks.

Neurological assessment is needed because similar pain may be secondary to multiple sclerosis, to posterior cerebral fossa lesions (particularly tumours), to neurosyphilis, AIDS or to other lesions. Patients with idiopathic trigeminal neuralgia show no abnormal neurological signs.

The cause of trigeminal neuralgia is unclear, but it may be due to a vascular malformation pressing on the roots of the trigeminal nerve.

Management of trigeminal neuralgia

It *must* be established that no abnormal neurological signs are present before drug treatment is started.

Carbamazepine (Tegretol) is the main treatment for trigeminal neuralgia. It is *not* an analgesic and, if given when an attack starts, will not relieve the pain; it must be given continuously prophylactically for long periods. The dose should be increased until symptoms are controlled unless side-effects become excessive. Most patients respond to 200–400 mg three times daily. Side-effects of carbamazepine include hypertension, ataxia, drowsiness and rashes, or rarely leucopenia, pancytopenia or facial dyskinesia. The blood pressure and blood picture should therefore be monitored and electrolytes checked from time to time. If carbamazepine fails, phenytoin is occasionally useful, but surgery may be required.

Local analgesic injections (for example using bupivicaine: Volume 1) will temporarily block the pain. Local cryosurgery to the trigeminal nerve branches involved (cryoanalgesia) can produce analgesia without permanent anaesthesia, but the benefit may only be temporary (Volume 1). Destruction of the trigeminal ganglion (radiofrequency ganglionolysis) or surgical decompression of the trigeminal nerve may be required in intractable cases but, with destructive surgical techniques, anaesthesia is exchanged for the pain and can cause such problems as anaesthesia of, and risk of damage to, the face and cornea and occasionally continuous pain (anaesthesia dolorosa).

Glossopharyngeal neuralgia

Glossopharyngeal neuralgia is *much* less common than trigeminal neuralgia. The pain is of a similar nature but affects the throat and ear, and typically is triggered by swallowing or coughing. Carbamazepine is usually less effective than for trigeminal neuralgia and adequate relief of pain can be difficult.

Occasionally glossopharyngeal neuralgia is secondary to lesions (often tumours) in the posterior cranial fossa or jugular foramen (jugular foramen syndrome) and there are then often lesions of the vagus (X) and accessory (XI) nerves.

Herpetic and post-herpetic neuralgia

Herpes zoster (shingles) is often preceded and accompanied by neuralgia (Chapter 16). Neuralgia may also persist after the rash has resolved. Post-herpetic neuralgia causes continuous burning pain that affects mainly elderly patients and may be so intolerable that suicide can become a risk. Facial pain occasionally follows zoster of the trigeminal nerve.

Treatment is difficult but antidepressants or chlorpromazine may possibly help if analgesics are not effective. Spontaneous improvement may follow, however, after about 18 months in some patients.

Raeder's paratrigeminal neuralgia

Severe persistent pain in and around the eye with an associated Horner's syndrome (Chapter 28) is often caused by a lesion at the base of the skull and requires neurological attention.

VASCULAR CAUSES OF OROFACIAL PAIN

Several disorders in which the most obvious organic feature is vascular dilatation or constriction cause facial pain. The pain is usually obviously in the face rather than in the mouth but occasionally can involve both, and can be difficult to differentiate from other causes or orofacial pain (Table 27.3).

Migraine

Migraine is a recurrent headache affecting women especially, but that which is described as 'migraine' by some patients often proves to be tension headache. The number, frequency, intensity and duration of migraine attacks vary widely and they tend to diminish in frequency and intensity with increasing age. Spontaneous remissions are not uncommon.

Migraine appears to be related to arterial dilatation. Attacks may be precipitated by alcohol, various foods such as ripe bananas or chocolate, or the contraceptive pill. Stress also seems to be a precipitating factor.

Classic migraine has the following features.

1. Preceding warning symptoms (an aura).
2. Headache which is severe, usually unilateral (hemicranial) and lasts for hours or days.
3. Photophobia, nausea or vomiting.

The aura may last about 15 minutes and consists of visual, sensory, motor or speech disturbances. Visual phenomena are often of zig-zag coloured lights (fortification spectra) or transient visual defects. Sensory phenomena include paraesthesia or anaesthesia—usually of the contralateral upper limb, or face and mouth. The headache often becomes throbbing and generalized and may be associated with facial pallor.

Migraine is usually managed by avoidance of precipitating factors and with drugs. If attacks are frequent, prophylaxis with clonidine is the treatment of choice, but sometimes pizotifen, ergotamine or methysergide are used.

In acute attacks aspirin or paracetamol may give some relief and patients usually prefer to lie in a quiet, dark room. Ergotamine given early may abort an attack.

Migrainous neuralgia (cluster headache)

Migrainous neuralgia is less common than migraine. Males are mainly affected and attacks often begin about middle age (Table 27.4). The pain is unilateral, occurs in attacks, is burning and 'boring' in character, and localized around the eye usually. It may spread to the upper teeth and very occasionally to the lower teeth. Generally, the attacks last less than 1 hour, commence and often termin-

Table 27.3
Differential diagnosis of orofacial pain

	Dental	Periodontal	Mucosal	Salivary glands	Neuralgic	Vascular	TMJ pain dysfunction	Psychogenic
Site	Mouth, ear, jaws, cheek	Tooth	Mucosa	Area of gland	Nerve distribution	Orbit or upper face	Temple, ear, jaws, teeth	Diffuse, deep, sometimes across midline
Localization	Poor, diffuse, radiating, does not cross midline	Good	Usually good	Usually good	Good	Usually good	Poor, but usually unilateral	Poor
Duration	Seconds to days	Hours to days	Hours to days	Hours to days	Seconds	Minutes to hours	Weeks to years	Weeks to years
Character of pain	Intermittent, sharp, paroxysmal	Steady, boring	Burning or sharp	Drawing, pulling	Lancinating, paroxysmal	Throbbing, deep	Dull, continuous	Dull, boring, continuous
Precipitating factors	Hot and cold	Chewing	Sour and spicy foods	Eating	Touch, wind	Alcohol	Yawning, chewing	Stress, fatigue
Associated signs	Caries, exposed dentine	Abscess	Erosions or ulcers	Salivary gland swelling	None usually	Lacrimation, injected eye, nasal discharge	Click in TMJ, trismus	None
Aetiological factors	Caries, trauma, gingival recession	Acute periodontitis	Varied	Saliva retention, infection	Idiopathic, multiple sclerosis	Vasomotor	Stress, parafunction	Depression
Treatment	Cracked tooth restoration, endodontics	Endodontics or extraction	According to cause	Drainage, antibiotics	Carbamazepine, nerve block, cryoanalgesia, neurosurgery	Clonidine, methysergide, or lithium carbonate	Antidepressants Other treatments	Antidepressants

Table 27.4
Differentiation of important types of facial pain

	Idiopathic trigeminal neuralgia	Atypical facial pain	Migraine	Migrainous neuralgia
Age (years)	50	30–50	Any	30–50
Sex	F > M	F > M	F > M	M > F
Site	Unilateral, mandible or maxilla	± Bilateral, maxilla	Any	Retro-orbital
Associated features	–	± Depression	± Photophobia ± Nausea ± Vomiting	± Conjunctival injection ± lacrimation ± nasal congestion
Character	Lancinating	Dull	Throbbing	Boring
Duration of episode	Brief (seconds)	Continual	Hours (usually day)	Few hours (usually night)
Precipitating factors	Trigger areas	None	± Foods	± Alcohol
Relieving factors	Carbamazepine	Antidepressants	Clonidine; ergot derivatives	Clonidine; ergot derivatives

ate suddenly, and often awaken the patient at night or in the early hours of the morning (2–3 a.m.).

This pain is associated on the affected side with profuse watering and 'congestion' of the conjunctiva, rhinorrhoea and nasal obstruction. During and after the attacks, marked tenderness is frequently found when pressing over the external carotid arteries.

Attacks are sometimes precipitated by alcohol. Migrainous neuralgia is managed with ergotamine, pizotifen or methysergide prophylactically. Sometimes corticosteroids or lithium carbonate are needed.

Cranial arteritis (temporal arteritis; giant-cell arteritis)

Cranial arteritis is a febrile, often self-limiting disease which affects the aged of both sexes. It is characterized by painful inflammation of the superficial temporal and other cranial arteries, malaise, weakness, weight loss, anorexia, fever, sweating and a raised erythrocyte sedimentation rate (or plasma viscosity).

The headache is intense, deep and aching, throbbing in nature and persistent. It is frequently made worse when the patient lies flat in bed and it may be exacerbated or reduced by digital pressure on the artery involved. Occasionally the artery may be enlarged, distended and extremely tender. Some patients suffer pain on mastication

or in the tongue. The symptoms may involve any of the divisions of the external carotid artery.

Up to one-half of patients with cranial arteritis are threatened with loss of vision, and urgent treatment with systemic corticosteroids (prednisolone) is indicated.

In cranial arteritis, biopsy shows the arterial elastic tissues to be fragmented, with giant cells numerous in the region of the deranged internal elastic lamina. There may be anticapillary antibodies in the serum, as well as deposits containing IgG localized to the arterial wall.

OTHER ORGANIC CAUSES OF HEADACHE AND FACIAL PAIN

Raised intracranial pressure

One of the most serious but also the least common cause of headache is raised intracranial pressure. This may be due to malignant hypertension, a tumour, abscess or haematoma. When no specific cause can be found it is termed benign intracranial hypertension.

The headache is severe, worse on waking and decreases during the day. It is aggravated by straining, coughing, sneezing or lying down. Nausea and vomiting are common. Neurological attention is essential.

Meningeal irritation

Severe headache with nausea, vomiting, neck pain or stiffness (with inability to touch the knees with the chin) or pain on raising the straightened legs (Kernig's sign) implies meningeal irritation. Urgent neurological attention is needed since it may indicate meningitis or subarachnoid haemorrhage.

Diseases of the skull

Headache is occasionally the presenting feature of bone metastases or Paget's disease (Chapters 7 and 8).

Medical diseases

Headache can be a feature in a range of diseases including fevers, hypertension, chronic obstructive airways disease and some endocrinopathies. Facial pain may occasionally be drug induced, for example by phenothiazines.

Headache can also be caused by exertion—even that associated with sexual intercourse (orgasmic headache). Rarely, the latter may lead to subarachnoid haemorrhage!

Chronic post-traumatic headache

Most people who have had head injuries have local pain or tenderness at the site of impact for a few hours or even for a few days, after which many become symptom free. However, up to one-half of all persons who injure their heads sufficiently to warrant hospitalization develop chronic post-traumatic headaches.

A small number of patients have pain due to bleeding in the epidural, subdural or subarachnoid spaces, which is potentially lethal and needs urgent neurological attention. The headache of subdural haematoma begins at the time of trauma or the regaining of consciousness and persists, often for weeks or months, until the haematoma is removed. Blood in the subarachnoid space may induce headache, as may adhesions after head injury involving pain-sensitive structures in the arachnoid.

However, most patients with post-traumatic headaches that persist or recur for long periods after head injury have no identifiable intracranial abnormalities to explain their pain and some of these have a 'compensation neurosis'—a psychogenic type of pain which appears in some persons awaiting financial compensation after an accident.

PSYCHOGENIC CAUSES OF OROFACIAL PAIN

The mouth and para-oral soft tissues have among the richest sensory innervation in the body. Furthermore, a large part of the sensory homunculus on the cerebral cortex receives information from orofacial structures. In addition, the muscles of emotional expression are mainly in and around the face and mouth. From the time of infancy, the mouth is concerned intimately with the psychological development of the individual, and disorders of structures such as the lips, teeth and oral mucosa can hold enormous emotional significance. Even *in utero* the fetus may place the thumb in the mouth.

It is hardly surprising, therefore, that there are a range of psychogenic types of orofacial pain, and that, in some studies, nearly 40% of the population have reported frequent headache and facial pain.

Four main groups of patient appear to suffer from psychogenic pain.

1. Normal individuals under extreme stress.
2. Those with a personality trait such as hypochondriasis.
3. Neurotic, often depressed persons.
4. Psychotic patients.

Tension headache

Tension headaches are very common, especially in young adults. The pain, which is caused by anxiety or stress-induced muscle tension, affects the frontal, occipital or temporal muscles, and is felt as a constant ache or band-like pressure. The pain is often worse by the evening, but does not waken the patient.

Reassurance may be effective, but the pain may be helped by benzodiazepines such as diazepam, as this is both anxiolytic and a mild muscle relaxant.

Atypical oral and facial pain

This is an ill-defined entity which includes the following.

1. Atypical facial pain (or 'neuralgia').
2. Burning or sore mouth (oral dysaesthesia).
3. Temporomandibular pain–dysfunction syndrome (facial arthromyalgia).
4. Atypical odontalgia.
5. The syndrome of oral complaints.

The following features are common to all types of atypical oral and facial pain.

1. Patients are often middle-aged or older.
2. Many are female.
3. Constant chronic discomfort or pain, often of a dull boring or burning type.
4. The location of the pain is ill-defined, may cross the midline to involve the other side, or may move to another site.
5. The symptoms do not waken the patient from sleep.
6. There is a total lack of objective signs.
7. All investigations are negative.
8. There are often recent adverse life-events, such as bereavement or family illness.
9. There are often multiple oral and/or other psychogenic related complaints, such as headaches, chronic back pains, irritable bowel syndrome or dysmenorrhoea.
10. Cure is uncommon in most, yet few seem to try or persist in using analgesics.

Atypical facial pain

Atypical facial pain is relatively common. It usually affects middle-aged women who complain of a dull, continuous ache, usually in the upper jaw, yet sleep and appetite are only rarely disturbed and analgesics rarely tried. Attempts at relieving pain by restorative treatment, endodontia or exodontia are usually unsuccessful.

Over 50% of such patients are depressed or hypochondriacal, and some have lost or been separated from parents in childhood. Many lack insight and will persist in blaming organic diseases (or the dentist!) for their pain. Some 70% respond to prothiaden, compared with a 50% response to placebo, and those who will respond invariably do so early in treatment. However, many refuse psychiatric help or medication.

Burning mouth (glossopyrosis; glossodynia; oral dysaesthesia)

Burning mouth 'syndrome' most frequently affects middle-aged and elderly females. Although the tongue is most frequently involved, the patient may also complain of burning lips, gums or palate. It is usually bilateral and often relieved by eating and drinking, in contrast to the pain associated with inflammatory lesions which is made worse by food.

Oral examination shows no abnormalities. Causalgia should be excluded (see below). Laboratory screening for anaemia, diabetes, a deficiency state or candidosis should be undertaken, but anxiety, depression or a cancero-

Table 27.5
Causes of burning mouth

Local causes	Candidosis
	Erythema migrans (geographical tongue)
	Lichen planus
Systemic causes	Psychogenic
	Cancerophobia
	Depression
	Anxiety states
	Hypochondriasis
	Deficiency states
	Vitamin B_{12} deficiency
	Folate deficiency
	Iron deficiency
	Diabetes
	Drugs (e.g. Captopril)

phobia is frequently the underlying cause (Table 27.5). Reassurance and occasionally psychiatric care are indicated.

Temporomandibular pain–dysfunction syndrome (myofacial pain–dysfunction; facial arthromyalgia)

This is discussed in Chapter 9.

Atypical odontalgia

This presents with pain and hypersensitive teeth in the absence of detectable pathology. The pain is typically indistinguishable from pulpitis or periodontitis but is aggravated by dental intervention. Probably a variant of atypical facial pain, it should be treated similarly.

The syndrome of oral complaints

Multiple pains and other complaints may occur simultaneously or sequentially, and relief is rarely found (or admitted). Patients may bring diaries of their symptoms to emphasize their problem (Fig. 27.7). This has been termed the 'malady of small bits of paper', and though there is not always a psychogenic basis, such notes characterize patients with non-organic complaints. An anecdotal example is a 35-year-old woman who sequentially 'developed' right submandibular gland pain, right glossopharyngeal neuralgia (her words!), left glossopharyngeal neuralgia, and left submandibular pain over a period of 15 years, during which time she appeared not to develop signs of neurological disease or to deteriorate physically. Occasional patients quite deliberately induce painful oral lesions (Fig. 27.8).

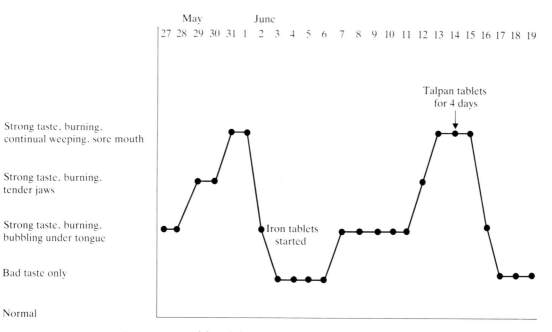

Fig. 27.7 *A graph brought by a patient who had multiple oral complaints.*

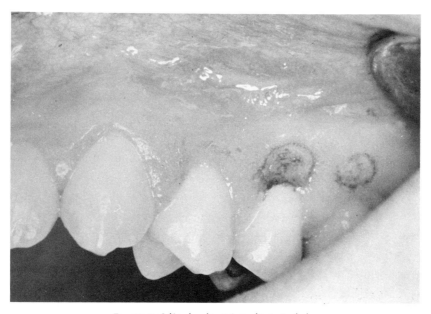

Fig. 27.8 *Self-induced (artefactual) gingival ulcers.*

REFERRED CAUSES OF OROFACIAL PAIN

Pain may occasionally be referred to the face or jaws from the neck (see above), lungs, or from the heart in patients with angina. The latter pain usually affects the mandible, is initiated by exercise (especially in the cold) and abates quickly on rest.

OTHER TYPES OF OROFACIAL PAIN

Causalgia

Causalgia is a persistent burning pain, often in the mandible, that follows surgery or trauma. The cause is unclear and there is no good evidence that it is related to a peripheral nerve lesion or to psychogenic causes.

If a local analgesic injection temporarily relieves causalgia, then cryoanalgesia may effect more permanent relief, but neurosurgery may be required.

Frey's syndrome (auriculotemporal syndrome)

This is a paroxysmal burning pain, usually in the temporal area or in front of the ear, associated with flushing and sweating on eating (see Chapter 30).

BRUXISM AND CLENCHING OF TEETH (PARAFUNCTIONAL HABITS)

Bruxism is the habit of grinding the teeth, and may occur during the day or night. Causes include occlusal factors, psychological stress, choreoathetosis (involuntary movements), some types of drug and mental handicap.

Bruxism and clenching habits may be of no consequence, but many produce attrition; may cause discomfort because of transient traumatic periodontitis; may contribute to periodontal damage; and may be associated with psychogenic oral disorders such as oral dysaesthesia and temporomandibular pain–dysfunction syndrome. Masseteric hypertrophy is an uncommon consequence.

Management is dealt with elsewhere (Volumes 3 and 4) but involves attention to the occlusion, possibly occlusal guards, and anxiolytic or antidepressant treatment.

FURTHER READING

Brooke R. I. (1980). Atypical odontalgia: a report of twenty two cases. *Oral Surg.*, **49**: 196–199.

Lazar M. L. (1980). Current treatment of tic douloureux. *Oral Surg.*, **50**: 504–508.

Lazar M. L., Greenlee R. G., Naarden A. L. (1980). Facial pain of neurologic origin mimicking oral pathologic conditions: some current concepts and treatment. *JADA*, **100**: 884–888.

Mitchell R. G. (1980). Pre-trigeminal neuralgia. *Br. dent. J.*, **149**: 167–170.

Mumford J. M. (1973). *Toothache and related pain.* Edinburgh: Churchill Livingstone.

Scully C. (1982). The mouth in general practice. 3. Oral and facial pain. *Dermatol. Practice*, **1**: 16–18.

Scully C., Cawson R. A. (1986). Oral medicine. *Med. Int.*, **28**: 1129–1151.

Sessle B. J. *et al.* (1988). Facial pain. *J. Canad. Dent. Assoc.*, **12**: 896–922.

Chapter
28 *Disorders of orofacial movement*

Movements of the facial muscles are controlled by the facial nerve. Lesions of this nerve (lower motor neurone lesions) or its central connections (upper neurone lesions), or muscle disease, can lead to facial weakness.

The facial (VIIth) cranial nerve is attached to the brainstem at the upper end of the medulla by a motor and a sensory root which cross the subarachnoid space above the vestibulocochlear nerve (VIIIth cranial) and enter the internal auditory meatus where they unite and enter the facial canal, winding through the petrous temporal bone between the semicircular canals of the inner ear behind, and the cochlea in front, to reach the medial wall of the middle ear. Here the facial nerve takes a sharp turn backward (the genu) and runs along the wall of the middle ear cavity.

At the genu is the sensory nucleus (geniculate ganglion), from where a branch containing secretomotor parasympathetic fibres, the greater superficial petrosal nerve, joins the internal carotid or deep petrosal nerve (sympathetic fibres from the superior cervical ganglion) to form the nerve of the pterygoid canal (Vidian nerve). In the pterygopalatine fossa this nerve joins the pterygopalatine (sphenopalatine) parasympathetic ganglion. In its course through the tympanic plexus, to which the glossopharyngeal nerve also contributes, the facial nerve gives off the chorda tympani branch which enters the middle ear cavity, crosses the tympanic membrane and leaves through the squamotympanic fissure to join the lingual nerve. The chorda tympani nerve contains taste fibres (sensory) from the anterior two-thirds of the tongue, and secretomotor parasympathetic fibres destined for the submandibular ganglion—which supplies submandibular and sublingual salivary glands.

The facial nerve passes through the middle ear to the stylomastoid canal to exit at the stylomastoid foramen, where it gives off motor branches to:

(a) the posterior auricular and occipitalis muscles;

(b) the posterior belly of the digastric muscle;
(c) the stylohyoid muscle.

The facial nerve then pierces the fascial sheath of the parotid gland and divides into an upper branch, giving rise to temporal, zygomatic and upper buccal branches, and a lower branch, giving rise to lower buccal, mandibular and cervical branches. The temporal branch supplies the anterior and superior auricular, frontalis, upper part of orbicularis oculi and corrugator supercilii muscles. The zygomatic branch supplies the orbicularis oculi. The buccal branches supply the buccinator muscle, muscles of the upper lip, risorius and muscles of the nose. The mandibular branch supplies the lower lip and mentalis muscles. The cervical branch supplies the platysma and may send a branch to join the mandibular branch. The facial nerve thus supplies the muscles of facial expression.

FACIAL PALSY

The common causes of facial paralysis are cerebrovascular accidents or strokes (upper motor neurone lesions) and Bell's palsy (lower motor neurone lesion) (Fig. 28.1). Occasionally, a temporary facial palsy follows the administration of an inferior alveolar local analgesic if the solution tracks through the parotid gland to reach the facial nerve. Other causes are shown in Table 28.1 and Figure 28.1, and features that differentiate upper motor neurone lesions from lower motor neurone lesions are outlined in Table 28.2.

The facial nerve neurones supplying the lower face receive upper motor neurones only from the contralateral motor cortex, whereas the neurones to the upper face receive bilateral upper motor neurone (UMN) innervation. Upper motor neurone facial palsy, therefore, is characterized by unilateral facial palsy, with some sparing of the frontalis and orbicularis oculi muscles because of the

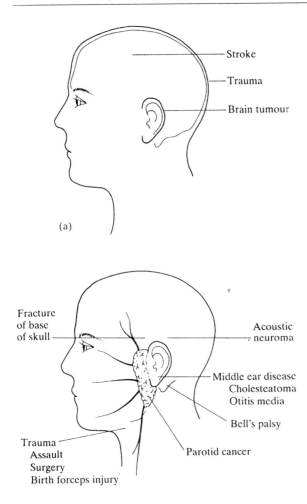

(a)

(b)

Fig. 28.1 *(a) Upper motor neurone lesions, (b) lower motor neurone lesions of the VIIth nerve causing facial palsy.*

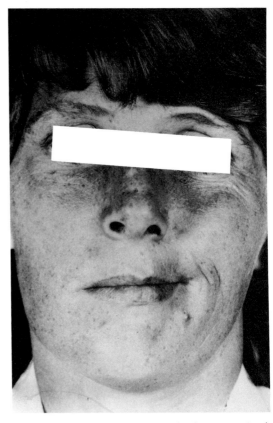

Fig. 28.2 *Lower motor neurone facial palsy, causing facial weakness on the right side of the patient.*

bilateral cortical representation. Furthermore, although voluntary movements are impaired, extrapyramidal influences can still act, and the face may still move with emotional responses, for example, on laughing. There may also be a paresis of the ipsilateral arm (monoparesis) or arm and leg (hemiparesis), or some aphasia, because of more extensive cerebrocortical damage.

In contrast, lower motor neurone (LMN) facial palsy is characterized by total unilateral paralysis of all muscles of facial expression, both for voluntary and emotional responses, but no hemiparesis.

In facial palsy, the forehead is unfurrowed and the patient unable to close the eye on that side. Upon attempted closure, the eye rolls upward (Bell's sign). Tears tend to overflow on to the cheek (epiphora). The corner of the mouth droops and the nasolabial fold is obliterated. Saliva may dribble from the commissure. Food collects in the vestibule on the affected side and plaque accumulates on the teeth. Depending on the site of the lesion, other features such as loss of taste may be associated (Table 28.1).

Diagnosis

Facial weakness is demonstrated by asking the patient to close the eyes against resistance, to raise the eyebrows, or to raise the lips to show the teeth or to try to whistle (Fig. 28.2). The following diagnostic tests are also necessary.

Table 28.1

Localization of site of lesion in and causes of unilateral facial palsy

Muscles paralysed	Lacrimation	Hyperacusis	Sense of taste	Other features	Probable site of lesion	Type of lesion responsible
Lower face	N	—	N	Emotional movement retained ± monoparesis or hemiparesis ± aphasia	Upper motor neurone (UMN)	Stroke (cerebrovascular accident) Brain tumour Trauma HIV infection
All facial muscles	↓	+	↓	± VIth nerve damage	Lower motor neurone (LMN) Facial nucleus	Multiple sclerosis Syphilis
All facial muscles	↓	+	↓	± VIIIth nerve damage	Between nucleus and geniculate ganglion	Fractured base of skull Posterior cranial fossa tumours Sarcoidosis
All facial muscles	N	±	N or ↓	—	Between geniculate ganglion and stylomastoid canal	Otitis media Cholesteatoma Mastoiditis
All facial muscles	N	—	N	—	In stylomastoid canal or extracranially	Bell's palsy Trauma Local analgesia (e.g. misplaced inferior dental block) Parotid malignant neoplasm Guillain–Barré syndrome
Isolated facial muscles	N	—	N	—	Branch of facial nerve extracranially	Trauma Local analgesia

N = normal;   + = present;   ↓ = reduced.

Table 28.2

Differentiation of upper (UMN) from lower motor neurone (LMN) lesions of the facial nerve

	UMN lesions	LMN lesions
Emotional movements of face	Retained	Lost
Blink reflex	Retained	Lost
Ability to wrinkle forehead	Retained	Lost
Drooling from commissure	Uncommon	Common
Lacrimation, taste or hearing	Unaffected	May be affected

1. A full neurological examination is required, looking particularly for V, VI and VII nerve signs, hemiparesis etc.

2. Test for hearing loss and look for discharge from the ear and other signs of middle ear disease.

3. Blood pressure should be measured and urinalysis performed to exclude diabetes and, in some areas Lyme disease should be excluded (tick-borne infection with Borrelia burgdorferi).

Bell's palsy

The common lower motor neurone lesion is Bell's palsy, caused by inflammation in the stylomastoid canal which may be immunologically mediated and associated with herpes simplex or another virus. The onset of paralysis is acute over a few hours, although pain in the region of the ear or in the jaw may precede the palsy by a day or two. There is usually facial palsy alone but, occasionally, heightened sense of hearing (hyperacusis) due to paralysis of the stapedius muscle that normally controls the stapes and dampens movements of the ossicles of the middle ear or loss of taste is noted.

Most patients recover within a few weeks, but the after-effects in others can be so severe and distressing that all patients should be treated with corticosteroids. The eye should be protected with a pad, since the corneal reflex is impaired and corneal damage may occur.

In chronic cases, where there is no recovery after months or years, surgical decompression of the nerve in the stylomastoid canal may be attempted or it may be necessary to use a splint or fascial graft to prevent drooping at the commissure, or other manoeuvres such as facial–hypoglossal nerve anastomosis in an attempt to overcome the cosmetic deformity.

Although most patients with Bell's palsy are otherwise healthy, there are occasional associations with diabetes mellitus, hypertension and lymphoma.

Ramsay–Hunt syndrome

Severe facial palsy with vesicles in the ipsilateral pharynx and external auditory canal (Ramsay–Hunt syndrome) may be due to herpes zoster affecting the geniculate ganglion of the VIIth nerve (Fig. 28.2).

Bilateral facial palsy

Bilateral facial palsy is rare, but may be seen in acute idiopathic polyneuritis (Guillain–Barré syndrome), sarcoidosis (Heerfordt's syndrome, uveoparotid fever), arachnoiditis (inflammation of the pia-arachnoid), and posterior cranial fossa tumours.

Other causes of facial weakness

An apparent facial palsy may be caused by myasthenia gravis, some myopathies or facial hemiatrophy. Other causes of palsy are shown in Table 28.1.

ABNORMAL FACIAL MOVEMENTS

Facial dyskinesias

Facial dyskinesias are abnormal movements of the tongue, facial or jaw muscles. They are usually associated with extrapyramidal disease such as athetosis or follow the use of drugs with extrapyramidal effects such as phenothiazines, butyrophenones or thioxanthenes (for example flupenthixol). Anti-Parkinsonian drugs such as benzhexol, orphenadrine or benztropine help to control these reactions.

Facial tics

Facial tics are benign spasms (habit spasms), worsened by emotion or tiredness. Most resolve spontaneously. Common tics are blinking, grimacing, shaking the head, clearing the throat, coughing or shrugging.

Hemifacial spasm

Hemifacial spasm (clonic facial spasm) typically affects the elderly. There is spasm of the angle of the mouth or the eyelid, worse towards evening. Many cases are idiopathic, but some indicate a cerebellopontine angle lesion.

Benign fasciculation

Benign fasciculation and myokymia (spontaneous twitching) of the lower eyelid are quite innocuous.

Facial myokymia

Facial myokymia is rare. It consists of continuous, fine, worm-like contractions of one or more of the facial muscles—especially around the mouth or eyes. It is frequently associated with multiple sclerosis or other neurological disorders and patients must therefore be referred for a neurological opinion.

DIPLOPIA AND STRABISMUS

Eye movements are controlled by the extraocular muscles

under neural control of the IIIrd, IVth and VIth cranial nerves.

Double vision (diplopia) is not uncommon following maxillofacial trauma and often resolves spontaneously within a few days, being caused by oedema. However, persistent diplopia after maxillofacial trauma can be caused by entrapment of, or damage to, the orbital muscles, or lesions of cranial nerves III, IV and VI. There are many other important causes of diplopia, mainly intracranial lesions.

Damage to the oculomotor (IIIrd) nerve causes the following.

1. Paralysis of internal, upward and downard rotation of the ipsilateral eye.
2. Double vision (the affected eye points downwards and laterally—'down and out') in all directions except when looking towards the affected side.
3. Ptosis (drooping ipsilateral upper eyelid).
4. Dilated pupil that fails to constrict if light is shone

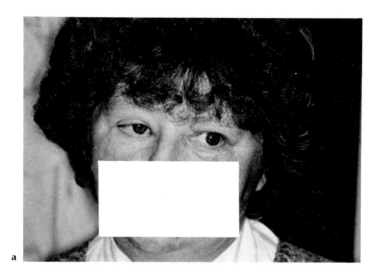

a

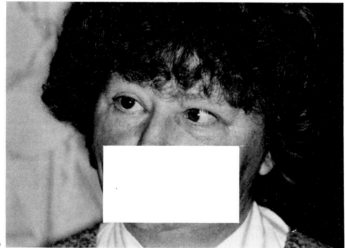

b

Fig. 28.3 Paralysis of the right abducens nerve: (a) no problem on looking to the left; (b) on looking to the right, the affected eye does not move but a pronounced squint appears.

in either the affected eye (negative direct light reaction), or the unaffected eye (negative consensual light reaction).

Damage to the trochlear (VIth) nerve causes serious disability because the superior oblique muscle that depresses the eye is paralysed and diplopia is maximal on looking down for reading, walking etc. The pupils and light reactions are normal.

Abducens (VIth) nerve lesions are characterized by:

(a) paralysis of the lateral rectus muscle and therefore paralysis of abduction of the ipsilateral eye;
(b) deviation of the affected eye towards the nose, and diplopia maximally on looking laterally towards the affected side (Fig. 28.3);
(c) normal pupils and light reactions.

Paralytic strabismus (squint) is the usual type of strabismus that follows maxillofacial injuries and is characterized by variable deviation of the ocular axes according to the position of gaze. The eye affected can be determined by noting in which direction of gaze the diplopia is maximal and then, while the patient looks in that direction, covering each eye in turn. The outermost image disappears when the affected eye is covered.

Diplopia or strabismus may be an occasional transient complication of inferior alveolar local analgesic injections, presumably because the analgesic tracks, for example, to the inferior orbital fissure, where it can block these nerves (Volume 1).

PUPILLARY ABNORMALITIES

The pupils are normally equal in size and constrict on exposure to bright light (light reflex) and on accommodation for near objects (convergence reflex). Light shone in one eye causes pupillary constriction both in that eye (direct light reflex) and in the unexposed eye (indirect or consensual light reflex). Pupil size is determined by dilator and constrictor fibres. The sympathetic supply to dilator muscles arises from the superior cervical ganglion, runs along the internal carotid artery and joins the ophthalmic division of the trigeminal nerve and the long ciliary nerves. The parasympathetic supply to the constrictor muscles of the iris runs with the oculomotor nerve.

The sympathetic nerve supply is partially responsible, with the oculomotor nerve, for contraction of the levator palpebrae superioris muscle (raising the upper eyelid) and a lesion of either will cause some drooping of the eyelid (ptosis).

Pupil constriction (miosis) can be caused by a lesion of the sympathetic supply or by cholinergic drugs (e.g. neostigmine) or opiates. The most important cause of pupil constriction is a rise in intracranial pressure, when the pupil also becomes non-reactive owing to pressure on the oculomotor nerve. Pupil dilatation (mydriasis) can be caused by a lesion of the parasympathetic fibres of the IIIrd nerve, by cholinergic blocking drugs (e.g. atropine), or by sympathomimetic drugs (e.g. adrenaline or cocaine). Other causes of unequal pupils include trauma and the following.

Adie's (Holmes–Adie) pupil

This is a benign condition in which one pupil is dilated and reacts only very slowly to light or convergence. There may be associated loss of knee or ankle jerks.

Argyll–Robertson pupil

This is characterized by small, irregular, unequal pupils which fail to react to light but still react to accommodation. Characteristically caused by neurosyphilis, the Argyll–Robertson pupil may also be seen in other conditions such as diabetes mellitus or multiple sclerosis.

Horner's syndrome

Horner's syndrome comprises usually unilateral:

(a) miosis (pupil constriction);
(b) ptosis (drooping of the upper eyelid);
(c) loss of sweating of the ipsilateral face;
(d) enophthalmos (retruded eyeball) sometimes.

It is caused by interruption of sympathetic nerve fibres peripherally as a result, for example, of trauma to the neck, or lung cancer infiltrating the superior cervical sympathetic ganglion.

RHYTHMIC EYE MOVEMENTS

A few irregular eye jerks are normal in some individuals, when the eyes are deviated far to one side, but jerking (nystagmus) may otherwise signify disease. Nystagmus is usually a rhythmic (jerk) nystagmus from side to side, fast in one direction. It can also be vertical or rotary. Causes of nystagmus include the following.

1. Drug intoxication (e.g. barbiturates).
2. Internal ear disease (vestibular disease).
3. Cerebellar disease.

4. Brainstem disease.

5. Positional nystagmus—on moving the head from side to side—may be caused by head injury, brain tumour, or vestibular disease.

6. Oscillating (pendular) nystagmus may result from ocular disease.

SWALLOWING

In normal swallowing, the activities of the striated muscle of the pharynx and upper oesophagus are integrated with those of the smooth muscle of the lower oesophagus.

The initial phase of swallowing is voluntary, under the control particularly of the glossopharyngeal nerve, with the vagus controlling further phases. Normal swallowing is dependent on adequate mastication of large food masses, lubrication with fluids and saliva, unobstructed lumens of the pharynx and oesophagus, and normal co-ordinated neuromuscular mechanisms of swallowing.

A sphincter formed by the cricopharyngeus prevents air from filling the oesophagus during respiration, while a lower oesophageal sphincter stops gastric reflux. The IXth and Xth cranial nerves are essential to swallowing.

The glossopharyngeal (IXth) cranial nerve

The glossopharyngeal cranial nerve is attached to the medulla, and passes through the jugular foramen where it has the jugular and petrosal ganglia. It then runs in the carotid sheath between the internal carotid artery and internal jugular vein. It leaves the carotid sheath and runs on the stylopharyngeus muscle deep to the external carotid and ascending palatine arteries to the upper border of the middle constrictor muscle, where it enters the oropharynx.

The following are the main branches of the glossopharyngeal nerve.

The *tympanic branch,* which joins with a branch of the facial nerve to form the tympanic plexus, from which arise sensory branches to the mucous membrane of the middle ear, the tympanic antrum and the Eustachian tube, and the lesser superficial petrosal nerve which contains secretomotor fibres derived from the glossopharyngeal nerve and destined for the otic ganglion and the parotid salivary gland.

The *carotid branch* descends to the carotid sinus and carotid body, carrying autonomic fibres involved in blood pressure regulation.

The *motor branch,* to the stylopharyngeus muscle.

Pharyngeal (sensory) branches, to the pharyngeal mucous membrane.

Tonsillar branches ascend to the upper part of the pharynx and Eustachian tube.

Lingual branches pass to the posterior third of the tongue.

Lesions of the glossopharyngeal nerve. These are rare in isolation but the gag reflex is usually impaired as may be taste sensation.

The vagus (Xth) cranial nerve

The vagus arises at the medulla and passes through the jugular foramen where it has a superior ganglion and lower down a large inferior ganglion. The cranial part of the accessory nerve (XI) joins the vagus at the inferior ganglion and fibres are distributed with the pharyngeal and laryngeal branches of the vagus. The ganglia also communicate with the facial, glossopharyngeal, hypoglossal and sympathetic nerves.

The vagus enters the carotid sheath between the internal jugular vein and the internal carotid artery to descend through the neck. On the right side the vagus enters the thoracic cavity after crossing the first part of the subclavian artery; on the left side, after descending between the left common carotid and subclavian arteries, it crosses in front of the aortic arch. On the right side the recurrent laryngeal branch loops around the subclavian artery; on the left side it passes around the arch of the aorta.

In the thorax, the vagus passes behind the hilum of the lung to form the oesophageal plexus, from which trunks pass through the diaphragm in front of (left vagus) and behind (right vagus) the oesophagus. The left vagus is distributed mainly to the anterior surface and lesser curvature of the stomach, to the liver, and to the gall bladder. The right vagus is distributed mainly to the stomach and midgut derivatives with branches to the coeliac, splenic and renal plexuses.

The branches of the vagus nerve in the neck are as follows.

A *recurrent meningeal branch* to the dura mater of the posterior cranial fossa.

The *auricular nerve (of Arnold)* supplies the mucous membrane of the external auditory canal and the outer surface of the tympanic membrane.

The *pharyngeal branch* contains motor fibres, mainly from the cranial part of the accessory nerve, to the constrictor muscles of the pharynx, and the palatopharyngeus, levator palati, palatoglossus and uvular muscles.

The *superior laryngeal nerve* consists mainly of fibres derived from the cranial part of the accessory nerve and gives an internal laryngeal (sensory) branch, and a motor branch (the external laryngeal) to the cricothyroid and inferior constrictor muscles.

Upper and lower cardiac branches supply autonomic (parasympathetic) control to the heart.

Recurrent laryngeal nerves are motor to the muscles of the larynx (except for the cricothyroid) and sensory to the laryngeal mucous membrane below the vocal folds, and the mucous membrane of the trachea. Some motor fibres to the lower part of the inferior pharyngeal constrictor may run in the recurrent laryngeal nerves.

Lesions of the vagus nerve

Lesions of the vagus are rare in isolation but cause a syndrome of dysphagia and dysphonia with the following features:

(a) impaired gag reflex;
(b) the soft palate moves towards the unaffected side when the patient is asked to say 'aah';
(c) hoarse voice;
(d) bovine cough.

The pharyngeal branches of the vagus were occasionally found to be affected in diphtheria (when this was common in the UK), giving the voice a nasal quality and allowing fluid to regurgitate through the nose during swallowing.

DYSPHAGIA

Difficulty in swallowing can be caused by the following (Table 28.3).

1. Attempting to swallow too large a bolus of food.
2. Inadequate lubrication of the food bolus (in xerostomia). Dry mouth is an uncommon cause of dysphagia, most obvious on eating biscuits (the 'cracker sign').
3. Pain or obstruction in the mouth, throat or oesophagus.

Tonsillitis is the most common cause of dysphagia. Oral causes include any painful condition such as infections or ulcers, particularly of the palate, fauces, tongue or floor of the mouth, and, importantly, carcinoma of the posterior lateral border of the tongue.

Infections involving the fascial spaces of the neck, particularly those of the parapharyngeal space, cause severe dysphagia.

Table 28.3
Causes of dysphagia

Inadequate lubrication of food
Xerostomia

Pain or obstruction in mouth or throat
Inflammatory lesions
Neoplasms

Neurological and neuromuscular causes
Achalasia
Syringobulbia
Cerebrovascular accidents
Cerebrovascular disease (pseudobulbar palsy)
Motor neurone disease
Guillain–Barré syndrome
Poliomyelitis
Diphtheria
Cerebellar disease
Myopathies
    Myasthenia gravis
    Muscular dystrophies
    Dermatomyositis

Obstruction in pharynx or oesophagus
Foreign bodies in pharynx
Sideropenic dysphagia (Paterson–Kelly syndrome)
Pharyngeal pouches
Benign stricture
Carcinoma
Scleroderma
External pressure, e.g. from mediastinal lymph nodes

4. Incoordination of any part of the act of swallowing—caused by neuromuscular disease or psychogenic disorders.

Neurological causes of dysphagia are rare but important. Achalasia is a progressive loss of oesophageal peristalsis with increased tension at the lower oesophageal sphincter. Dysphagia may be particularly important in disorders of the medulla. Lesions of the glossopharyngeal nerve are usually associated with lesions of the vagus, accessory and hypoglossal nerves (bulbar palsy). Symptoms resulting from a IXth nerve lesion include impaired pharyngeal sensation so that the gag reflex may be impaired.

Psychogenic causes include hysteria (globus hystericus).

Bulbar palsy is the term given to weakness or paralysis of muscles supplied by the medulla (bulb), namely the tongue, pharynx, larynx, sternomastoid and upper trapezius (cranial nerves IX–XII inclusive). Poliomyelitis, diphtheria or HIV infection can cause acute bulbar palsy.

Chronic causes are progressive bulbar palsy, tumours or aneurysms of the posterior cranial fossa or nasopharynx, or strokes.

5. Narrowing of the pharyngeal or oesophageal lumen, for example by foreign body, stricture or tumour.

Management

The history is often the most important factor in the diagnosis of dysphagia. If liquids cannot be drunk rapidly, a neurological cause or achalasia is likely. If there is dysphagia but fluids can be drunk rapidly, then a stricture is more likely. In psychogenic dysphagia the patient complains of dysphagia even when not trying to swallow.

Chest radiography, oesophagoscopy and barium swallow examination are usually required if the lesion is not in the mouth, unless there are indications of neuromuscular disease. Videofluorescopy is a useful diagnostic aid. Treatment can be difficult; a surgical opinion is often required, particularly in the case of oesophageal impacted foreign bodies, strictures, pouches, achalasia or carcinoma.

The ACCESSORY (XIᵀᴴ) CRANIAL NERVE

The cranial part of the accessory nerve arises from the medulla and the spinal part from the spinal cord. The spinal portion enters the foramen magnum and unites with the cranial part to form a common trunk which passes through the jugular foramen between the internal jugular vein and the internal carotid artery. The cranial part then separates to join the vagus and is distributed through the pharyngeal and laryngeal branches of the vagus to pharyngeal, soft palatal and laryngeal muscles.

The spinal part passes backwards to supply sternomastoid and trapezius muscles.

Lesions of the accessory nerve

Lesions of the accessory nerve are often associated with damage to the IXth and Xth nerves and cause weakness of:

(a) the sternomastoid—weakness on trying to turn the head away from the affected side;
(b) the trapezius, on shrugging the shoulders.

Testing this nerve is useful in differentiating patients with genuine palsies from those with palsies of non-organic cause since in a true palsy the head cannot be turned *away* from the affected side.

The HYPOGLOSSAL (XIIᵀᴴ) CRANIAL NERVE

The hypoglossal nerve arises from the medulla and leaves the cranial cavity through the anterior condylar canal to enter the carotid sheath, where it is joined by branches from the first and second cervical nerves and from the superior cervical sympathetic ganglion. The nerve turns forwards, looping around the origin of the occipital artery and lying superficial to the external carotid, facial and lingual arteries in the carotid triangle. It leaves the carotid triangle deep to the digastric and stylohyoid muscles and enters the floor of the mouth between the mylohyoid and hyoglossus muscles, communicating with the lingual nerve and penetrating the genioglossus muscle to enter the tongue below the sublingual gland. Within the tongue it supplies all muscles, except the palatoglossus.

Lesions of the hypoglossal nerve

Lesions of the hypoglossal nerve are rare but produce:

(a) dysarthria (difficulty in speaking)—particularly for lingual sounds;
(b) deviation of the tongue towards the affected side on protrusion.

Lower motor nerve lesions also cause ipsilateral wasting of the tongue.

FURTHER READING

Groher M. E. (1984). Ed. Dysphagia: diagnosis and management. Boston: Butterworths.
Leading article (1982). Bell's palsy. *Lancet*, **i**: 663.
Ludman H. (1981). Facial palsy. *Br. med. J.*, **282**: 545–547.
Scully C. (1980). Orofacial manifestations of disease. 6. Neurological, psychiatric and muscular disorders. *Hospital Update*, **6**: 135–145.
Sonies B. C., Weiffenbach J., Atkinson, J. C., *et al.* (1987). Clinical examination of motor and sensory functions of the adult oral cavity. *Dysphagia*, **1**: 178–186.

Chapter
29
Disorders of orofacial senses

The senses of taste and smell are intimately related.

SMELL

Bipolar olfactory receptors for the sense of smell are scattered through the mucous membrane in the roof of the nasal cavities. The peripheral processes of the olfactory cranial nerves (cranial nerve I) end in the mucous membrane as hair-like structures. Mucus from small nasal mucous glands keeps the epithelial surface moist, a feature necessary for the efficient sense of smell. The central processes pass through the ethmoidal cribriform plate to the olfactory bulb of the brain and, from there, the central olfactory projections are predominantly to the primitive cerebral cortex—the archipallium and paeleopallium (the hippocampus and pyriform lobe respectively)—and to the hypothalamus.

Olfactory function is demonstrated by the ability to smell substances such as orange or peppermint oil. Microencapsulated odorants mounted on card are now available for testing the sense of smell (*Scratch and sniff* booklet: Sensonics Inc., 155 Hadden Avenue, Huddersfield, New Jersey 08033, USA). Ammoniacal solutions must *not* be used as they stimulate the trigeminal rather than the olfactory nerve.

TASTE

The special sense of taste is mediated by taste buds found in the mucous membrane of the tongue, soft palate, fauces and pharynx, and, in the newborn, on the lips and in the cheeks. Taste buds are oval bodies made up of groups of neuroepithelial and supporting cells. The neuroepithelial cells are rod shaped with a peripheral hair-like process projecting into the taste pores at the surface of the overlying mucous membrane. The terminal branches of the nerve fibres subserving taste end in close relationship to these special cells. Several different mechanisms are involved in taste perception. For example, salts depolarize receptor cells by passing through channels in the cell membrane; acids by blocking potassium channels; and bitter substances by effects on an inositol phospholipid pathway. Cyclic nucleotides may also be involved as intracellular messengers—especially in perception of sugars. The cells of the taste buds undergo continual renewal, with a life span of about 10 days. Renewal is altered by nutrition, hormonal status, age, drugs, radiation and other factors.

Taste buds on the tongue are on the fungiform, circumvallate and foliate, but not on the filiform, papillae. The four fundamental varieties of taste sensation (sweet, bitter, sour and salt) do not appear to be detected by structurally different taste buds (Chapter 11).

Taste sensation from the anterior two-thirds of the tongue and the palate is mediated by the lingual and palatine nerves respectively (Fig. 29.1). The taste fibres pass into the brainstem along the chorda tympani and greater superficial petrosal branches of the facial nerve. The central processes of the chorda tympani nerve bringing taste impulses from the anterior two-thirds of the tongue pass,

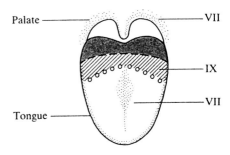

Fig. 29.1 *Cranial nerves in which sense of taste projects centrally.*

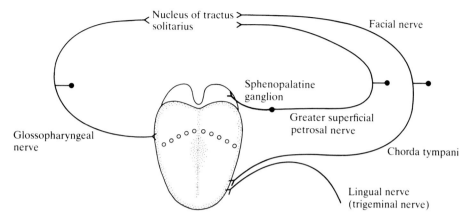

Fig. 29.2 *Neurological connections in relation to sense of taste.*

as the nervus intermedius, to the solitary tract, through which the taste impulses are carried to the nucleus solitarius (Fig. 29.2).

Taste fibres from the posterior third of the tongue pass in the glossopharyngeal nerve and to the nucleus solitarius. The taste buds of the epiglottis are innervated by the vagal nerve fibres, whose cell bodies are situated in the nodose ganglion and whose central processes terminate once again in the nucleus solitarius.

These various 'taste' fibres passing to the nucleus solitarius form the solitary tract (tractus solitarius). The secondary neurones of the pathway for taste (from the nucleus solitarius to the thalamus) cross to be included in the medial lemniscus of the opposite side and, on reaching the level of the thalamus, end along with other secondary fibres from the head region. Tertiary, or third-order, taste fibres project to the inferior part of the postcentral gyrus and the adjacent cortex of the insula. Pontine neurones also project to the 'feeding area' in the hypothalamus.

Studies of taste thresholds in human subjects commonly use sucrose for the sweet taste, vinegar or citric acid to produce sour taste sensations, and sodium chloride for the taste of salt. Detection and recognition thresholds can be measured by applying the selected solution to precise regions of the oral mucosa or asking them to rinse the mouth with the solution dissolved in water. The tongue is most sensitive for salt and sweet tastes. Sour and bitter tastes can also be recognized on the tongue but not as well as by the palatal mucosa. Salt and sweet tastes can be appreciated on the palate also, but higher concentrations of solution are required. Commercial kits are available (Kit for screening taste function: Westport Pharmaceuticals, Westport, Connecticut 06881, USA).

The flavour of food results from chemical stimulation of both taste buds and olfactory neurones. Free nerve endings in the nose, mouth and throat also contribute to an appreciation of food and there is also a strong element from higher centres.

DISTURBANCES OF SENSES OF SMELL AND TASTE

Taste and olfaction are both susceptible to the general sensory phenomenon known as adaptation, i.e. the progressive reduction in the appreciation of a stimulus during the course of continual exposure to that stimulus, and can be distorted by various factors.

The terminology of the various dysfunctions is shown in Table 29.1.

Disorders can result mainly from (Table 29.2; Fig. 29.3):

(a) modification of the local environment of the receptors;

Table 29.1
Terminology of disorders of smell and taste

Dysfunction	Terminology	
	Sense of smell	Sense of taste
Absence	Anosmia	Ageusia
Diminished	Hyposmia	Hypogeusia
Distorted	Dysosmia	Dysgeusia
Heightened	Hyperosmia	Hypergeusia

Table 29.2

Disorders affecting taste

Local disorders
Xerostomia
Sepsis
Various foods

Disorders affecting taste buds
Irradiation or burns
Zinc and other deficiencies
Cytotoxic drugs

Disorders affecting cranial nerves
Damage to lingual nerve
Bell's palsy
Damage to chorda tympani or intracranial VIIn.

Cerebral disorders
Frontal lobe tumours
Psychogenic disorders

Others
Smoking
Old age
Cancer
Cirrhosis
Drugs
  Penicillamine
  Captopril
  Metronidazole
  Antirheumatic drugs
  Solvent abuse
  Cytotoxic drugs

(b) damage to sensory receptors;
(c) damage to the cranial nerves involved;
(d) cerebral cortical disorders.

Probably the most common causes of loss of senses of taste and smell are viral upper respiratory tract infections which affect olfaction but also, thereby, decrease the appreciation of food. Olfaction may be impaired after head injuries, due to tearing of olfactory fibres, and in ageing.

Dry mouth for any reason can distort taste, as can drugs (particularly penicillamine and captopril), nutritional deficiencies (especially of zinc), ageing, and various disorders.

Lesions in the nose (especially respiratory infections) or in the olfactory pathway may cause anosmia. Other causes of anosmia include some endocrine disorders (especially hypothyroidism), Parkinson's disease, and some other cerebral disorders. Unilateral anosmia is often unnoticed by the patient.

Both olfaction and taste are susceptible to genetic and hormonal factors. For example, sensitivity to the bitter taste of phenylthiourea is genetically determined and some other patients are genetically unable, for example, to smell fish. There appear to be no significant differences in the senses of olfaction and taste between sexes, but both senses vary through the menstrual cycle and may be distorted during pregnancy, often with the appearance of cravings for unusual foods.

Disorders of these senses can be distressing and sometimes incapacitating, and can cause anorexia and depression.

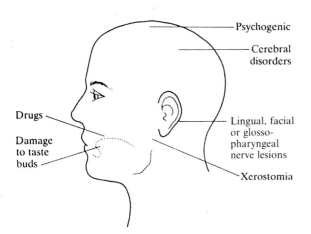

Fig. 29.3 *Causes of disturbed sense of taste.*

Psychogenic
Cerebral disorders
Drugs
Damage to taste buds
Lingual, facial or glosso-pharyngeal nerve lesions
Xerostomia

SIGHT

The rods and cones of the retina of the eye respond to light sensation, and the resultant nerve impulses from them pass through the optic nerve (IInd cranial nerve), optic tract and optic radiation to the visual cortex in the occipital lobe of the brain.

Blindness (or defects of the visual field) is caused by lesions of the eye, optic nerve, or cortex. If there is a complete lesion of one optic nerve, then that eye is totally blind, there is no direct reaction of the pupil to light (loss of constriction) and, if a light is shone into the affected eye, the pupil of the unaffected eye also fails to respond (loss of the consensual reflex). However, the nerves responsible for pupil constriction run in the IIIrd cranial nerve and are thus intact, and therefore if a light is shone into the *unaffected* eye, the pupil of the blind eye will still constrict.

Lesions of the optic tract, chiasma, radiation or cortex cause bilateral visual field defects. Visual fields are tested by 'confrontation'—comparing the patient's visual fields with one's own. Visual acuity is tested with Snellen charts.

FACIAL SENSORY LOSS

Lesions of a sensory branch of the trigeminal nerve may cause anaesthesia in the distribution of the affected branch. Lesions involving the ophthalmic division cause corneal anaesthesia, which is tested by gently touching the cornea with a wisp of cotton wool twisted to a point. Normally, this procedure causes a blink, but if the cornea is anaesthetic (or if there is facial palsy), no blink follows, provided that the patient does not actually see the cotton wool. Lesions of the sensory part of the trigeminal nerve initially result in a diminishing response to pin-prick of the skin and, later, complete anaesthesia. It is important in patients complaining of facial anaesthesia to test all areas but particularly the corneal reflex. *If the patient complains of complete facial or hemifacial anaesthesia, but the corneal reflex is retained or there is apparent anaesthesia over the angle of the mandible (an area **not** innervated by the trigeminal nerve), then the symptoms are probably functional (non-organic).*

Facial sensory loss may be caused by intracranial or, more frequently, by extracranial lesions of the trigeminal nerve. It may lead to corneal, facial or oral ulceration (Fig. 29.4).

Extracranial causes of sensory loss

Common extracranial causes of facial sensory loss are shown in Table 29.3. The mandibular division or its branches may be traumatized by inferior alveolar local analgesic injections, fractures or surgery (particularly osteotomies (Volume 4) or surgical extraction of lower third molars). Occasionally the mental foramen is close beneath a lower denture and there is anaesthesia of the lower lip on the affected side, as a result of pressure from the denture. The mental nerve may be damaged by surgery, such as removal of impacted second premolars. The lingual nerve is fairly often damaged, especially during removal of lower third molars, particularly when the lingual split technique is used. Osteomyelitis or tumour deposits in the mandible may affect the inferior alveolar nerve to cause labial anaesthesia.

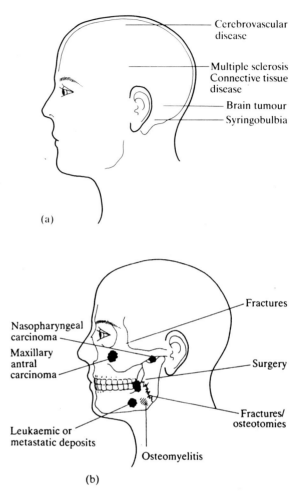

Fig. 29.4 *Causes of facial sensory loss: (a) intracranial, and (b) extracranial.*

Nasopharyngeal carcinomas may invade the pharyngeal wall to infiltrate the mandibular division of the trigeminal nerve, causing pain and sensory loss and, by occluding the Eustachian tube, deafness (Trotter's syndrome: Chapter 15).

Damage to branches of the maxillary division of the trigeminal may be caused by trauma (middle-third facial fractures) or a tumour such as carcinoma of the maxillary antrum.

Intracranial causes of facial sensory loss

Common intracranial causes of facial sensory loss (Table 29.3) are multiple sclerosis, cerebral tumours (especially

Table 29.3
Causes of sensory loss in the trigeminal area

Extracranial		
	Trauma	To inferior alveolar, lingual, mental or infra-orbital nerves
	Inflammatory	Osteomyelitis
	Neoplastic	Malignant disease in jaws, antrum or nasopharynx Metastatic tumours Leukaemic deposits
Intracranial		
	Syringobulbia Inflammatory	Multiple sclerosis Neurosyphilis HIV infection Sarcoidosis Connective tissue disease
	Neoplastic	Cerebral tumours
	Vascular	Cerebrovascular disease Aneurysms
	Trauma	e.g. surgical treatment of trigeminal neuralgia
	Drugs	Labetalol
	Bone disease	Paget's disease
	Idiopathic	Benign trigeminal neuropathy
	Psychogenic	Hysteria Hyperventilation syndrome

acoustic neuroma) and syringobulbia (cavitation of the spinal canal). Since other cranial nerves are anatomically close, there may be associated neurological deficits.

In posterior or middle cranial fossa lesions, there may be other features (p. 331).

Benign trigeminal neuropathy

This is a transient sensory loss in one or more divisons of the trigeminal nerve which seldom occurs until the second decade. The corneal reflex is not affected. The aetiology is unknown, though some patients prove to have a connective tissue disorder, and the benign nature of the condition can only be confirmed by the exclusion of organic disease and the passage of time.

Psychogenic causes

Hysteria, and particularly hyperventilation syndrome, may underlie some cases of facial anaesthesia.

Management of patients with facial sensory loss

In view of the potential seriousness of facial sensory loss, care should be taken to exclude local causes and a full neurological assessment should be undertaken. Examination of the postnasal space may be essential, as may radiography of the base of the skull (for erosion of foramina), maxillary sinuses and jaws, and serological tests

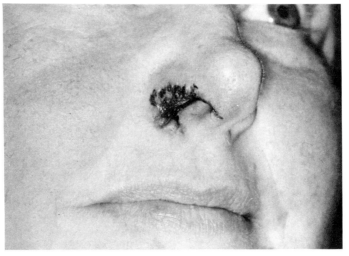

Fig. 29.5 *Repeated damage to the nose in a patient who has anaesthesia of the right trigeminal nerve.*

for syphilis connective tissue disease and HIV infection. If the aetiology is not established, a neurological opinion and prolonged follow-up are necessary.

In any event, the patient should be careful not to traumatize the skin or mucosa (Fig. 29.5). If the cornea is anaesthetic, a protective eye pad should be worn and a tarsorrhaphy (an operation to unite the upper and lower eyelids) may be indicated since the protective corneal reflex is lost and the cornea may be traumatized.

FURTHER READING

Fielding A. F., Reck S. F. (1986). Bilateral lingual nerve anaesthesia following mandibular third molar extractions. *Oral Surg.*, **62**: 13–16.

Henkin R. I. (1986). Taste. In *Pharmacology in medicine: principles and practice* (S. N. Pradhan *et al.*, eds.) pp. 748–753. Bethesda: SP Press.

Moore-Gillon V. (1987). Testing the sense of smell. *Brit. med. J.*, **294**: 793–794.

Nelson L. W., Johnson W. T., Blaha D. A. (1986). Mandibular paresthesia secondary to cerebrovascular changes. *Oral Surg.*, **62**: 17–19.

Rollin H. (1978). Drug related gustatory disorders. *Ann. Atol. Rhinol. Laryngol.*, **87**: 37–42.

Schiffman S. S. (1983). Taste and smell in disease. *N. Engl. J. Med.*, **308**: 1275–1279.

Speirs R. L. (1988). The sense of taste. *Dental Update*, March: 82–87.

Teeter J., Gold G. H. (1988). A taste of things to come. *Nature*, **331**: 298–299.

Weiffenbach J. M., Fox P. C., Baum B. J. (1986). Taste and salivary function. *Proc. Natl. Acad. Sci. (USA)*, **83**: 6103–6106.

Ziporyn T. (1982). Taste and smell: The neglected senses. *JAMA*, **247**: 277–285.

Chapter
30

Miscellaneous relevant neurologically related disorders

SPEECH

The act of speaking involves a highly coordinated sequence of movements of the muscles of respiration, larynx, pharynx, palate, tongue and lips. Articulation and phonation therefore are under direct control of the vagus (and adjacent cranial nerves), facial and hypoglossal nerves. As with all muscle activity, phonation and articulation are under higher control from pyramidal and extrapyramidal influences.

Speech disorders

Speech involves a wide range of acquired skills, deficiencies of which impede interpersonal communication irrespective of any other impairment in language usage.

Disturbances of language use are referred to as dysphasias (or aphasias), and disorders may be caused by the following.

1. Brain disease such as stroke or after head injury, in which there is loss of production and comprehension of speech and language (dysphasia).

2. Deranged speech due to central nervous system disorders, as in delirium or dementia, or the use of various drugs (including alcohol).

3. Defects in articulation because of paralysis, rigidity, or involuntary movements of tongue or palate (dysarthria).

4. Loss of voice due to laryngeal disease or paralysis (dysphonia).

Dysphasia and derangements of speech are outside the province of the dentist, but dysarthria and dysphonia are of some relevance.

Dysarthria

1. Dysarthria may be caused by painful or neoplastic lesions, swelling, paralysis, rigidity or tremor of the tongue in particular.

2. Paralytic dysarthria may be caused by disease of the medulla oblongata (bulbar palsy); lesions affecting cranial nerves VII, IX, X, XI or XII; or myopathies such as myasthenia gravis.

3. Spastic dysarthria is more common and usually is caused by cerebrovascular disease affecting the motor cortex (causing *pseudo*bulbar palsy). Extrapyramidal disease such as Parkinsonism or drugs such as phenothiazines that can cause extrapyramidal abnormalities may cause rigid dysarthria.

4. Tremor of the tongue is seen in basal ganglia and cerebellar disease and causes choreic or ataxic dysarthria, respectively.

Patients with persistent dysarthria should be referred for a neurological opinion.

Dysphonia

The most obvious cause of dysphonia is laryngitis, but it may also be due to paralytic disorders, extrapyramidal disease, some psychogenic disorders and endocrine disorders—notably hypothyroidism and acromegaly.

If one vocal cord becomes paralysed, the voice becomes low pitched, hoarse and rasping, though similar changes can arise with heavy smoking, singing, chronic laryngitis, polyps, neoplasms etc.

Patients with dysphonia should be referred for an ear, nose and throat opinion.

SWEATING

Sweating is a sympathetic nervous system function. Nevertheless, the postganglionic secretomotor fibres are cholinergic. Preganglionic fibres destined for the head and neck arise from T1 and T2 spinal cord levels, from the intermediolateral columns, synapse in the superior cervical ganglia with postsynaptic fibres that join branches of the trigeminal to innervate facial sweat glands.

Gustatory sweating

Facial sweating associated with eating (gustatory sweating) is commonly due to spicy foods, cheese or chocolate. Atropine, or anaesthetizing the *posterior* third of the tongue, can block the sweating.

Hemifacial gustatory sweating is uncommon but may follow trauma, surgery (thoracic sympathectomy; thyroid surgery), syringomyelia, mediastinal tumours, or is sometimes idiopathic. Hemifacial gustatory sweating in the distribution of the auriculotemporal nerve usually arising after parotid surgery, is termed Frey's syndrome (or auriculotemporal syndrome).

Frey's syndrome

Following damage to the auriculotemporal nerve which carries parasympathetic secretomotor fibres to the parotid as well as sympathetic vasomotor and secretomotor fibres to the overlying skin, regenerating parasympathetic fibres become misdirected and come to innervate structures normally supplied by the sympathetic system. Frey's syndrome manifests with sweating and flushing in the pre-auricular and temporal areas associated with any stimulus to salivation. It may follow any trauma to, or inflammation of, the parotid glands and usually appears within 2 months to 2 years. An analogous syndrome (the chorda tympani syndrome) may follow damage to the submandibular gland.

Creams containing atropinics or antiperspirants (aluminium hexahydrate) usually control the symptoms, but anticholinergic drugs such as poldine methyl sulphate may be needed. Rarely is avulsion of the auriculotemporal nerve indicated.

EPILEPSY

Epilepsy is discussed in Volume 1.

THE UNCONSCIOUS PATIENT

Causes of loss of consciousness are discussed in Volume 1, and include drug overdose and reactions, head injury, meningitis, rising intracranial pressure, and diabetes.

Management

In the absence of a known cause, call for medical help and undertake the following.

(a) Clear and maintain the airway and place the patient in the head-injury position to avoid inhalation of vomit (Fig. 3.12).

(b) Check pulse and blood pressure and respiration and put up an intravenous infusion of 0.9% saline after taking blood for glucose levels, urea, electrolytes and full blood picture.

(c) Give 50 ml of 50% glucose intravenously since the cause may be hypoglycaemia.

(d) Try not to extend the neck, in case there is damage to the cervical spine.

(e) Collect as much information from relatives, witnesses, or ambulance staff.

(f) Full physical examination is required, but this necessitates medical expertise.

The Glasgow Coma scale is now often used to record and monitor the conscious state and this is the best way to assess prognosis (Table 30.1).

HEAD INJURY

Many patients with maxillofacial injuries have head injuries (see Chapter 3). Emergency care is as under 'The unconscious patient' (above) and also involves the following.

1. Clear the airway: keep the patient in the head-injury position.

2. Put up an intravenous line and take blood for the haemoglobin level; record pulse rate (PR), blood pressure (BP) and respiration. In severe haemorrhage, PR rises and BP falls; in rising intracranial pressure such as may result from intracranial bleeding, PR falls and BP rises (when an urgent neurological opinion is required).

3. Record the history, particularly with regard to any loss of consciousness and amnesia; record the level of consciousness.

4. Neurological clinical assessment. Record pupil dilatation reactivity to light and whether the pupils are

Table 30.1
Glasgow Coma Scale

Best *motor* response	Grade	Best *verbal* response	Grade	*Eye* opening	Grade
Obeys command	1	Orientated	1	Spontaneous	1
Localizing response to pain	2	Confused conversation	2	In response to speech	2
Flexor response to pain	3	Inappropriate speech (no conversational exchange)	3	In response to pain	3
Extensor response to pain	4	Incomprehensible (moaning)	4	None	4
No response to pain	5	None	5		

equal. Record visual fields. Check power, tone, reflexes. Examine for cerebrospinal fluid leaks from ears or nose. Check for skull injury and eye injury.

5. Investigations: skull radiographs, CT scans, and other radiographs as indicated.

6. Control infection: antitetanus vaccine if none in last 5 years; antimicrobials as indicated, e.g. compound fracture or contaminated wound.

7. Admit to ward if any loss of consciousness, amnesia, severe headache, vomiting, skull fracture, neurological signs, serious injuries or bleeding, any danger to the airway of if the patient is a child or an adult living alone.

Deteriorating consciousness, headache, neck stiffness or vomiting are all danger signs.

FURTHER READING

Scully C. (1985). *Hospital dental surgeons guide*. London: British Dental Journal.

Section V
The Neck

Chapter
31

Neck lumps

A wide range of diseases may present with lesions in the neck. The most common lesions are swelling and/or pain in the lymph nodes (Table 31.1). Occasionally the salivary glands (Table 31.2; Chapter 24), thyroid gland or other structures may swell. More diffuse swelling of the neck may be caused by infection, haematoma oedema, surgical emphysema or, rarely, a neoplasm. This chapter concentrates mainly on lymph node disease.

Lymph node swellings

Swollen lymph nodes in the neck are common and they constitute an important part of the examination of the dental patient. Most frequent is an enlarged jugulo-digastric (tonsillar) lymph node, inflamed secondary to a viral upper respiratory tract infection. Nodes also enlarge in oral infections or local infections in the drainage area

Table 31.1
Causes of cervical lymph node enlargement

Inflammatory	Infective	Local	Bacterial	Local infections (Head and Neck)
			Viral	Viral respiratory infections
				Simplex
				Zoster
				Herpangina
		Systemic	Bacterial	Syphilis
				Tuberculosis
				Cat scratch fever
				Brucellosis
			Viral	Glandular fever syndromes (EBV, CMV, HIV)
			Protozoal	Toxoplasmosis
			Other	Mucocutaneous lymph node syndrome
	Non-infective	Sarcoidosis Crohn's disease Connective tissue diseases		
Malignancy	Primary	Leukaemias Lymphomas		
	Secondary	Metastases		
Other	Drugs, e.g. Phenytoin			

Table 31.2

Causes of salivary gland swellings

Inflammatory	Infective	Mumps Bacterial sialadenitis
	Non-infective	Sjögren's syndrome Sarcoidosis
Neoplastic	Benign Malignant	
Others	Obstructions Sialosis Drugs, e.g. chlorhexidine (rarely)	

(virtually anywhere in the head and neck). Enlarged cervical lymph nodes may also be related to malignant disease in the drainage area (e.g. carcinoma) or may be a manifestation of *systemic* disease (e.g. AIDS, leukaemia or lymphoma). Many of these disorders have been discussed in Chapters 14–17; others are covered here.

Lymph nodes that are increasing in size and are hard or rubbery may be malignant; those that are tender may be inflammatory. Lymphadenopathy in the anterior triangle of the neck alone is often due to local disease, especially if the nodes are enlarged on only one side. Generalized lymphadenopathy with or without enlargement of other lymphoid tissue such as liver and spleen (hepatosplenomegaly), however, suggests a systemic cause.

The site of a lump in the neck will give a good indication of the tissue of origin, and the age of the patient may suggest the most likely diagnoses (Table 31.3). The duration of the lesion is clearly relevant: one that has been present since an early age is likely to be of congenital origin, while a lump appearing in later life and persisting may be malignant.

The dental surgeon should examine the neck as part of the examination of every patient.

Anatomy

The lymphoid system (Fig. 31.1) is the essential basis of immune defences (see Chapter 13) and comprises predominantly the bone marrow, spleen, thymus and lymph nodes. Tissue fluid drains into lymph nodes which act as 'filters' of antigens and, after processing in the nodes, lymph containing various immunocytes drains from the nodes to lymph ducts and then to the circulation. A lymph node consists of a cortex, paracortex and medulla and is enclosed by a capsule (Fig. 31.2). Lymphocytes and antigens (if present) pass into the node through the afferent lymphatics, are 'filtered' and lymphocytes pass out from the medulla through the efferent lymphatics. The cortex contains B cells aggregated into primary follicles; following stimulation by antigen these develop foci of active proliferation (germinal centres) and are termed secondary follicles. These follicles are in intimate contact

Table 31.3

Swellings in the neck at different ages

Age	Most common causes of swelling
Child (first decade)	Lymphadenitis due to viral respiratory tract infection
Adolescent and teenager (second decade)	Lymphadenitis due to viral respiratory tract infection Bacterial infection Glandular fever syndromes HIV infection
Adult (third and fourth decades)	Lymphadenitis Glandular fever syndromes HIV infection Malignancy
After fourth decade	Lymphadenitis Malignancy

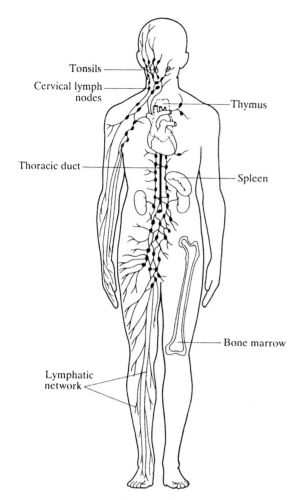

Fig. 31.1 The lymphoid system.

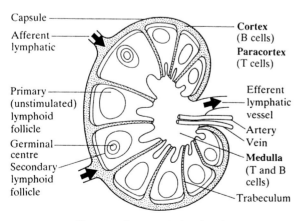

Fig. 31.2 Structure of a lymph node.

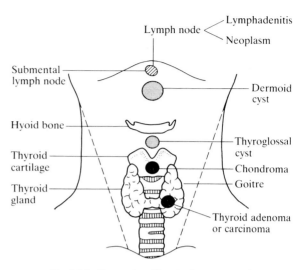

Fig. 31.3 Causes of swellings in the anterior neck.

with antigen-presenting dendritic cells (Chapters 11 and 13). The paracortex contains T cells, and the medulla contains both T and B cells.

Many diseases present in the lymph nodes can most easily be detected in the anterior triangle of the neck, which is bounded superiorly by the mandibular lower border, posteriorly and inferiorly by the sternomastoid muscle, and anteriorly by the midline of the neck (Figs. 31.3 and 31.4). Nodes in this site drain most of the head and neck except the occiput and back of the neck.

Examination

Visual inspection of the neck, looking particularly for swellings (Fig. 31.5) or sinuses (Fig. 31.6), should be followed by careful palpation of all the lymph nodes (Fig. 31.7) and the thyroid gland, searching for swelling or tenderness. Lymph nodes swell usually because they are involved in an immune response to an infectious agent in the area of drainage; such nodes are usually firm, discrete and tender, but are mobile (lymphadenitis). The focus of inflammation can usually be found in the drainage area, which is anywhere on the face, scalp and nasal cavity, sinuses, ears, pharynx and oral cavity. However, lymph nodes may also swell because of reactive hyperplasia to a malignant tumour in the drainage area, or because of metastatic tumour. The latter may cause the node to feel distinctly hard, and it may become bound down to adjacent tissues (fixed), may not be discrete, and may even, in advanced cases, ulcerate through the skin.

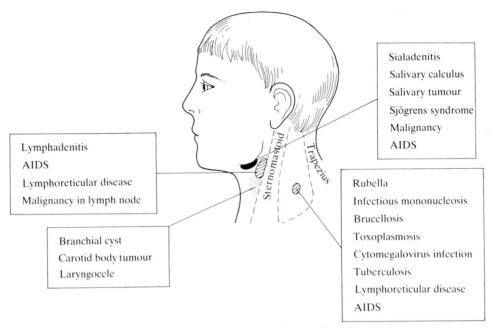

Fig. 31.4 *Causes of swellings in the side of the neck.*

Sialadenitis
Salivary calculus
Salivary tumour
Sjögrens syndrome
Malignancy
AIDS

Lymphadenitis
AIDS
Lymphoreticular disease
Malignancy in lymph node

Branchial cyst
Carotid body tumour
Laryngocele

Rubella
Infectious mononucleosis
Brucellosis
Toxoplasmosis
Cytomegalovirus infection
Tuberculosis
Lymphoreticular disease
AIDS

Sternomastoid

Trapezius

The local cause of lymph node enlargement may not always be found despite a careful search. For example, children occasionally develop a *Staphylococcus aureus* lymphadenitis (usually in a submandibular node) in the absence of any obvious portal of infection (Fig. 31.8). More serious is the finding of an enlarged node suspected to be malignant but where the primary neoplasm cannot be found. Nasopharyngeal carcinoma is a classic cause of this, and an ear, nose and throat specialist opinion should therefore be sought.

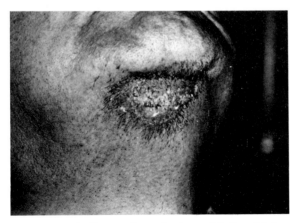

Fig. 31.5 *Swelling in submental region: an infection related to lower incisor teeth.*

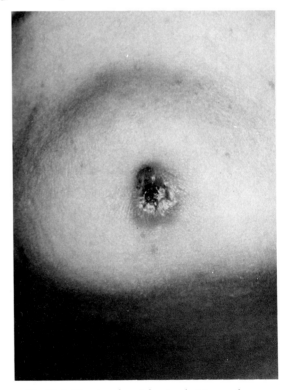

Fig. 31.6 *Sinus in submental region draining an abscess on a lower incisor.*

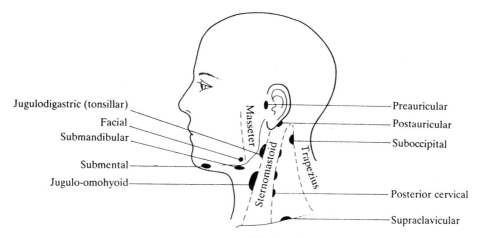

Fig. 31.7 *Cervical lymph nodes.*

Lymph nodes may also swell when there are disorders involving the immune system more generally, such as the glandular fever syndromes, AIDS and related syndromes, various other viral infections; bacterial infections such as syphilis and tuberculosis; parasites such as toxoplasmosis; non-infective lesions such as sarcoidosis; connective tissue diseases; mucocutaneous lymph node syndrome; and neoplasms such as lymphomas and leukaemias (Table 31.1; Fig. 31.9). In these instances, there is usually enlargement of many or all cervical lymph nodes and in some there is involvement of the whole reticuloendothelial system, with generalized lymph node enlargement (detectable clinically in neck, groin and/or axilla) and enlargement of the liver and spleen (hepatosplenomegaly). In the systemic infective disorders the nodes are usually firm, discrete, tender and mobile. In the lymphomas, particularly, the nodes may be rubbery, matted together and fixed to deeper structures.

About one-third of all the lymph nodes in the body are in the neck and the dental surgeon can often detect serious disease through examination of it. The anterior and posterior cervical nodes should be examined as well as other nodes, liver and spleen if systemic disease is a possibility.

Investigations

Investigations that may be indicated in patients with swellings in the neck are discussed under the relevant diseases below and in Volume 1, but diagnosis is based primarily on the history and clinical examination (Fig. 31.10).

ENLARGED CERVICAL LYMPH NODES

Most enlarged cervical lymph nodes are associated with

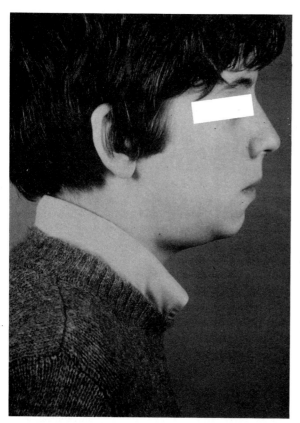

Fig. 31.8 *Submandibular staphylococcal lymphadenitis.*

Generalized enlarged lymph nodes

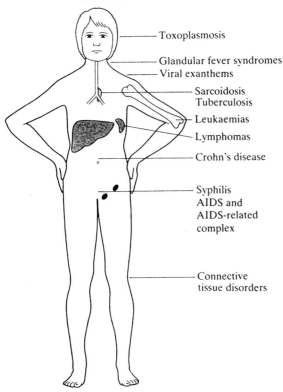

Toxoplasmosis

Glandular fever syndromes
Viral exanthems

Sarcoidosis
Tuberculosis

Leukaemias

Lymphomas

Crohn's disease

Syphilis
AIDS and
AIDS-related
complex

Connective
tissue disorders

Fig. 31.9 *Causes of generalized enlarged lymph nodes.*

viral upper respiratory infections, though sometimes the cause is a bacterial infection in the drainage area (basically anywhere in the head and neck), and occasionally it may be due to a more serious disorder.

Other causes are summarized in Table 31.1.

Infective inflammatory conditions

Viral infections with predominantly upper respiratory and oral manifestations

Any viral upper respiratory infection such as the common cold or viral tonsillitis can be responsible for enlarged cervical nodes (Table 31.1; Fig. 31.11).

Oral viral infections that may cause cervical lymph node infection are mainly those that also produce mouth ulcers, i.e. herpes simplex stomatitis, herpangina, and occasionally herpes zoster of the trigeminal nerve (Chapter 16).

Usually, several anterior triangle nodes—especially the jugulodigastric nodes—are enlarged, often bilaterally. Posterior triangle nodes are not enlarged and there is, of course, no generalized lymph node enlargement nor hepatosplenomegaly unless there are systemic complications or lesions elsewhere.

Non-bacterial infections with multiple systemic manifestations

These include mainly hand, foot and mouth disease (Chapter 16); viral exanthemata (chickenpox, measles, rubella); glandular fever syndromes (Epstein–Barr virus and cytomegalovirus infections and toxoplasmosis); and acquired immune deficiency syndrome and related syndromes (AIDS, human immunodeficiency virus (HIV) infection). In these disorders there are usually several anterior and often posterior triangle nodes enlarged, with generalized lymph node enlargement and, in some instances, hepatosplenomegaly.

1. *Hand, foot and mouth disease* (see Chapter 16).
2. *Chickenpox* (see Chapter 16).
3. *Measles.* Measles is an infection predominantly of childhood, caused by the measles virus. A maculopapular rash, conjunctival infection, acute respiratory symptoms, cervical lymphadenopathy and fever are the main features. During the prodrome, small white spots (Koplik's spots) may be seen in the buccal mucosa and are almost pathognomonic of measles (Fig. 31.12). They should not be confused with the yellowish ectopic sebaceous glands (Fordyce spots) seen in the buccal mucosa of healthy adults (Chapter 12), or with thrush (which will wipe off the mucosa).
4. *Rubella* (German measles). Rubella is a highly infectious viral disease that causes cervical lymphadenopathy, a macular rash starting on the face and behind the ears, mild fever, sore throat and, occasionally, palatal petechiae.

Transplacental infection may cause high-tone deafness of the fetus or, in more severe instances, mental handicap, blindness, cardiac defects or death. The deciduous dentition may be hypoplastic. Affected children excrete the virus for months or years after birth.

Because of the danger to the fetus, non-immune females should be immunized against rubella before childbearing age, and pregnant patients suspected of contracting rubella should have serological investigation to confirm immunity. Unfortunately, rashes resembling rubella (rubelliform rashes) are not uncommon, particularly with enterovirus infections, and therefore a

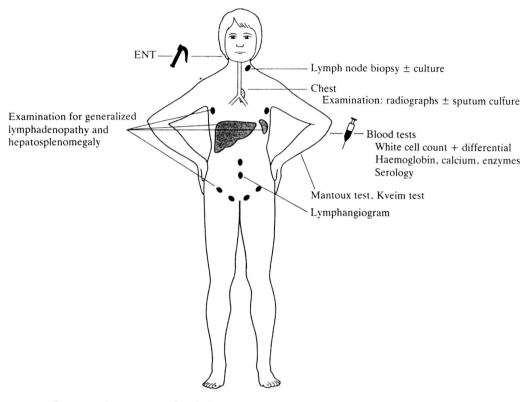

Fig. 31.10 *Investigations in lymphadenopathy that may be indicated if there is no obvious local disease.*

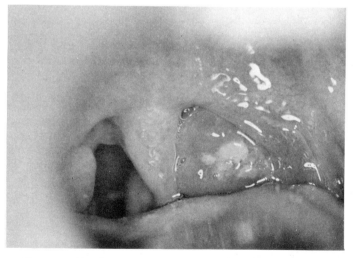

Fig. 31.11 *Tonsillitis: a common cause of cervical lymph node enlargement.*

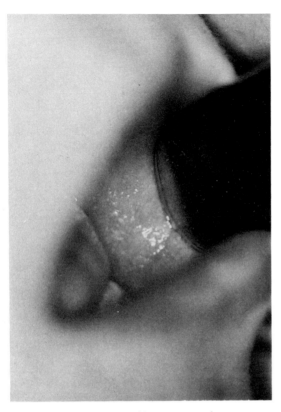

Fig. 31.12 *Koplik's spots in measles.*

clinical diagnosis of rubella may not always be accurate unless supported by serological data. Females who think they have had rubella may in fact not be immune, and if they become pregnant, their fetus may therefore be at risk.

5. *Glandular fever syndromes.* Glandular fever syndromes are characterized by fever, malaise and lymph node enlargement. Several infectious agents, including Epstein–Barr virus, cytomegalovirus, *Toxoplasma gondii* and HIV, can cause a similar syndrome. At present, the most frequent cause is the Epstein–Barr virus (EBV), one of the herpesvirus group.

(a) *EBV infection (infectious mononucleosis).* Infection with EBV appears to be spread by close oral contact, such as kissing. EBV is latent in pharyngeal epithelium and appears in the saliva from patients with infectious mononucleosis and for several months after clinical recovery. The incubation period extends over several weeks. Infection is common among young adults (especially students) and is often subclinical.

Clinical features

Infectious mononucleosis is protean in its clinical manifestations, which include mainly lymphadenopathy, sore throat, fever, malaise and rashes. Particular features predominate in some patients. In the anginose type of infectious mononucleosis (sore-throat type), the throat is sore,

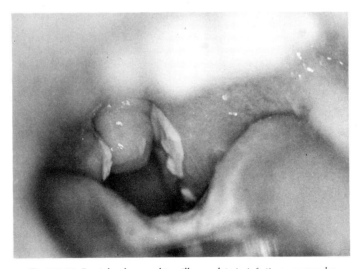

Fig. 31.13 *Faucial oedema and tonsillar exudate in infectious mononucleosis.*

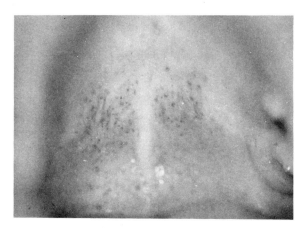

Fig. 31.14 *Palatal petechiae in infectious mononucleosis.*

with soft palate petechiae and a whitish exudate on oedematous tonsils (Figs. 31.13 and 31.14). Pharyngeal oedema may threaten the airway. The glandular type of infectious mononucleosis is characterized by general lymph node enlargement and splenomegaly; the febrile type by fever (Fig. 31.15).

Recovery can take weeks or months and the virus thereafter remains latent, in pharyngeal and/or salivary epithelial cells. Chronic infection may cause persistent malaise.

Ampicillin and amoxycillin very frequently cause a maculopapular rash of a non-allergic nature affecting the extensor surfaces of the limbs in patients with infectious mononucleosis.

Immunocompromised individuals may also be infected with EBV or the virus may be reactivated leading to recurrence of infectious mononucleosis or, rarely, producing lymphoma. EBV is also implicated in Burkitt's lymphoma, and nasopharyngeal carcinoma and in the hairy leukoplakia of HIV-infected patients (Volume 1 and Chapter 19).

Diagnosis

Characteristics of infectious mononucleosis are large numbers of atypical mononuclear cells in the blood and a

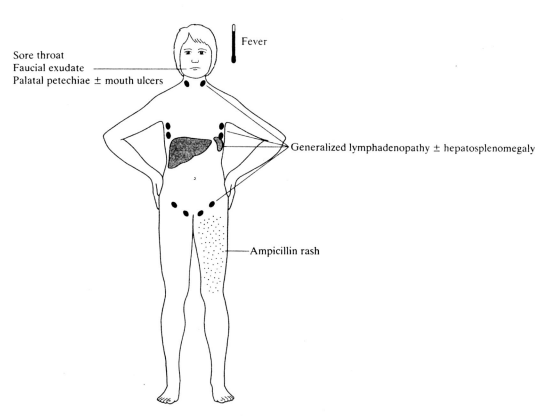

Fig. 31.15 *Features of infectious mononucleosis.*

Table 31.4
Glandular fever syndromes

	Infectious mononucleosis	Infectious lymphocytosis	Toxoplasmosis	AIDS and related syndromes
Fever	+	+	+	+
Lymphadenopathy	+	+	+	+
Other clinical features	Sore throat	–	Chorioretinitis	Opportunistic infections, neoplasms
Groups at high risk	Adolescents and young adults	Adolescents and young adults	Contracted from cat excreta or infected meat	Adult males mainly
Causal agent	Epstein–Barr virus (EBV)	Cytomegalovirus (CMV)	*Toxoplasma gondii*	Human immune deficiency viruses (HIV)
Paul–Bunnell test	+	–	–	–
Other tests	EBV antibody titres	CMV antibodies	Sabin–Feldman dye test Specific IgM antibodies	HIV antibody titres Lymphopenia T4 (CD4) cell numbers

wide variety of serological changes. Heterophil antibodies—human antibodies which agglutinate animal (sheep and horse) erythrocytes—are detectable by the Paul–Bunnell or Monospot tests, usually during the first or second week of the illness. The antibody levels decline and disappear over 3–6 months. Although several other antibodies against EBV appear during the course of infectious mononucleosis, the one most frequently tested for is the antibody to viral capsid antigen (VCA), the titre of which reaches a peak at about 4 weeks and persists for many years.

Patients who have a glandular fever type of syndrome but a negative Paul–Bunnell test are usually suffering not from EBV but from CMV, HIV or *Toxoplasma* infection (Table 31.4).

Management

No specific treatment is available, but supportive care should be given. Systemic corticosteroids are required if there is pharyngeal oedema severe enough to hazard the airway.

(b) *Cytomegalovirus infection.* Cytomegalovirus (CMV) is a ubiquitous herpesvirus that infects most people at some time during their lives. Transmission appears to be by sexual or intimate contact with persons excreting

CMV in saliva, urine and other secretions. The CMV can also be transmitted via blood, and transplacentally.

Clinical features

Infection in normal children or adults is usually asymptomatic, but the virus thereafter remains latent in the body. Transplacental infection may cause mental handicap or defects, and the affected child excretes CMV in urine for months or years after birth and is a major reservoir of the virus.

Immunocompromised patients, such as those with renal transplants and those with AIDS, may also be infected with CMV, or latent CMV may be reactivated. They also excrete the virus. In these patients, CMV acts as an opportunistic infection and may cause serious disease involving the lungs, liver, gastrointestinal tract, CNS and eyes. CMV may also be implicated in the aetiology of Kaposi's sarcoma and it is of interest therefore that Kaposi's sarcoma can affect patients with AIDS or who are immunocompromised for other reasons, e.g. after renal transplant because of immunosuppressive drugs.

Symptomatic CMV infection in otherwise apparently healthy children and adults causes the CMV mononucleosis syndrome of headache, back and abdominal pain, sore throat, fever and atypical lymphocytosis, but with a negative Paul–Bunnell test (infectious lympho-

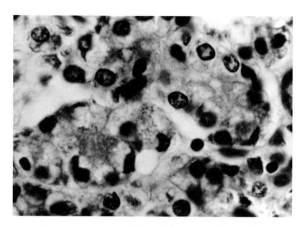

Fig. 31.16 *Cytomegalovirus inclusions in salivary gland.*

cytosis). Of particular interest, but uncertain significance, is the presence of CMV (the salivary gland inclusion virus) in salivary glands (Fig. 31.16). A relationship has been suggested between CMV and Sjögren's syndrome.

Diagnosis

Virus isolation and serology may be of value in the diagnosis.

Management

Treatment is usually symptomatic, though antivirals such as acyclovir are indicated in the immunocompromised host.

(c) *Toxoplasmosis.* Toxoplasmosis is another cause of a Paul–Bunnel-negative glandular fever syndrome. The causal parasite, *Toxoplasma gondii*, infests members of the cat family who excrete it in faeces. *T. gondii* survives in soil for up to 1 year, and infection is generally by ingestion of its cysts or oocysts, which are present in up to 10% of lamb and 25% of pork used for human consumption. The parasite may also be picked up directly from infected soil.

In normal patients, symptomatic toxoplasmosis manifests in one of the following ways.

(i) Glandular fever syndrome: with generalized lymphadenopathy, malaise, fever, sore throat, maculopapular rash, atypical lymphocytosis and a negative Paul–Bunnell test.

(ii) Ocular toxoplasmosis with chorioretinitis.

Transplacental transmission may result in mental handicap and other fetal defects.

Immunocompromised patients such as those with AIDS are at particular risk from *T. gondii* and many develop CNS involvement.

Diagnosis

Toxoplasmosis is diagnosed by:

(i) detection of serum antibodies by the Sabin–Feldman dye test, indirect haemagglutination test, or IgM fluorescent antibody test;

(ii) isolation of *T. gondii*;

(iii) histological demonstration of trophozoites.

Management

Toxoplasmosis is usually treated with pyrimethamine plus sulphadiazine.

(d) *AIDS and related syndromes* (Volume 1).

Acute non-specific bacterial infections

Any bacterial infection in the area of drainage, such as a dental abscess, pericoronitis, sinusitis, or a boil in the nose, can cause enlargement of anterior cervical lymph nodes (Fig. 31.17). Most of these infections are nonspecific. Usually only one or two nodes are enlarged, often unilaterally and only in the anterior triangle in most instances.

However, lesions on the back of the scalp or neck may cause enlargement of posterior cervical nodes.

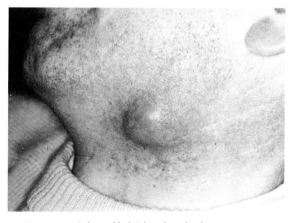

Fig. 31.17 *Submandibular lymph node abscess consequent to a periapical infection on the mandibular canine.*

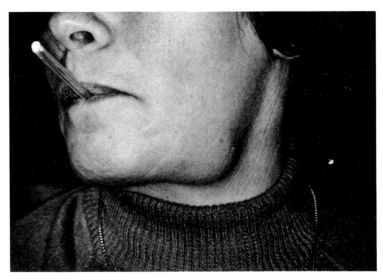

Fig. 31.18 *Facial node lymphadenitis. The source of infection was never identified.*

Acute specific bacterial infections

Occasionally, specific acute bacterial infections involve lymph nodes, particularly in young children who can develop acute lymphadenitis caused by *Staphylococcus aureus* in the absence of any detectable entry point for the organism. These infections, usually of a submandibular lymph node, should be treated with antibiotics—usually flucloxacillin because the *S. aureus* is often penicillinase producing. If the lesion is fluctuant and pointing, surgical drainage is needed (Figs. 31.8 and 31.18; see also Volume 1).

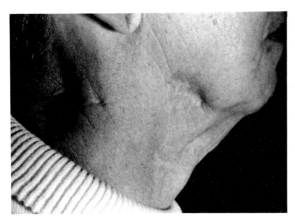

Fig. 31.19 *Tuberculous lymphadenitis often causes scarring on healing.*

Cat scratch disease

Cat scratch disease is almost always, but not invariably, acquired from a scratch or close contact with a cat. The infection, with an unidentified Gram-negative bacterium, is characterized by indolent, sometimes suppurative, regional lymphadenitis. Most cases are children who develop a primary, 'tender' non-pruritic papule, usually at the site of the scratch, after 3–10 days and then, within a few days to a few weeks, unilateral regional lymphadenitis, sometimes with mild fever and malaise. The disease is self-limiting.

The history together with an intradermal skin test and occasionally biopsy facilitate the diagnosis. There is often a mild leucocytosis and raised erythrocyte sedimentation rate (or plasma viscosity).

No treatment is available or needed, apart from supportive care.

Chronic bacterial infections

1. Syphilis (Chapter 16).
2. Tuberculosis (Fig. 31.19; see also Chapter 16).
3. Atypical mycobacterial infections (Chapter 16).
4. Brucellosis.

Chronic granulomatous disease

Chronic granulomatous disease is a rare genetic immune defect of leucocyte function in which neutrophils and macrophages fail to kill catalase-positive bacteria such as staphylococci. Patients suffer from recurrent, pyogenic infections and may develop suppurating cervical lymph nodes, showing granulomas on biopsy.

Mucocutaneous lymph node syndrome (Kawasaki disease)

This uncommon childhood disease of apparently infectious aetiology, initially reported from Japan, manifests with generalized lymphadenopathy, a rash with desquamation of hands and feet, oedematous lips and pharyngitis, and may be complicated by myocarditis. There is no specific diagnostic test or treatment.

Non-infective inflammatory conditions

Sarcoidosis (see also Chapter 26)

Sarcoidosis is a multisystem granulomatous disorder of unknown aetiology affecting Blacks ten times more frequently than Caucasians, twice as frequent in females as males, and affecting mainly young adults.

Sarcoidosis typically causes bilateral hilar lymphadenopathy, pulmonary infiltration and skin or eye lesions, but may present with cervical lymph node enlargement, oral swellings or salivary gland enlargement or dry mouth (Fig. 31.20). It is protean in its manifestations and can involve virtually any tissue.

Pulmary involvement is the most common and important lesion and causes cough and dyspnoea. Acute uveitis can progress to blindness. Hypercalcaemia is common and can cause kidney damage.

Diagnosis

Chest radiography (which often shows hilar lymph node enlargement), laboratory investigations (looking for raised serum levels of adenosine deaminase and angiotensin-converting enzyme), and sometimes the Kveim test are needed.

Biopsies of sarcoid lesions show granulomas (Fig. 31.21) and these must be differentiated from tuberculosis, Crohn's disease, and various foreign body reactions—particularly to zirconium and beryllium.

A gallium scan may be positive in the involved lymph nodes, salivary and lacrimal glands; gallium is taken up by macrophages in the granulomas.

The Kveim test is carried out by an intracutaneous injection of a heat-sterilized suspension of human lymphoid tissue affected with sarcoidosis. After 4–6 weeks the area is biopsied and, if positive, shows well-formed epithelioid non-caseating granulomas. The test is positive in about 80% of patients with sarcoidosis.

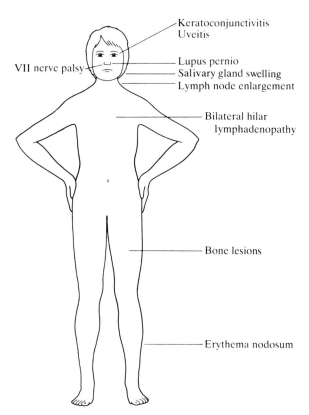

Fig. 31.20 *Features of sarcoidosis.*

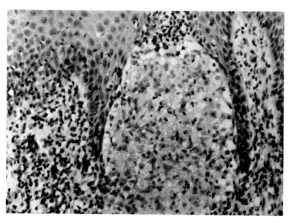

Fig. 31.21 *Photomicrograph from an oral mucosal lesion of sarcoidosis showing non-caseating granuloma.*

Management

Patients with only minor symptoms of sarcoidosis often require no treatment. Corticosteroids are used if there is active disease of the lungs or eyes, cerebral involvement, or other serious complications.

Crohn's disease (Chapter 16)

Connective tissue diseases

Cervical lymph nodes may be enlarged in rheumatoid arthritis or lupus erythematosus.

Neoplastic

Metastatic malignancy (other than lymphoid)

The usual neoplasms that metastasize to cervical lymph nodes are oral squamous carcinoma (Chapter 15), naso-pharyngeal carcinoma, and thyroid tumours. Usually one or more anterior cervical nodes are involved, often uni-laterally in oral neoplasms anteriorly in the mouth. Nodes on both sides of the neck may be involved (Fig. 31.22).

1. *Nasopharyngeal carcinoma.* Nasopharyngeal carcinoma is not a common tumour in the UK but is most prevalent in Chinese (and North Africans and Eskimos). It is almost certainly associated with Epstein–Barr virus and other co-factors (environmental and genetic). The tumour usually starts high in the nasopharynx and, because it does not occlude the pharynx to produce symptoms and is very inaccessible to casual inspection, frequently presents late and with a poor prognosis. The tumour usually presents in one or a combination of the following ways (Trotter's syndrome).

(a) Causing unilateral loss of hearing on the same side (ipsilateral) by invading and blocking the Eustachian tube.
(b) Causing pain, paraesthesia, or sensory loss in the ipsilateral face—by infiltrating the mandibular division of the trigeminal nerve.
(c) With cervical lymph node enlargement—metastatic (Fig. 31.23).

Nasopharyngeal carcinoma is a common cause of a malignant cervical node where no primary tumour is obvious, and therefore a lymph node biopsy and thorough ENT examination are required.

2. *Other metastatic neoplasms.* Rare causes include metastases from stomach or even testicular tumours to

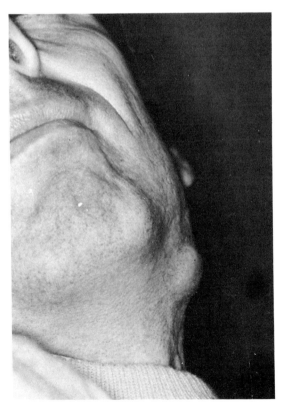

Fig. 31.22 *Metastasis of oral squamous carcinoma in cervical lymph node.*

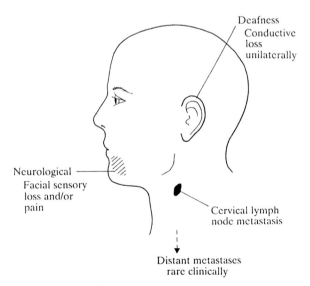

Deafness
Conductive loss unilaterally

Neurological
Facial sensory loss and/or pain

Cervical lymph node metastasis

Distant metastases rare clinically

Fig. 31.23 *Presentation of nasopharyngeal carcinoma.*

lower cervical nodes. In some patients with a malignant cervical lymph node, the primary tumour is *never* located. Lymph node biopsy may well be needed to help the diagnosis.

Lymphoid malignancies

In lymphoid malignancies there is usually swelling both of anterior and posterior cervical lymph nodes, together with generalized lymph node enlargement and often hepatosplenomegaly.

1. *Leukaemias*

(a) *Acute lymphoblastic leukaemia.* Acute lymphoblastic leukaemia (ALL), the most common leukaemia of childhood, has a peak incidence at 3–5 years of age.

Malignant lymphoblasts proliferate and infiltrate the viscera, skin and central nervous system. Marrow infiltration causes granulocytopenia (predisposing to infections), thrombocytopenia (causing a bleeding tendency), and anaemia—'there is no leukaemia without anaemia'—(Fig. 31.24; see also Chapter 16, and Volume 1).

Diagnosis of this and other leukaemias is confirmed by a blood film (shows blasts), white cell count (raised) and differential platelet count (reduced) and bone marrow biopsy. Treatment is mainly by chemotherapy—remarkably successful in acute lymphoblastic leukaemia.

(b) *Acute myeloblastic leukaemia.* Acute myeloblastic leukaemia (AML) is the most common acute leukaemia of adults. The features are similar to those of ALL except that central nervous system involvement is rare.

Orofacial features of the acute leukaemias

Cervical lymph node enlargement is almost invariable in acute leukaemias, oral bleeding and petechiae being the other common manifestations. Sometimes there is gingival swelling and mucosal ulceration (Fig. 31.25). Other findings include paraesthesia (particularly of the lower lip), extrusion of teeth, painful swellings over the mandible and parotid swelling (Mikulicz's syndrome). Since there is a secondary immunodeficiency, oral fungal infections, especially candidosis, are common and there is a predisposition to herpes simplex and herpes varicella–zoster lesions (Chapter 16). Many of the oral lesions are aggravated or caused by local factors and chemotherapy, and are readily infected by opportunistic micro-organisms. Such infections may lead to serious or fatal consequences.

Management of oral lesions

Microbiological investigations, with care to obtain specimens for anaerobic culture, are essential. Oral hygiene should be carefully maintained with 0.2% chlorhexidine mouthwashes and the use of a soft toothbrush. Prophylactic antifungal therapy (nystatin mouthwashes, 10 ml of 100 000 units of nystatin per millilitre used four times daily, nystatin pastilles (same dose), or amphotericin lozenges 10 mg four times daily) is also indicated. Viral infections should be treated with topical or systemic acyclovir (Chapter 15).

Many of the chemotherapeutic agents can cause oral ulceration. Methotrexate is a major offender, but ulceration may be prevented or ameliorated by concomitant intravenous administration of folinic acid ('leucovorin rescue'). Topical folinic acid may also be useful.

Dental treatment should only be carried out after consultation with the responsible physician. Conservative treatment is indicated where possible. Surgery, except for emergencies such as fractures, haemorrhage, potential airways obstruction or dangerous sepsis, should be deferred

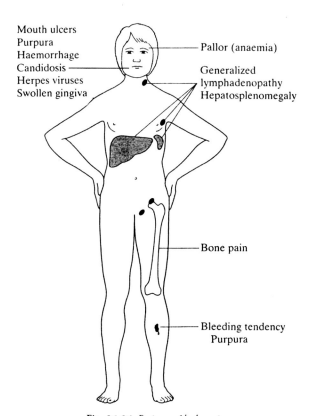

Mouth ulcers
Purpura
Haemorrhage
Candidosis
Herpes viruses
Swollen gingiva

Pallor (anaemia)

Generalized lymphadenopathy
Hepatosplenomegaly

Bone pain

Bleeding tendency
Purpura

Fig. 31.24 *Features of leukaemia.*

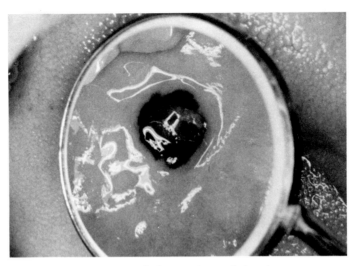

Fig. 31.25 *Oral purpura in acute leukaemia.*

until a remission phase because of the bleeding tendency and liability to infections.

Regional local analgesia injections may be contra-indicated because of the bleeding tendency. Extractions should be avoided because of the dangers of haemorrhage and infections such as osteomyelitis or septicaemia. Before surgery, platelet infusions or blood may be needed, and antibiotics should be given until the wound has healed.

(c) *Chronic lymphocytic leukaemia.* Chronic lymphocytic leukaemia (CLL) is the most common type of chronic leukaemia and mainly affects the elderly. Some patients are asymptomatic, while in others the disease is insidious with fever, weight loss, anorexia, haemorrhage and infections. Other effects are anaemia and thrombocytopenia. Lymph node enlargement is early and may be detected in the neck.

(d) *Chronic myeloid leukaemia.* Chronic myeloid leukaemia (CML) is characterized by proliferation of myeloid cells in the bone marrow, peripheral blood and other tissues, and mainly affects those over 40 years of age. Splenomegaly and hepatomegaly are common but lymphadenopathy is not. Anaemia, weight loss and joint pains are not uncommon.

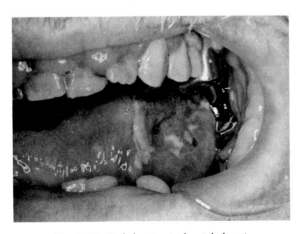

Fig. 31.26 *Oral ulceration in chronic leukaemia.*

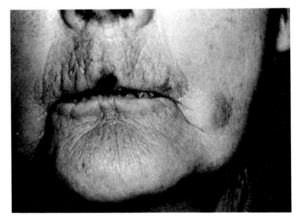

Fig. 31.27 *Recurrent herpes labialis in leukaemia. (Note haematoma in cheek.)*

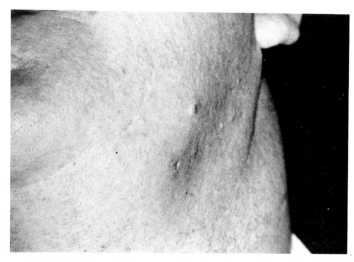

Fig. 31.28 *Enlarged rubbery cervical lymph nodes in Hodgkin's lymphoma.*

The prognosis is variable, but sooner or later there is transformation to an acute phase similar to AML (blast crisis).

Orofacial features of the chronic leukaemias

Gingival swelling is seen less commonly than in the acute leukaemias. Palatal mucosal swelling (submucosal leukaemic nodules), gingival bleeding, oral petechiae or oral ulceration may also be features (Fig. 31.26). Herpes simplex, zoster or candidosis may be seen (Fig. 31.27). Leukaemic infiltration of lacrimal and salivary glands can cause swelling—Mikulicz's syndrome.

Drug treatment of chronic leukaemia can also cause oral complications.

2. *Lymphomas.*

Lymphomas are malignant tumours that originate in lymph nodes and lymphoid tissue; they can originate from any type of lymphocyte but usually arise from B cells. Diagnosis is made from clinical findings (generalized lymph node enlargement and hepatosplenomegaly), radiography (hilar and abdominal lymph node enlargement), lymphangiography, and lymph node or lesional biopsy.

(a) *Hodgkin's disease.* Nearly one-half of all lymphomas are Hodgkin's disease, which can affect any age group, particularly males in middle age. There is progressive involvement of lymphoid tissue, often beginning in the neck (Fig. 31.28). The lymph nodes become enlarged, discrete and rubbery. Pain, fever, night sweats, weight loss, malaise, bone pain and pruritus are common. Drinking alcohol may cause pain in affected lymph nodes.

Treatment by chemotherapy and radiotherapy is now remarkably successful.

(b) *Non-Hodgkin's lymphoma.* Lymphomas other than Hodgkin's disease have a variable but generally poor prognosis, and occur primarily in the gastrointestinal tract and CNS. Often enlargement of cervical lymph nodes is the first sign but non-Hodgkin's lymphomas may occur in the faucial region (Fig. 31.29). Lymphomas, including those affecting the mouth, are a recognized complication of HIV infection.

(c) *Burkitt's lymphoma.* Lymphomatous deposits in many tissues, especially the jaws (in 50% of patients) characterize this lymphoma, which is most prevalent in children in Uganda and Kenya. Cervical lymph node enlargement is uncommon. The disease appears to be caused by Epstein–Barr virus in patients from endemic malaria areas, and responds well to chemotherapy.

Orofacial aspects of lymphomas

Painless enlarged cervical lymph nodes are the initial complaint in 50% of cases, but a lymphoma may occasionally produce primary or secondary tumours in the oral cavity. Involvement of Waldeyer's ring is more common in non-Hodgkin's lymphomas than in Hodgkin's disease. AIDS predisposes to oral lymphomas.

Lymphomas may appear as swellings, often of the pharynx, palate, tongue, gingiva or lips. Herpes zoster,

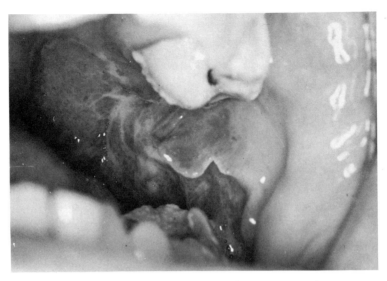

Fig. 31.29 *Non-Hodgkin's lymphoma in the fauces—a typical site.*

herpetic stomatitis and oral candidosis may be seen, since these patients develop a secondary immunodeficiency.

ENLARGED SALIVARY GLANDS

These are discussed in Chapter 24 and their causes listed in Table 31.2.

ENLARGED THYROID GLANDS

Thyroiditis, hyperthyroidism and hypothyroidism may be associated with a goitre, but more discrete lumps are often neoplastic. Patients should be referred to the relevant specialist.

OTHER LUMPS IN THE NECK

Cystic hygroma

Cystic hygroma is a developmental anomaly of the lymphatics presenting as a swelling of the neck seen before the age of 2 years. It may extend into the mediastinum and/or tongue.

Since it is unsightly and prone to infection or internal haemorrhage, cystic hygroma is usually surgically removed.

Branchial cyst

This is a lymphoepithelial cyst which may arise from enclavement of salivary tissue in a lymph node or from the cervical sinus. It usually becomes apparent in the third decade as a cyst, and requires excision.

Carotid body tumour

Carotid body tumour is a slow-growing but malignant neoplasm of chromaffin cells that both invades locally and metastasizes. It presents as a mass over the internal carotid and transmits the carotid pulsation. It should be resected.

Dermoid cyst

This is a developmental cyst lined by epidermis and cutaneous appendages, which commonly arises above the mylohyoid muscle in the midline of the neck. The dermoid cyst usually becomes clinically obvious in the second decade of life and causes elevation of the tongue. Occasionally dermoid cysts become infected. Dermoid cysts should be removed surgically.

Thyroglossal cyst

The thyroglossal cyst arises from remnants of the thyroglossal duct and is therefore midline at any point between the tongue and thyroid gland, and moves up on protrusion of the tongue. The cyst may cause dysphagia or become infected; it should be surgically removed.

Pharyngeal pouch

This is a rare evagination from the pharynx (pulsion diverticulum) that appears because of a potential weakness in the pharyngeal muscles. Dysphagia characterized by regurgitation of food results and may cause aspiration into the lungs.

CAUSES OF DIFFUSE SWELLING OF THE NECK

Oedema

Oedema from trauma, infective lesions, angioedema or, rarely, in nephritis or superior vena cava obstruction may present with diffuse swelling of the neck and often the face. Fascial space infections are discussed in Volume 1; these may produce a hazard to the airway which can asphyxiate the patient.

Superior vena cava obstruction

Obstruction of venous return to the heart, usually by an infiltrating lung cancer, may produce oedema and cyanosis of face, neck and arms.

Surgical emphysema

Escape of air into the tissues, usually as a consequence of operative intervention, may result in diffuse swelling which characteristically is painless but gives rise to crepitus on palpation. This usually resolves spontaneously but it may be prudent to give an antimicrobiotic.

Neoplasms infiltrating

Rarely, neoplasms present as a diffuse swelling.

FURTHER READING

Eisenbud L., Scuibba J. J., Mir R., Sachs S. A. (1984). Oral presentations in non-Hodgkins lymphoma: a review of thirty one cases. *Oral Surg.*, **57**: 272–280.
Ioachim H. L., Cooper M. C., Hellman G. C. (1985). Lymphomas in men at high risk for acquired immune deficiency syndrome (AIDS); a study of 21 cases. *Cancer*, **56**: 2831–2842.
Scully C., Cawson R. A. (1987). *Medical problems in dentistry*, 2nd edn. Bristol: Wright.

Section VI
Oral Manifestations of Systemic Disease

Oral lesions are usually the result of local disease but may be the early signs of, or in some instances may be responsible for, the main symptoms in patients with systemic disease.

Many systemic diseases can produce oral manifestations, but the most significant are infective, haematological, gastrointestinal, connective tissue, dermatological, bone and endocrine disorders. Constant exposure of mucosal lesions to moisture, trauma, and a complex flora presumably explains why many different lesions break down to produce mouth ulcers.

The most common and important systemic diseases are discussed at greater length in the earlier chapters of this volume, and in other volumes of the series. The next two chapters are only a brief summary, designed mainly for revision for examinations.

Chapter 32 summarizes oral manifestations of systemic disease by considering those diseases which affect specific oral tissues. Chapter 33 tabulates the oral manifestations of specific systemic diseases.

Diseases affecting specific orofacial tissues

DENTAL MANIFESTATIONS OF SYSTEMIC DISEASE

Loosening and early loss of teeth

Early loss of teeth is usually caused by trauma, dental caries or destructive periodontal disease. Congenital disorders such as Down's syndrome (mongolism: Fig. 32.1) or acquired disorders such as diabetes mellitus or immune defects including AIDS may predispose to periodontal disease. Teeth are lost early in other systemic disorders, for example hypophosphatasia (Table 32.1).

Retarded eruption of teeth

Congenital hypopituitarism, congenital hypothyroidism (cretinism), Down's syndrome, cleidocranial dysplasia, cytotoxic drugs and radiotherapy may cause retarded eruption, but most cases are of local aetiology.

Dental aplasia

Wisdom teeth, second premolars and upper lateral incisors are sometimes absent in otherwise normal individuals, probably because of some unidentified genetic

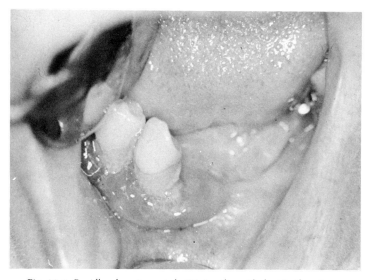

Fig. 32.1 *Rapidly advancing periodontitis together with short tooth roots causes early tooth loss in Down's syndrome.*

Table 32.1
Pathological causes of loosening of the teeth

Local causes
Periodontitis
Trauma
Neoplasms

Systemic causes
Early onset (accelerated) periodontitis in:
    Down's syndrome
    Diabetes mellitus
    Leucopenia or leucocyte defects
    AIDS-related disorders
    Rapidly progressive periodontitis
    Juvenile periodontitis

Genetic syndromes
    Hypophosphatasia
    Papillon– Lefevre syndrome (Volume 3)
    Ehlers–Danlos syndrome (type VIII)

Neoplasms
Eosinophilic granuloma

Table 32.2
Causes of discoloration of teeth

Extrinsic stains	Poor oral hygiene
	Smoking
	Beverages/foods
	Drugs, e.g. iron, chlorhexidine
	Black stain
	Green stain
Intrinsic stains	Trauma
	Caries
	Restorative material, e.g. amalgam
	Pink spot (internal resorption)
	Drugs—mainly tetracyclines
	Fluorosis
	Kernicterus (severe neonatal jaundice)
	Congenital disorders: amelogenesis imperfecta, dentinogenesis imperfecta
	Porphyria

variance. Absence of several teeth may indicate cleido-cranial dysplasia or ectodermal dysplasia (Fig. 32.2).

Extra teeth

Extra teeth are rare and the cause is usually unknown, but they are common in cleidocranial dysplasia.

Malformed and discoloured teeth

Local infection or trauma, or unknown factors, may cause malformation of single (or a few) teeth. The lower premolars are usually affected because there is infection of their deciduous predecessors—such hypoplastic permanent teeth are termed Turner's teeth. The upper incisors may be malformed if there is trauma to the deciduous incisors. Radiotherapy involving the jaws may also be implicated, as may cytotoxic drugs. Enamel hypoplasia may be seen in children with congenital rubella or cytomegalovirus infection, but the classical Hutchinsonian incisors and Moon's (or mulberry) molars of congenital syphilis are extremely rare in the UK (Fig. 32.3). Hypoplasia is seen in malabsorption syndromes and in some forms of epidermolysis bullosa and peg-shaped teeth may be found in ectodermal dysplasia.

Erosion of teeth may occur because of the use of acidic drinks or as a feature of gastric regurgitation in bulimia or anorexia nervosa.

Most dental discoloration is of local aetiology and caused by food and beverages (such as tea), medicines such as chlorhexidine, or poor oral hygiene (Table 32.2). Tetracyclines given to a pregnant or lactating mother may discolour the child's teeth and, if given to a child, particularly those under the age of 8 years, may cause significant brown intrinsic staining (Fig. 32.4).

Fluoride, at the concentrations present in water supplies in Western countries, or given prophylactically, may occasionally produce inconsequential minute white flecks in the teeth. Concentrations over 2 p.p.m. may produce clinically significant fluorosis which at high concentrations may be dramatic (Fig. 32.5).

Dentinogenesis imperfecta may be seen in some patients with osteogenesis imperfecta (Fig. 32.6; see also Chapter 1). Amelogenesis imperfecta is not usually associated with any systemic disease (Fig. 32.7).

PERIODONTAL MANIFESTATIONS OF SYSTEMIC DISEASE

Gingival swelling

Gingival swelling is seen in some inflammatory periodontal disease and may be produced by drugs such as phenytoin (an anticonvulsant), cyclosporin (an immunosuppressive agent), nifedipine (an antihypertensive drug), diltiazem (an anti-anginal) and by various systemic disorders (Table 32.3).

A degree of gingival swelling may be seen in herpetic stomatitis (Fig. 32.8), pregnancy, leukaemia (Fig. 32.9), Crohn's disease, scurvy, Wegener's granulomatosis, sar-

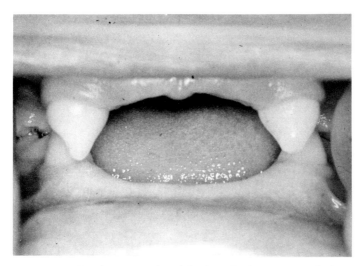

Fig. 32.2 *Hypodontia in ectodermal dysplasia. Teeth present may also be peg-shaped.*

coidosis, amyloidosis and mucopolysaccharidoses, and various localized swellings (epulides) may be manifestations of systemic disease (Chapter 21 and Table 21.2).

Gingival bleeding

Bleeding from the gingival margins is common and almost invariably a consequence of gingivitis (Table 32.4). The tendency to gingivitis is slightly increased in some patients taking oral contraceptives and in some pregnant women (especially during the second trimester).

Gingival haemorrhage, however, may be a premonitory feature in platelet or some vascular disorders and is commonly a problem in leukaemics.

Pigmentation

Gingival pigmentation is usually seen in certain races

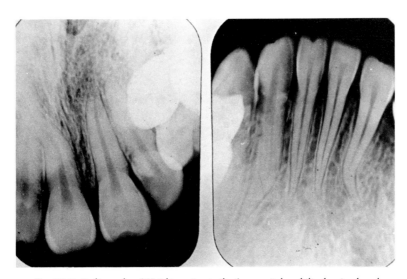

Fig. 32.3 *Radiographs of Hutchinsonian teeth of congenital syphilis showing barrel-shaped incisors with notched edge but otherwise normal structure.*

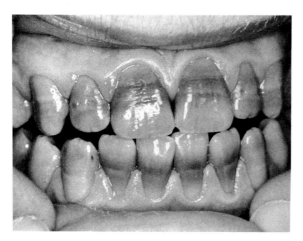

Fig. 32.4 *Tetracycline discoloration, showing the severe cosmetic deformity that may result.*

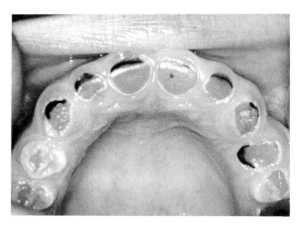

Fig. 32.6 *Dentinogenesis imperfecta: the normal enamel chips away from the abnormal dentine but secondary dentine formation usually prevents exposure of the pulp.*

(and can be seen even in those who are not black) (Fig. 32.10).

Addison's disease and melanoma are the most important acquired causes of pigmentation (Chapter 20; see also Volume 3).

Redness

Gingivitis is the usual cause of gingival redness—and then is usually restricted to the gingival margins and interdental papillae.

More widespread erythema, particularly if associated with soreness, is usually caused by desquamative gingivitis—usually due to lichen planus or mucous membrane pemphigoid (Chapter 16), rarely by pemphigus. Red lesions may also represent erythroplasia, or neoplasms such as carcinoma, Wegener's granulomatosis or Kaposi's sarcoma.

Ulcers

Acute ulcerative (necrotizing) gingivitis (Fig. 32.11; see also Volume 3), or a similar type of disorder, in rare in-

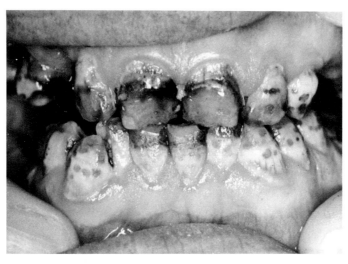

Fig. 32.5 *Severe fluorosis in an immigrant from an area with an extremely high natural fluoride level in the water.*

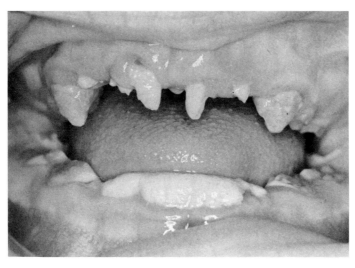

Fig. 32.7 *Amelogenesis imperfecta.*

stances is a complication of AIDS, neutropenia or leukaemia, and in the malnourished or some immunosuppressed patients may spread to the cheek (noma;
cancrum oris). Aphthae (sometimes) and other causes of
mouth ulcers (rarely) involve the gingiva (Table 32.5).
Gingival ulcers are sometimes self-induced (artefactual) in
psychologically disturbed or mentally handicapped
patients (Fig. 32.12).

ORAL MUCOSAL MANIFESTATIONS OF SYSTEMIC DISEASE

Blisters

The most important vesiculobullous disorders affecting
the oral mucosa are pemphigoid and pemphigus. The bullae of pemphigus break down rapidly to produce ulcers.

Table 32.3
Causes of gingival swelling

	Generalized swelling	Localized swelling
Local causes	Gingivitis Hyperplastic gingivitis due to mouth breathing	Abscesses Cysts Pyogenic granuloma Neoplasms

Systemic causes	Hereditary gingival fibromatosis
	Drugs: Phenytoin
	      Cyclosporin
	      Nifedipine
	      Diltiazem
	Pregnancy
	Sarcoidosis and Crohn's disease
	Leukaemia
	Wegener's granulomatosis
	Scurvy
	Amyloidosis
	Rare inborn errors of metabolism,
	e.g. mucopolysaccharidoses
		Pregnancy
		Sarcoidosis
		Wegener's granulomatosis
		
		Amyloidosis
		Neoplasms

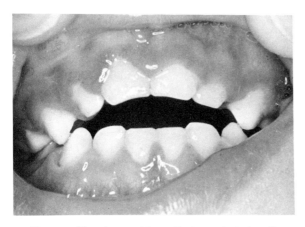

Fig. 32.8 *Herpetic stomatitis manifesting as gingival swelling.*

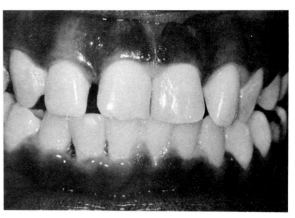

Fig. 32.10   *Racial gingival pigmentation.*

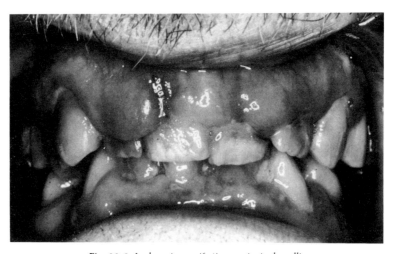

Fig. 32.9 *Leukaemia manifesting as gingival swelling.*

Table 32.4
Causes of gingival bleeding

Local causes
Chronic gingivitis
Chronic periodontitis
Acute ulcerative gingivitis

Systemic causes
Any condition causing exacerbation of gingivitis (e.g.
pregnancy)
Leukaemia
Other causes of purpura
Clotting defects
Drugs, e.g. anticoagulants

The bullae of mucous membrane pemphigoid may or may not be bloodfilled and, in the former case, a bleeding tendency must be excluded. Bloodfilled blisters may be caused by localized oral purpura (angina bullosa haemorrhagica). The gingival bullae of pemphigus and pemphigoid break down rapidly to produce desquamative gingivitis. Epidermolysis bullosa and erythema multiforme may present with bullae or vesicles, but ulcers are more common (Chapter 16).

Blisters on the lips are usually a manifestation of recurrent herpes simplex infection. In the immunocompromised, widespread herpes simplex infection may involve the lips and face and oral tissues (Chapter 16).

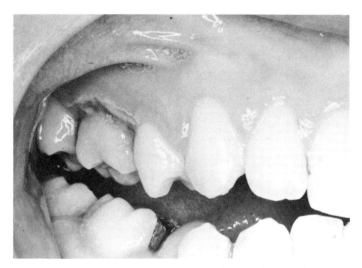

Fig. 32.11 *Acute necrotizing gingivitis may be a manifestation of AIDS.*

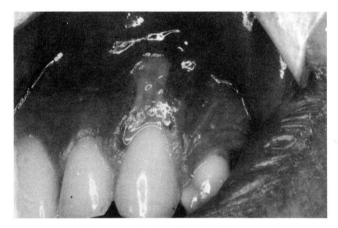

Fig. 32.12 *Artefactual gingival ulceration.*

Purpura

Oral purpura is most frequently a manifestation of a bleeding tendency caused by thrombocytopenia (Fig. 32.13) and may also be seen in infectious mononucleosis, rubella or AIDS. Petechiae may also occur in amyloidosis or scurvy. Bloodstained crusting on the lips is characteristic of erythema multiforme.

Pigmentation

Race is the most important cause of pigmentation. Addison's disease, melanoma, pigmentary incontinence and other causes (Chapter 20) must be excluded. Peutz–Jeghers syndrome is the association of circumoral melanosis with small intestine polyposis.

Red areas (see also Chapter 18)

Telangiectasia may be a manifestation of hereditary haemorrhagic telangiectasia or systemic sclerosis, or may follow radiotherapy. Haemangiomas may occasionally extend deeply and rarely involve the ipsilateral meninges, producing a facial angioma and epilepsy, sometimes with mental handicap (Sturge–Weber syndrome).

Localized red areas may represent erythroplasia, car-

Table 32.5

Main causes of ulcers associated with systemic disease

Microbial diseases
   Herpetic stomatitis
   Chickenpox
   Herpes zoster
   Hand, foot and mouth disease
   Herpangina
   Infectious mononucleosis
   Acute ulcerative gingivitis
   Tuberculosis
   Syphilis
   AIDS
Rarely fungal infections

Malignant neoplasms

Cutaneous disease
   Erosive lichen planus
   Pemphigus
   Pemphigoid
   Erythema multiforme

Blood disorders
   Anaemia
   Leukaemia
   Neutropenia

Gastrointestinal diseases
   Coeliac disease
   Crohn's disease
   Ulcerative colitis

Connective tissue disease
   Lupus erythematosus

Drugs
   Cytotoxic and other agents

Others
   Behcet's syndrome
   Reiter's syndrome

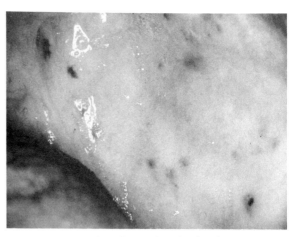

Fig. 32.13 *Oral petechiae in idiopathic thrombocytopenia.*

Various infections or systemic disorders, particularly those of blood, gastrointestinal tract or skin, also produce mouth ulcers, as may drugs (Table 32.5).

Angular stomatitis (see Chapter 16)

This is usually associated with denture-induced stomatitis and is then of local aetiology. In other instances a haematinic deficiency state, sometimes caused by malabsorption, and occasionally AIDS, should be excluded.

White patches (Chapter 19)

Thrush is a 'disease of the diseased' and produces white patches. An increasingly important cause, especially in high-risk groups, is HIV infection (Fig. 32.14; Chapter 19;

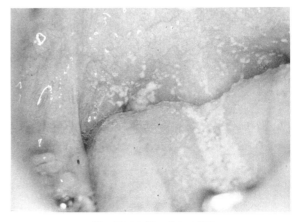

Fig. 32.14 *Thrush in AIDS.*

cinoma, lichen planus or lupus erythematosus. Kaposi's sarcoma may present as a red, purple, brown or bluish macule or nodule. Lingual depapillation in deficiencies of iron, folate or vitamin B12 may produce the red tongue termed glossitis. Erythema migrans may also produce red patches (Chapters 17 and 18).

   Xerostomia predisposes to candidosis (Chapter 25). Irradiation-induced mucositis is a further cause of a red sore mouth (Volume 1).

Ulcers (Chapter 14, 15 and 16)

Oral ulcers are often caused by trauma or are recurrent aphthae. Malignant neoplasms may present as ulcers.

Table 32.6
Main causes of oral white lesions

Local causes
Frictional keratosis
Smoker's keratosis
Idiopathic keratosis
Carcinoma
Burns
Skin grafts

Systemic causes
White sponge naevus
Candidosis
Lichen planus
Lupus erythematosus
Hairy leukoplakia (AIDS)
Syphilitic keratosis
Chronic renal failure

Table 32.7
Causes of facial swelling

Inflammatory
   Oral infections
   Cutaneous infections
   Insect bites
   Crohn's disease
   Melkersson–Rosenthal syndrome
   Sarcoidosis

Traumatic
   Oedema or haematoma
   Surgical emphysema

Immunologically mediated (non-inflammatory)
   Allergic and hereditary angioedema

Endocrine and metabolic
   Obesity
   Systemic corticosteroid therapy
   Cushing's syndrome
   Myxoedema
   Acromegaly
   Nephrotic syndrome

Superior vena cava syndrome (*obstruction to SVC*, e.g. bronchial carcinoma)

Cysts

Hamartomas

Neoplasms

Foreign bodies

Volume 1). Leukoplakia may be associated with smoking, occasionally with syphilis, candidosis, or chronic renal failure. Hairy leukoplakia is a feature of AIDS. Lichen planus and lupus erythematosus may present as white lesions (Table 32.6). Lichenoid lesions are rarely associated with liver disease or graft versus host disease.

Swelling of the lips or face

This is usually caused by inflammatory oedema associated with trauma or dental abscess, but may be allergic in nature or caused by a complement pathway anomaly

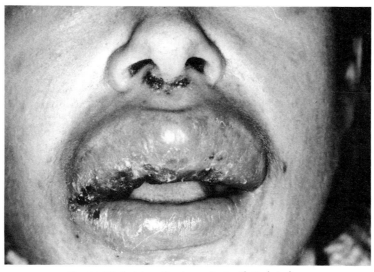

Fig. 32.15 *Facial swelling in a patient with Crohn's disease.*

(angioedema) or may be seen in sarcoidosis or Crohn's disease of the mouth (Table 32.7; Fig. 32.15; Chapter 22).

Swelling of the tongue may be traumatic, inflammatory or allergic in origin. A chronically enlarged tongue may also be a feature of Down's syndrome, cretinism, acromegaly, multiple endocrine adenoma type III (IIb), and amyloid disease.

SALIVARY MANIFESTATIONS OF SYSTEMIC DISEASE

Dry mouth (Chapter 25)

The complaint of a dry mouth (xerostomia) is by no means always supported by objective evidence—and not infrequently has a psychogenic basis. Drugs with anticholinergic or sympathomimetic activity are the most common cause of xerostomia (Table 32.8). Tricyclic anti-

Table 32.8
Causes of dry mouth

Drugs with anticholinergic effects
Atropine and analogues
Tricyclic antidepressants
Antihistamines
Antiemetics
Phenothiazines
Antihypertensives

Drugs with sympathomimetic effects
Ephedrine
Decongestants
Bronchodilators
Amphetamines and appetite suppressants

Dehydration
Diabetes mellitus
Diarrhoea and vomiting
Severe haemorrhage

Organic disease of glands
Sjögren's syndrome
Irradiation damage
Mumps and other infections (temporary)
Sarcoidosis
Graft versus host disease

Psychogenic
Anxiety states
Depression
Hypochondriasis

Others
HIV infection

depressants, phenothiazines and lithium are most commonly implicated.

Sjögren's syndrome (Chapter 25) and sarcoidosis are the systemic disorders most commonly associated with this complaint. Severe dehydration from any cause, irradiation of the major salivary glands and *rarely* graft versus host disease may produce xerostomia.

Salivary gland swelling (Chapter 24)

Mumps is the most common cause of salivary gland swelling, particularly in children. Duct obstruction, Sjögren's syndrome, sarcoidosis and sialoadenosis (sialosis) usually affect adults (Table 32.9). Sialosis may be a feature of, for example, diabetes or alcoholic cirrhosis.

Sialorrhoea (Chapter 26)

Painful oral lesions, or foreign bodies (e.g. new dentures), may cause sialorrhoea (ptyalism), as may cholinergic drugs such as anticholinesterases and the analgesics buprenorphine and meptazinol.

Drooling of saliva may occur in normal infants, in teething, and in those with pharyngeal obstruction in various disorders in which there is poor neuromuscular

Table 32.9
Causes of salivary gland swelling

Local causes	
Inflammatory	Ascending sialadenitis
Neoplasms	
Others	Duct obstruction
Systemic causes	
Inflammatory	Mumps
	Sjögren's syndrome
	Sarcoidosis
	Actinomycosis
	HIV infection
Others	Sialosis
	Mikulicz's disease (lymphoepithelial lesion and syndrome)
Drug associated	Chlorhexidine
	Phenylbutazone
	Iodine compounds
	Thiouracil
	Catecholamines
	Sulphonamides
	Phenothiazines
	Methyldopa

co-ordination (mentally handicapped, Parkinsonism, facial palsy) and, *rarely*, rabies.

JAW AND TEMPOROMANDIBULAR JOINT MANIFESTATIONS OF SYSTEMIC DISEASE

Acquired swellings of the jaw are usually cysts, neoplasms (primary or metastatic) or fibro-osseous lesions (see below and Chapters 5–8). The mandible may become protrusive in acromegaly.

Pain in the jaw

Infection, fractures, cysts or neoplasms are the common causes of pain in the jaw, but occasionally pain is related to neurological disease (e.g. trigeminal neuralgia), psychogenic disease (e.g. atypical facial pain), vascular disease (e.g. bone infarcts such as in sickle cell anaemia), drugs such as vinca alkaloids, or is referred (e.g. angina pectoris—see Orofacial pain: Chapter 27).

Jaw radiolucencies

Cystic lesions (Chapter 5 and 6)

The vast majority of jaw cysts are benign dental cysts at the apices of non-vital teeth. Some other benign cysts— dentigerous cysts—are associated with unerupted teeth. More aggressive in terms of their recurrence are ameloblastomas and odontogenic keratocysts (primordial cysts). The latter may be associated with basal cell naevi, widely spaced eyes (hypertelorism), calcified falx cerebri, and skeletal anomalies in Gorlin's syndrome (Fig. 32.16).

Non-cystic lesions

Brown tumours in osteitis fibrosa cystica are now rare in hyperparathyroidism; loss of the lamina dura is more typical (Chapter 2). Fibrous dysplasia and Paget's disease may have osteolytic phases (Chapter 8).

Inflammatory disorders, especially osteomyelitis, may produce jaw radiolucencies particularly in the mandible; some of these patients have reduced host resistance because of alcoholism or, occasionally, immune defects.

Oral malignant neoplasms, predominantly squamous carcinoma, may invade the jaw bone, but there may also be neoplastic deposits in histiocytoses, myelomatosis, leukaemia, or metastases—particularly from breast, bronchus and stomach (Fig. 32.17; Chapter 7).

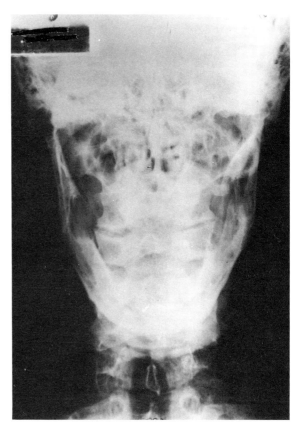

Fig. 32.16 *Odontogenic keratocysts in both mandibular rami in Gorlin's syndrome.*

A few patients with systemic sclerosis have widening of the periodontal ligament space visible on radiographs.

Jaw radio-opacities

Radio-opacities are predominantly caused by retained elements of dental hard tissues, foreign bodies or lesions unassociated with systemic disease. Osteomas are usually seen in isolation but may, with desmoid tumours and colonic polyps (which may undergo malignant change), be a manifestation of Gardner's syndrome. Fibrous dysplasia and Paget's disease may cause radio-opaque lesions (Fig. 32.18; Chapter 8), and some metastases (e.g. prostatic) are osteoblastic and cause radio-opacities.

Temporomandibular joint (Chapter 9)

Systemic disorders only rarely produce symptoms in the temporomandibular joints. The most common cause of

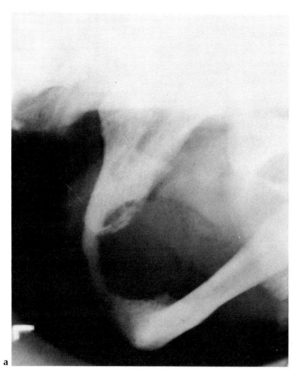
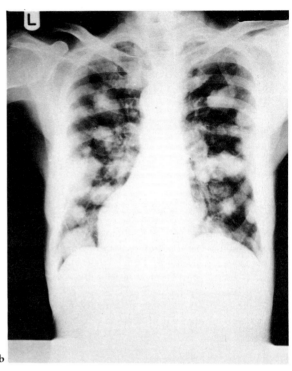

a   b

Fig. 32.17 *(a) Osteolytic metastasis in mandible in a patient with carcinomatosis. (b) Chest radiograph shows widespread metastases.*

pain is the mandibular pain–dysfunction syndrome (Chapter 9).

Juvenile rheumatoid arthritis may involve the joint and produce ankylosis. In contrast, adult rheumatoid arthritis frequently produces *asymptomatic* radiographic changes in the joint. Prolonged steroid treatment occasionally causes aseptic necrosis in the joint. Infective arthritides affecting the temporomandibular joint are rare.

CHANGES IN OROFACIAL SENSATION AND MOVEMENT AS MANIFESTATIONS OF SYSTEMIC DISEASE

Burning mouth (oral dysaesthesia: Chapter 27)

The complaint of a burning sensation in the mouth—especially affecting the tongue—is common. Most patients are middle-aged or elderly women.

Occasionally the sensation is associated with obvious disease such as erythema migrans, candidosis, lichen planus or glossitis due to a deficiency state. More frequently, the mucosa appears normal.

A deficiency state (deficiency of vitamin B12, folic acid or iron) and occasional causes such as denture-related

Table 32.10
Causes of burning mouth

Local lesions
Candidosis
Erythema migrans (geographic tongue)
Lichen planus
Others

Systemic causes
Drugs (e.g. Captopril)
Psychogenic
   Cancerophobia
   Depression
   Anxiety states
   Hypochondriasis
Deficiency states
   Pernicious anaemia
   Folate deficiency
   Iron deficiency
Diabetes

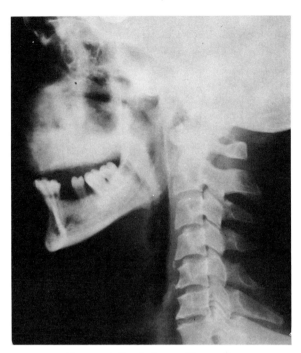

Fig. 32.18 *Paget's disease of the maxilla.*

problems and diabetes must be excluded, but many patients seem to have this complaint as a result of anxiety states, depression or cancerophobia (Table 32.10).

Cacogeusia and halitosis (Chapter 22)

Cacogeusia (an unpleasant taste in the mouth) and halitosis are usually a consequence of poor oral hygiene and oral or nasal infections, starvation, xerostomia, drugs, or psychogenic disorders, but may appear in various systemic disorders such as suppurative respiratory infections, hepatic or renal failure, diabetic ketosis and gastrointestinal disease (Table 32.11).

Loss of taste (Chapter 29)

Anosmia commonly produces an apparent loss of sense of taste. Lingual nerve damage, xerostomia, some drugs such as penicillamine, psychotic disorders, and neurological disease such as cerebral metastases and lesions affecting the chorda tympani (including some facial nerve lesions) may be responsible for a loss of the sense of taste.

Table 32.11
Causes of unpleasant taste and mouth odour

Local causes
Dental infections
    Chronic periodontitis
    Acute ulcerative gingivitis
    Pericoronitis
    Chronic dental abscesses
    Dry socket
Nasal disease
    Chronic sinusitis
    Oro-antral fistula
    Foreign body in nose

Systemic causes
Salivary gland disorders causing xerostomia
    Sjögren's syndrome
    Irradiation damage
    Mumps
Psychogenic causes
    Depression
    Anxiety states
    Psychoses
    Hypochondriasis
Drugs
    Drugs causing dry mouth (see Table 32.8)
    Metronidazole, lithium, gold, etc.
Foods
    Garlic
    Curries
    Onions
Drugs
    Solvent abuse
    Alcohol
    Chloral hydrate
    Nitrites and nitrates
    Dimethyl sulphoxide
    Cytotoxic drugs
    Phenothiazines
    Amphetamines
    Smoking
Respiratory tract infections
Liver failure and cirrhosis
Renal failure
Diabetic ketosis
Gastrointestinal disease

Pain (Chapter 27)

Nearly all oral and dental pain is of local aetiology—usually a consequence of caries, trauma or infections (Table 32.12). Oral pain may also be neurological in origin, particularly idiopathic trigeminal neuralgia; vascular in origin, such as migraine or giant-cell arteritis; psycho-

Table 32.12
Causes of orofacial pain

Local causes
Disease of the teeth and supporting tissues
  Trauma
  Pulpitis
  Periapical periodontitis
  Lateral periodontal abscess
  Acute ulcerative gingivitis
  Pericoronitis
Diseases of the jaws
  Trauma
  Fractures
  Osteomyelitis and dry socket
  Infected cysts
  Malignant neoplasms
Diseases of the temporomandibular joint
Disease of the maxillary antrum
  Sinusitis
  Malignant neoplasms
Diseases of salivary glands
  Acute sialadenitis
  Calculi
  Malignant neoplasms
Diseases of eyes
  Glaucoma
  Iritis

Systemic causes
Vascular disorders
  Migrainous neuralgia
  Migraine
  Temporal arteritis
Neurological disorders
  Trigeminal neuralgia
  Intracranial tumours
  Post-herpetic neuralgia
  Herpes zoster
  Multiple sclerosis
  Bell's palsy (occasionally)
Psychogenic pain
  Atypical facial pain and other oral symptoms associated with
    anxiety or depression
  Mandibular pain–dysfunction syndrome depression
Referred pain
  Angina and myocardial infarction
  Lung cancer

Table 32.13
Causes of paraesthesia and sensory loss of lips

Local causes
Nerve injury
Fracture of the mandible
Osteomyelitis
Malignant neoplasms
Pressure by a lower denture on mental nerve

Systemic causes
Tumour deposits in mandible or pterygomandibular space
Intracranial disease
  Multiple sclerosis
  Tumours
  Syringomyelia
  Surgical treatment of trigeminal neuralgia
Psychogenic
  Hyperventilation syndrome
  Hysteria
Drugs
  Labetalol
  Sulthiame
Benign trigeminal sensory neuropathy

damage to the lingual or inferior alveolar nerves during removal of wisdom or other teeth, jaw fractures, or orthognathic surgery. However, peripheral or central neuropathies may be responsible (Table 32.13). Mandibular osteomyelitis, leukaemic deposits and metastases may all give rise to lower labial anaesthesia, as may nasopharyngeal carcinoma or other neoplasm invading the pterygomandibular space or jaws. Antral carcinoma may involve the maxillary division of the trigeminal nerve.

Intracranial lesions such as tumours, disseminated sclerosis, syringobulbia, sarcoidosis and Paget's disease may also cause sensory disturbances, as may, in some cases, drugs such as labetalol. Other patients may have benign trigeminal sensory neuropathy, sometimes related to a connective tissue disorder.

Sensory disturbances may also be due to hyperventilation, hysteria or other psychogenic causes.

genic, particularly atypical facial pain; and (rarely) referred, particularly angina.

Sensory disturbances (Chapter 29)

Sensory disturbances about the mouth usually result from

Facial palsy (Chapter 4)

Upper motor neurone facial palsy is usually a consequence of a stroke. Lower motor neurone facial palsy is usually idiopathic (Bell's palsy), but occasionally HIV or other infections, disease of the middle ear or parotid gland, or trauma are responsible (Table 32.14). Operations in the region of the parotid and submandibular

Table 32.14
Causes of facial palsy

Peripheral	Neurological disease
	Bell's palsy
	Trauma to facial nerve or its branches
	Middle ear disease
	Cholesteatoma
	Mastoiditis
	Parotid
	Parotid cancer and surgery
Central	Neurological disease
	Stroke
	Cerebral tumour
	Head injury
	Multiple sclerosis
	Infection (HIV, Leprosy, Lyme disease)
	Ramsay–Hunt syndrome
	Guillain–Barré syndrome
Others	Melkersson–Rosenthal syndrome
	Sarcoidosis (Heerfordt syndrome)

salivary glands carry the risk of damage to branches of the facial nerve.

FACE AND LIPS

Swellings in or of the lips are not uncommon and are usually of local cause, but angioedema, sarcoidosis and Crohn's disease are systemic causes that should be excluded (see Table 32.7).

FURTHER READING

Jones J. H., Mason D. K. (Eds.) (in press). *The oral manifestations of systemic disease*, 2nd edn. London: Ballière Tindall and Cox.

Scully C., Cawson R. A. (1986). Oral medicine. *Med. Int.,* **28**: 1129–1151.

Scully C., Cawson R. A. (1987). *Medical problems in dentistry*, 2nd edn. Bristol: Wright.

Scully C., Cawson R. A. (1988). *Colour aids to oral medicine.* Edinburgh: Churchill Livingstone.

Chapter
33
Oral manifestations of disorders of specific systems

This chapter tabulates the oral manifestations of disorders of specific systems; further details are found elsewhere in this and other volumes of the series. Oral manifestations are by no means invariable nor even common in some disorders.

Oral manifestations in haematological disease

Disease	Oral manifestations
Deficiency of the haematinics—iron, folic acid or vitamin B12	Burning mouth sensation Glossitis Ulcers Angular stomatitis
Sickle cell anaemia	Jaw deformities caused by marrow expansion *Rarely*, osteomyelitis or pain
Thalassaemia major	Jaw deformities caused by marrow expansion
Aplastic anaemia	Ulcers Bleeding tendency
Haemolytic disease of newborn	Tooth pigmentation (rarely) Enamel defects
Any leukocyte defect	Infections, especially herpetic and candidal Ulcers
Any cause of purpura	Bleeding tendency Purpura
Leukaemia/lymphoma	Infections Ulcers Bleeding tendency and purpura (in leukaemias only) Gingival swelling in myelomonocytic leukaemia Cervical lymph node enlargement
Multiple myeloma	Bone pain Tooth mobility Amyloidosis
Amyloid disease	Enlarged tongue Purpura

Oral manifestations in cardiovascular disease

Disease	Oral manifestations
Any disorder causing right-to-left shunt, e.g. Fallot's tetralogy	Cyanosis Delayed tooth eruption
Angina pectoris	Pain referred to jaw (rarely)
Hereditary haemorrhagic telangiectasia	Telangiectasia that may bleed profusely
Giant-cell arteritis (cranial or temporal arteritis)	Pain usually over the temple Rarely, tongue pain or ischaemic necrosis
Polyarteritis nodosa	Ulcers
Any disorder in which anticoagulants are used	Bleeding tendency
Hypertension	Dry mouth and other problems caused by some antihypertensives, e.g. gingival hyperplasia (nifedipine); lichenoid lesions (methyldopa)

Oral manifestations in renal disease

Disease	Oral manifestations
Chronic renal failure of any cause	Xerostomia Halitosis/taste disturbance Leukoplakia Dental hypoplasia in children Renal osteodystrophy Bleeding tendency (especially if anticoagulated)
Post-renal transplant (immunosuppressed)	Infections, particularly herpetic and candidal Bleeding tendency if anticoagulated Gingival hyperplasia if on cyclosporin
Nephrotic syndrome	Dental hypoplasia
Renal rickets (vitamin D resistant)	Delayed tooth eurption Dental hypoplasia (rarely) Enlarged pulp

Oral manifestations in gastrointestinal and liver disease

Disease	Oral manifestations
Pernicious anaemia	Ulcers Glossitis Angular stomatitis
Any cause of malabsorption	Ulcers Glossitis Angular stomatitis
Any cause of regurgitation	Tooth erosions Halitosis
Crohn's disease	Facial swelling Mucosal tags or gingival hyperplasia Cobblestoning of mucosa Ulcers Glossitis Angular stomatitis
Coeliac disease	Ulcers Glossitis Angular stomatitis Dental hypoplasia in severely affected children
Peutz–Jegher's syndrome (small intestinal polyps)	Melanosis
Chronic pancreatitis	Sialosis (rarely)
Cystic fibrosis	Salivary gland swelling
Most liver diseases with jaundice	Bleeding tendency Jaundice
Alcoholic cirrhosis	Bleeding tendency Sialosis
Chronic active hepatitis	Lichen planus
Primary biliary cirrhosis	Sjögren's syndrome Lichen planus
Gardner's syndrome (familial colonic polyps)	Osteomas

Oral manifestations in connective tissue diseases

Disease	Oral manifestations
Any connective tissue disease	Sjögren's syndrome Lymph node enlargement
Lupus erythematosus	White lesions Ulcers Sjögren's syndrome in SLE
Rheumatoid arthritis	Temporomandibular arthritis, rarely Sjögren's syndrome Drug reactions (e.g. lichenoid) Ulcers because of neutropenia in Felty's syndrome
Systemic sclerosis	Stiffness of lips, tongue, etc. Trismus Telangiectasia Sjögren's syndrome Periodontal ligament widened on x-ray

Oral manifestations of skin diseases

Disease	Oral manifestations
Ectodermal dysplasia	Hypodontia Dental anomalies (peg-shaped teeth)
Epidermolysis bullosa	Blisters, erosions and scarring Dental hypoplasia
Lichen planus	White lesions Erosions in some Desquamative gingivitis
Pemphigoid	Blisters Ulcers Desquamative gingivitis
Pemphigus	Ulcers Blisters (rarely) Desquamative gingivitis, rarely
Erythema multiforme	Ulcers Bloodstained crusting of lips
Dermatitis herpetiformis and linear IgA disease	Ulcers

Oral manifestations in viral diseases

Virus	Oral manifestations
Herpes simplex	Ulcers in primary infection Gingivitis in primary infection Vesicles on lips in recurrence (rarely—oral ulcers) Lymph node enlargement
Herpes zoster–varicella	Ulcers in chickenpox, or in zoster of maxillary or mandibular divisions of the trigeminal nerve Pain in maxillary or mandibular zoster Facial palsy in the rare Ramsay–Hunt syndrome of zoster of the geniculate ganglion
Coxsackie and Echo viruses	Ulcers in herpangina and hand–foot and mouth disease
Epstein–Barr virus (in infectious mononucleosis)	Sore throat Tonsillar exudate Palatal petechiae Cervical lymph node enlargement Recurrent parotitis (possibly) in children Hairy leukoplakia (AIDS)
Measles	Koplik's spots
Mumps	Salivary gland swelling
Papillomaviruses	Warts and papillomas
HIV (human immunodeficiency virus causing AIDS)	Lymph node enlargement Infections, particularly herpetic and candidal Ulcers Kaposi's sarcoma Carcinoma or lymphoma Hairy leukoplakia Parotitis Xerostomia Periodontitis, gingivitis Cranial nerve lesions Purpura

Oral manifestations in other infections

Disease	Oral manifestations
Syphilis	Chancre Mucous patches Ulcers Gumma Pain from neurosyphilis Leukoplakia Lymph node enlargement Hutchinson's teeth in congenital syphilis
Gonorrhoea	Pharyngitis (occasionally) Gingivitis (occasionally) Temporomandibular arthritis (rarely)
Tuberculosis (including atypical mycobacteria)	Ulcers (rarely) Cervical lymph node enlargement
Leprosy	Cranial nerve palsies (rarely)
Lyme disease	Facial palsy
Cat scratch disease	Cervical lymph node enlargement
Toxoplasmosis	Lymph node enlargement
Candidosis	White lesions Red lesions Angular stomatitis
Histoplasmosis	Ulcers (especially in immune defects)
Mucormycosis Aspergillosis	Antral infections or ulcers (especially in immune defects)

Oral manifestations of skeletal disorders

Disease	Oral manifestations
Osteopetrosis (Albers–Schonberg disease)	Cranial neuropathies Delayed tooth eruption Osteomyelitis after tooth extractions
Cherubism	Jaw swellings
Osteogenesis imperfecta	Dentinogenesis imperfecta in some
Cleidocranial dysplasia	Delayed tooth eruption Multiple supernumerary teeth Dentigerous cysts Short tooth roots

Craniofacial dysostosis (Crouzon's syndrome)	Maxillary hypoplasia Cleft palate
Mandibulofacial dysostosis (Treacher–Collins syndrome)	Mandibular hypoplasia Cleft palate
Fibrous dysplasia	Expansive jaw lesions
Paget's disease	Expansive jaw lesions Hypercementosis Osteomyelitis, rarely after tooth extractions Post-extraction bleeding

Oral manifestations in endocrine disorders

Disease	Oral manifestations
Pituitary dwarfism	Microdontia Retarded tooth eruption
Congenital hypothyroidism	Macroglossia Retarded tooth eruption
Congenital hypoparathyroidism	Dental hypoplasia May be chronic candidosis if there is associated immune defect
Gigantism/acromegaly	Spaced teeth Mandibular prognathism Macroglossia Megadontia (in gigantism)
Hyperparathyroidism	Loss of lamina dura Osteitis fibrosa cystica, rarely
Hypoadrenocorticism	Mucosal hyperpigmentation
Diabetes mellitus	Periodontal disease, accelerated in severe diabetes Xerostomia Candidosis Sialosis Lichen planus
Pregnancy	Gingivitis Epulis, occasionally
Precocious puberty	Accelerated eruption (fibrous dysplasia in Albright's syndrome)

Oral manifestations in neurological disorders

Disease	Oral Manifestations
Facial palsy of any cause	Palsy and poor natural cleansing of mouth on same side
Trigeminal neuralgia	Pain
Bulbar palsy	Fasciculation of tongue
Parkinsonism	Drooling Tremor of tongue Dysarthria
Neurosyphilis	Pain, rarely Dysarthria Tremor of tongue
Cerebral palsy	Spastic tongue Dysarthria Attrition Periodontal disease
Choreoathetosis	Green staining of teeth in kernicterus Hypoplasia of deciduous dentition in congenital rubella
Epilepsy	Trauma to teeth/jaws/mucosa Gingival hyperplasia if on phenytoin
Down's syndrome (mongolism)	Delayed tooth eruption Macroglossia Scrotal tongue Maxillary hypoplasia Anterior open bite Hypodontia Periodontal disease

Oral manifestations of immunodeficiencies

Disease	Oral manifestations
Severe combined immunodeficiency	Candidosis Viral infections Oral ulceration Absent tonsils Recurrent sinusitis
Sex-linked agammaglobulinaemia	Cervical lymph node enlargement Oral ulceration Recurrent sinusitis Absent tonsils
Common variable immunodeficiency	Recurrent sinusitis Candidosis
Selective IgA deficiency	Tonsillar hyperplasia Oral ulceration Viral infections Parotitis
Di George syndrome	Abnormal facies Candidosis Viral infections Bifid uvula
Ataxia telangiectasia	Recurrent sinusitis Oral ulceration Facial and oral telangiectasia Cervical lymphomas Mask-like facial expression
Wiskott–Aldrich syndrome	Candidosis Viral infections Purpura
Hereditary angioedema	Swellings of face, mouth and pharynx
Chronic benign neutropenia	Oral ulceration Severe periodontitis
Cyclic neutropenia	Oral ulceration Severe periodontitis Eczematous lesions of the face
Chronic granulomatous disease	Cervical lymph node enlargement and suppuration Candidosis Enamel hypoplasia Acute gingivitis Oral ulceration
Myeloperoxidase deficiency	Candidosis

Chediak Higasi syndrome	Cervical lymph node enlargement Oral ulceration Periodontitis
Job's syndrome	Abnormal facies
Secondary immune defects including HIV infection (see p. 000)	Oral ulceration Periodontitis Candidosis Viral infections Malignant neoplasms (rarely)

(see p. 000)

Oral manifestations in psychiatric disease

Disease	Oral manifestations
Depression, hypochondriasis and various psychoses	Various complaints such as dry mouth, discharges, pain, disturbed taste and sensation Drug reactions Often multiple complaints Artefactual ulcers
Anxiety states	Cheek biting Bruxism
Bulimia	Tooth erosion

Oral manifestations of metabolic disorders

Disease	Oral manifestations
Congenital hyperuricaemia (Lesch–Nyhan syndrome)	Self-mutilation
Mucopolysaccharidoses	Spaced teeth Retarded tooth eruption Temporomandibular joint anomalies Enamel defects
Niemann–Pick disease	Retarded tooth eruption Loosening of teeth Mucosal pigmentation
Hypophosphatasia	Loosening and loss of teeth (hypoplastic cementum)
Erythropoietic porphyria	Reddish teeth Bullae/erosions Dental hypoplasia
Amyloidosis	Macroglossia Purpura
Vitamin B12 or folic acid deficiency	Ulcers Glossitis Angular stomatitis
Scurvy	Gingival swelling Purpura Ulcers
Rickets (vitamin D dependent)	Dental hypoplasia Large pulp chambers Delayed tooth eruption

Oral side-effects of drugs

Tissue	Drug effect	Drugs commonly implicated
Teeth	Discoloration	Tetracyclines Chlorhexidine
	Root anomalies	Phenytoin
Gingiva	Swelling	Phenytoin Cyclosporin Nifedipine
Salivary glands	Dry mouth	Tricyclic antidepressants Phenothiazines Antihypertensives Lithium
Taste	Disturbed	Metronidazole Penicillamine
Facial movements	Dykinesias	Phenothiazines Metoclopramide
Mucosa	Thrush	Broad-spectrum antimicrobials Corticosteroids Cytotoxic drugs
	Ulcers Lichenoid lesions	Cytotoxic drugs Non-steroidal anti-inflammatory agents
	Erythema multiforme	Barbiturates Sulphonamides

Oral manifestations in miscellaneous disorders

Disease	Oral manifestations
Myasthenia gravis and other myopathies	Facial weakness Lingual weakness Dysarthria
Sarcoidosis	Xerostomia Salivary gland swelling Heerfordt syndrome (parotid swelling, lacrimal swelling, facial palsy) rarely
Behçet's syndrome	Ulcers
Reiter's syndrome	Ulcers
Langerhan's histiocytosis (histiocytosis X)	Loosening of teeth Jaw radiolucencies
Wegener's granulomatosis	Gingival swellings Ulcers
Kawasaki's disease (mucocutaneous lymph node syndrome)	Cervical lymph node enlargement Sore tongue Cheilitis
Ehlers–Danlos syndrome	TMJ hypermobility Pulp stones Periodontitis (rarely)
Ellis–van Creveld syndrome (chondroectodermal dysplasia)	Multiple fraena Short roots Hypodontia
Tuberous sclerosis	Enamel defects
Preterm infants	Enamel defects Palatal grooving

FURTHER READING

Jones J. H., Mason D. K. (Eds.) (in press). *The oral manifestations of systemic disease,* 2nd edn. London: Ballière Tindall and Cox.
Scully C., Cawson R. A. (1986). Oral medicine. *Med. Int.,* **28**: 1129–1151.
Scully C., Cawson R. A. (1987). *Medical problems in dentistry,* 2nd edn. Bristol: Wright.
Scully C., Cawson R. A. (1988). *Colour aids to oral medicine.* Edinburgh: Churchill Livingstone.

Index